Research Integrity

Research Integrity

Best Practices for the Social and Behavioral Sciences

Edited by

LEE J. JUSSIM,
JON A. KROSNICK,
AND
SEAN T. STEVENS

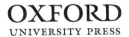

OXFORD
UNIVERSITY PRESS

Oxford University Press is a department of the University of Oxford. It furthers
the University's objective of excellence in research, scholarship, and education
by publishing worldwide. Oxford is a registered trade mark of Oxford University
Press in the UK and certain other countries.

Published in the United States of America by Oxford University Press
198 Madison Avenue, New York, NY 10016, United States of America.

© Oxford University Press 2022

All rights reserved. No part of this publication may be reproduced, stored in
a retrieval system, or transmitted, in any form or by any means, without the
prior permission in writing of Oxford University Press, or as expressly permitted
by law, by license, or under terms agreed with the appropriate reproduction
rights organization. Inquiries concerning reproduction outside the scope of the
above should be sent to the Rights Department, Oxford University Press, at the
address above.

You must not circulate this work in any other form
and you must impose this same condition on any acquirer.

Library of Congress Cataloging-in-Publication Data
Names: Jussim, Lee J., editor. | Krosnick, Jon A., editor. | Stevens, Sean T., editor.
Title: Research integrity : best practices for the social and behavioral sciences /
Lee J. Jussim, Jon A. Krosnick, and Sean T. Stevens, (editors).
Description: New York, NY : Oxford University Press, [2022] |
Includes bibliographical references and index.
Identifiers: LCCN 2021050776 (print) | LCCN 2021050777 (ebook) |
ISBN 9780190938550 (hardback) | ISBN 9780190938574 (epub) |
ISBN 9780190938581
Subjects: LCSH: Psychology—Research—Methodology. |
Social sciences—Research—Methodology.
Classification: LCC BF76.5 .R4627 2022 (print) | LCC BF76.5 (ebook) |
DDC 150.72—dc23/eng/20211221
LC record available at https://lccn.loc.gov/2021050776
LC ebook record available at https://lccn.loc.gov/2021050777

DOI: 10.1093/oso/9780190938550.001.0001

1 3 5 7 9 8 6 4 2

Printed by Integrated Books International, United States of America

This book is dedicated to every person who ever aspired to a career in academic science or social science, who was committed to truthseeking, and who was forced out of such a career because they could not successfully compete with the superstars who produced highly funded, highly cited, highly influential but ultimately invalid research.

Contents

Preface — ix
Contributors — xi

1. Science Reform — 1
   Annabell Suh, Jon A. Krosnick, Lee J. Jussim, Sean T. Stevens, and Stephanie Anglin

2. Improving Research Transparency in the Social Sciences: Registration, Preregistration, and Multiple Testing Adjustments — 36
   Garret Christensen and Edward Miguel

3. What Can We Do About Our (Untrustworthy) Literature? — 70
   Harold Pashler and Christine R. Harris

4. Is Science in Crisis? — 93
   Daniele Fanelli

5. Accuracy and Completeness in the Dissemination of Classic Findings in Social Psychology — 122
   David A. Wilder and Thomas E. Cuthbert

6. Strengths and Weaknesses of Meta-Analyses — 150
   Katherine S. Corker

7. Statistical Inference in Behavioral Research: Traditional and Bayesian Approaches — 175
   Alexander Etz, Steven N. Goodman, and Joachim Vandekerckhove

8. Stimulus Sampling and Research Integrity — 203
   James J. Cummings and Byron Reeves

9. Questionable Interpretive Practices: Data (Mis)Interpretation and (Mis)Representation as Threats to Scientific Validity — 224
   Lee J. Jussim, Sean T. Stevens, and Stephanie Anglin

10. Questionable Research Practices — 260
    Ernest H. O'Boyle and Martin Götz

11. P-hacking: A Strategic Analysis 295
    Robert J. MacCoun

12. The Importance of Type III and Type IV Epistemic
    Errors for Improving Empirical Science 316
    Charlotte Ursula Tate

13. Publication Bias in the Social Sciences: A Threat to
    Scientific Integrity 338
    Neil Malhotra and L. J. Zigerell

14. Let's Peer Review Peer Review 357
    Simine Vazire

15. Impact and Influence of the Institutional Review Board:
    Protecting the Rights of Human Subjects in Scientific
    Experiments 370
    Alison Dundes Renteln

16. Viral Science and the Tragedy of the Scientific Commons 396
    Tanya Menon and Christopher Winship

Index 423

Preface

Knowing what is true is hard. Discovering new truths is even harder. How do we know when some new scientific discovery should be accepted as true? In the physical sciences, new discoveries can usually be checked against physical realities. If global warming is predicted to produce more hurricanes in the future, this will either occur or not. Yet, even if it does not occur, this does not mean that claims that the Earth is warming are false; but it does mean that more frequent hurricanes has not been a consequence.

In the social and behavioral sciences, identifying new truths is more difficult. Meteorologists have widely-agreed upon, objective standards as to what constitutes a hurricane (a rotating storm system with winds of at least 74mph). Biomedical researchers working on vaccines to prevent infectious diseases can determine whether new vaccines are effective by comparing illness rates among those administered and not administered vaccines, especially if they are randomly assigned. People either get sick or they don't; they are either hospitalized or they are not; they either die or they do not.

Such objectively measurable outcomes in social science are rare. Social scientists have no similarly objective standards for determining what constitutes high self-esteem, prejudice, or motivation. This is not to say they cannot study these phenomena—but the absence of objective standards against which to test their theories and hypotheses heightens the uncertainty surrounding whatever is found, and introduces more subjectivity when attempting to interpret whatever is found.

This problem is compounded when scientists underestimate the uncertainty of their findings. Many incentives align to encourage scientists to drape their findings in the trappings of rigor (complex statistics, sophisticated models, arcane theories, etc.) and confidently proclaim "Eureka!" to a world that mostly lacks the training necessary to understand why they might not want to trust those findings. It often takes years, maybe decades, of intense skeptical vetting by other scientists before claims of new scientific discoveries are either clearly confirmed or debunked. As Mark Twain probably never actually said, but is a good point nonetheless, "It ain't what you don't know that gets you in trouble. It's what you know for sure that just ain't so."

This book was inspired by a growing recognition in many social and behavioral science fields that what we knew for sure just isn't so. The results of famous studies were not replicated. Dubious methodological practices were endorsed and used far more widely than was good for us. Peer review's reputation for insuring quality vastly exceeded its track record.

One consequence of this growing recognition of the extent of uncertainty in the social and behavioral sciences has been a nascent movement to reform and improve scientific practices. Thus, this book has two connected purposes. The first is to identify, describe and expose known suboptimal scientific practices so that future generations of scientists and science consumers can more deeply understand the limitations of research and more effectively skeptically vet it so that fewer mistakes enter the scientific canon in the future. The second purpose is to identify and describe practices that have emerged from exposés of suboptimal practices that offer considerable hope of reducing the uncertainty around, and improving the validity of, research in the social and behavioral sciences.

Contributors

Stephanie Anglin, PhD
Assistant Professor
Department of Psychological Science
Hobart and William Smith Colleges
Geneva, NY, USA

Garret Christensen, PhD
Senior Financial Economist
Department of FDIC
Yucca Valley, CA, USA

Katherine S. Corker, PhD
Associate Professor
Department of Psychology
Grand Valley State University
Allendale, MI, USA

James J. Cummings, PhD
Assistant Professor
Division of Emerging Media, College of Communication
Boston University
Boston, MA, USA

Thomas E. Cuthbert, BA
Learning Centers
Rutgers University
New Brunswick, NJ, USA

Alexander Etz, MS, PhD
Assistant Professor of Instruction
Department of Psychology
University of Texas at Austin
Irvine, CA, USA

Daniele Fanelli, PhD
Fellow in Quantitative Methodology
Department of Methodology
London School of Economics and Political Science
London, UK

Steven N. Goodman, MD, MHS, PhD
Professor, Associate Dean
Department of Epidemiology & Population Health, and Medicine
Stanford University School of Medicine
Stanford, CA, USA

Martin Götz, PhD
Research Associate
Department of Psychology, Social and Business Psychology
University of Zurich
Zurich, Switzerland

Christine R. Harris, PhD
Professor
Department of Psychology
University of California—San Diego
La Jolla, CA, USA

Lee J. Jussim, PhD
Distinguished Professor
Department of Psychology
Rutgers University
New Brunswick, NJ, USA

Jon A. Krosnick, PhD
Professor
Department of Communication, Political Science, Psychology
Stanford University
Stanford, CA, USA

Robert J. MacCoun, PhD
James & Patricia Kowal Professor of Law
Law School
Stanford University
Stanford, CA, USA

Neil Malhotra, PhD
Edith M. Cornell Professor of Political
Economy
Graduate School of Business
Stanford University
Stanford, CA, USA

Tanya Menon, PhD
Professor
The Ohio State University
Columbus, IL, USA

Edward Miguel, PhD
Professor
Department of Economics
University of California, Berkeley
Berkeley, CA, USA

Ernest H. O'Boyle, PhD
Associate Professor
Department of Management and
Entrepreneurship
Indiana University
Bloomington, IN, USA

Harold Pashler, PhD
Distinguished Professor
Department of Psychology
University of California, San Diego
La Jolla, CA, USA

Byron Reeves, PhD
Professor
Department of Communication
Stanford University
Stanford, CA, USA

Alison Dundes Renteln
Professor
Political Science, Anthropology, Public
Policy and Law
University of Southern California
Los Angeles, CA, USA

Sean T. Stevens
Senior Research Fellow
Foundation for Individual Rights in
Education
Philadelphia, PA, USA

Annabell Suh
Academic Research Associate
Department of Academic Research
Noom, Inc.
New York, NY, USA

Charlotte Ursula Tate, PhD
Professor
Department of Psychology
San Francisco State University
San Francisco, CA, USA

Joachim Vandekerckhove, PhD
Professor
Department of Cognitive Sciences
University of California, Irvine
Irvine, CA, USA

Simine Vazire, PhD
Professor
Melbourne School of Psychological
Sciences
University of Melbourne
Melbourne, Australia

David A. Wilder, PhD
Professor
Department of Psychology
Rutgers University
New Brunswick, NJ, USA

Christopher Winship, PhD
Diker-Tishman Professor of Sociology
Department of Sociology
Harvard University
Cambridge, MA, USA

L. J. Zigerell, PhD
Associate Professor
Department of Politics and Government
Illinois State University
Normal, IL, USA

1
Science Reform

*Annabell Suh, Jon A. Krosnick, Lee J. Jussim,
Sean T. Stevens, and Stephanie Anglin*

This paper reports the content and implications of discussion of issues in best practices in science during a conference on maximizing scientific integrity, funded by the Fetzer Franklin Fund, and held at the Center for Advanced Study in the Behavioral Sciences at Stanford University.

Widespread concern about scientific methodology presents an opportunity for meta-research on how the process of scientific inquiry works. Much of this chapter was inspired by discussions held during a conference held at Stanford regarding scientific integrity. In it, we identify potentially useful directions for research on how behavioral science goes wrong and how to improve it. We review known problematic practices, identify several others, and review the potential causes of such behaviors. We also review existing solutions to these problems and identify additional potential solutions. We argue that far more empirical research on the nature of scientific processes is necessary, in order to maximize the efficiency of scientific inquiry and the validity of scientific conclusions.

Introduction

Scientific discoveries often build on—and are inspired by—previous discoveries. If the scientific enterprise were a tower of blocks, each piece representing a scientific finding, scientific progress might entail making the tower bigger and better block by block, discovery by discovery.

Annabell Suh, Jon A. Krosnick, Lee J. Jussim, Sean T. Stevens, and Stephanie Anglin, *Science Reform* In: *Research Integrity*. Edited by: Lee J. Jussim, Jon A. Krosnick, and Sean T. Stevens, Oxford University Press. © Oxford University Press 2022. DOI: 10.1093/oso/9780190938550.003.0001

Rather than strong wooden blocks, imagine the blocks, or scientific findings, can take on shape based on scientific accuracy. The most accurate pieces are the strongest and sturdiest, while the least accurate are soft and pliable. Building a tower of the scientific enterprise with a large number of inaccurate blocks will cause the tower to start to wobble, lean over, and potentially collapse, as more and more blocks are placed upon weak and faulty pieces.

Unlike in the simple world of block towers, where the problematic pieces would be easy to remove and replace, it can be difficult to ascertain where to begin in locating the sources of, and correcting, major and widespread problems in science in recent years. One issue is the astounding and extensive non-replicability of published scientific studies. For example, pharmaceutical companies such as Amgen and Bayer conducted replications of studies in medical journals and could only replicate as few as 11% and 25% of studies, respectively. The problem is not limited to the biosciences. Recent attempts to replicate more than 100 social psychological studies have also replicated many fewer studies than would be expected (Open Science Collaboration, 2015).

Problems in science in recent years are not limited to studies not replicating. Other pervasive problems that decrease the accuracy of scientific findings include, but are not limited to, errors leading to inaccurate findings, questionable research practices in which researchers are motivated to report certain types of findings that are significant while excluding mention of others, misleading generalizations and interpretations of findings, and doing many studies or analyses until a significant effect is found.

This report aims to provide a path forward, illuminating where the problems are and how they might be solved for the betterment of scientific progress. It is split into two main sections. The first is an overview, in which we explain the source of inspiration for the ideas in this report and provide a broad overview of suboptimal behaviors on the part of scientists, their causes, and effects, as well as solutions that have been raised for some of these behaviors and issues. We explain why empirical research is necessary, setting the stage for the second main section. In this second section, we provide testable empirical research questions for suboptimal behaviors, their causes, and solutions. We conclude by providing some study designs that could be used to examine these research questions.

Overview

Conference Overview

While in recent years there has been wide public debate and discussion over major and obviously problematic issues in scientific practice, such as outright fraud, the Center for Advanced Study in the Behavioral Sciences (CASBS) Scientific Integrity Group from Stanford University and Rutgers University recognized the need for systematic empirical research and thorough discussions about best practices in science as a whole. Behaviors that are not, at face value, unethical, but nonetheless lead to inaccurate scientific findings, especially require thoughtful analysis and behavioral science insights. Such behaviors have not been adequately studied or analyzed.

To fill that gap, the group, led by Professors Jon Krosnick, Lee Jussim, and Simine Vazire with advisers/consultants Jonathan Schooler, Brian Nosek, and Leif Nelson, convened experts from various fields at the Best Practices in Science Conference, on June 18–19, 2015. These experts engaged in detailed discussions on problematic behaviors or issues, what may cause those behaviors or issues, and potential solutions, with a focus on exploring how to empirically examine the extent of the problems and the best solutions.

Participants ranged from academics who have studied specific problematic behaviors or issues to government officials working in the area of scientific integrity. Discussions spanned the spectrum from specific, focused on one specific issue and all of its potential causes and effects, to broad, exploring the complexities of the scientific world and its players and incentive structure.

The ideas in this chapter have been inspired by the discussions that took place.

Overview of Issues in Scientific Practice

On September 7, 2011, Diederik Stapel was suspended from Tilburg University after fabricating the data behind no less than 55 published papers (Levelt et al., 2012). Stapel was not the only researcher to make headlines for making up data: Dirk Smeeters, Lawrence Sanna, and Marc Hauser soon followed.

These cases of outright fraud harm science in many ways, yet the damage can be traced and targeted with solutions. For instance, the papers can be retracted and word can be spread so that young investigators are aware of the inaccurate papers and data.

Even trickier, however, are behaviors that are not as serious as falsifying data but nonetheless lead to inaccurate scientific findings. Following the trail of these behaviors to their causes, in order to determine solutions, is difficult and involves parsing the complicated webs of causes, incentives, and cultures. There is often not a simple one-to-one relationship between behaviors and causes, making it difficult to quickly understand which solutions will help.

Even unambiguously problematic behaviors, such as p-hacking by manipulating statistics or data to find significant p-values, or selectively publishing only successes and not failures, have many potential causes that might have other causes. For instance, researchers are able to hide such questionable research practices due to a lack of transparency, which might arise from powerful incentives to publish compared to small incentives to be transparent, or lack of knowledge, whether practical or cultural, preventing people from trying transparency measures. That lack of knowledge may be caused or exacerbated by cultural norms, or even basic human tendencies, of following the procedures, rules, and knowledge structure of others.

Even what may seemingly be a quick fix, such as increasing transparency, is complicated. An academic culture comprising many different kinds of parties, from graduate students to professors to journal editors and reviewers, has multiple layers of differing and perhaps competing incentives. Researchers, for instance, may want transparency only if they receive rewards for doing so, but not if there are no rewards and it takes time away from working on other papers to be published. Journal editors, on the other hand, may not want to require transparency because they might lose submissions that would be sent to other journals that were less stringent about transparency, or need to keep page counts to certain limits for financial purposes. Or they might adopt transparency requirements if researchers submit stronger and better research as a result of having to be transparent.

Other causes of these behaviors may be difficult or complicated to address. An overreliance on p-value cutoffs in certain fields may make people fish for significant p-values, but it may not be possible to ban the use of p-value thresholds from a practice and culture of science that uses them and conceives of scientific problems in relation to them.

An additional challenge arises when examining behaviors that at first glance do not seem unethical, but still decrease the accuracy of scientific work. Exploring the impact of these behaviors requires the additional steps of ascertaining whether the behavior is in fact detrimental to science and at which point it becomes harmful.

For example, the "chrysalis effect" describes the tendency for published studies to differ markedly from a prior, unpublished version of the same study (see O'Boyle & Götz, this volume). Behaviors that apply include changing hypotheses to fit the data and adding or dropping participants or variables. If these behaviors were done for legitimate reasons (e.g., removing extreme outliers that are distorting the data), they are not necessarily problematic. But they, some argue, become an issue when researchers engage in these behaviors solely to find significant results.

Some may argue, though, that changing the hypothesis after the fact is not a problem, because social learning works in such a way that the human brain is designed to invent theoretical models when results are unexpected. Thus, the argument goes, the best kind of theorizing and learning might occur after the fact, and changes in the direction of hypotheses or theories may be essential for scientific progress.

When thinking about these kinds of behaviors, causes, and effects, the following questions are important: Is the behavior actually problematic? Does it hinder science and make it less accurate? Does it also help science? These are the types of questions that need to be answered for behaviors that can in some cases be acceptable and in other cases suboptimal, and the answers are not always clear-cut.

Examinations of best practices in science also need to extend beyond behaviors of individual researchers to take into account the scientific world at large. Other problematic behaviors, for instance, center on how the scientific finding is interpreted or perceived. For example, sometimes a researcher might find no effect overall, but find an effect when the sample is divided in a certain way. When this is published, based on accurate data and hypotheses, the media might tell the wrong story about the study. Even if the study did not find the effect overall, it might be reported as such, which becomes common knowledge in the field as it makes its way into textbooks and other material.

Sometimes researchers themselves engage in questionable interpretative practices in order to reach a certain conclusion. Questionable interpretive practices are conceptual and narrative tools for reaching one's preferred conclusions, regardless of the actual evidence. Researchers engage in these questionable interpretive practices even when the data contradict those conclusions, contributing to inaccurate perceptions of science.

Lack of or inaccurate knowledge of research also may abound. Textbooks for college students do not update their material with newer studies that are conducted more stringently, but instead refer to the same classic studies over and over again, even if those studies are problematic in some way. Textbooks also inaccurately portray the work that has been done in a field since the original "classic" study, for example by referring to an effect as existing when work since then has shown that it does not. This increases inaccurate perceptions of a field's knowledge and research.

In addition, journals do not have a system for allowing comments on journal papers quickly and in an accessible place. Thus, errors are not corrected in a timely manner or at all, increasing the amount of inaccuracy in scientific literature. For instance, researchers who are not aware of the errors of original papers might try to replicate or expand results that are inaccurate.

Thus, problems in scientific practice cannot be isolated to one particular behavior, one cause, one effect, and one solution. There are interrelated and interacting behaviors, causes, and effects. Assumptions based on merely observing these issues may not lead to helpful solutions due to their complexity. Thus, the literature so far lacks, but urgently needs, a comprehensive understanding of which aspects are important and which are not.

Overview of Possible Solutions

Some purported solutions, which are research procedures that are designed to minimize biases and problematic behaviors, are currently being implemented. For example, biases, such as publication bias, can distort meta-analyses, which are based on a number of studies, some problematic and some not. Thus, some techniques help to identify the extent of the biases, correct for them in some way, and understand what effect they have on estimates(see Corker, this volume, for a review of some of those newer techniques)

Other solutions, however, particularly those that are not new research techniques, are not simple to isolate and implement. Some proposed solutions, for example, have to do with culture, which often has many different components. One proposed solution about culture assumes that the scientific culture of stigmatizing retractions and admission of fraudulent or unethical behavior may decrease transparency and motivate researchers to keep any mistakes hidden. Taking steps to change that culture, such as encouraging researchers to take pride in retractions or in being open and transparent, might help to increase transparency. Students will imitate the culture they see around them, so setting the bar for scientific integrity will make students work in ways that are high in integrity. But the question of how to change that culture, and what aspects may be helpful or not, needs to be answered.

Other broad-level solutions might impact the way people think about research. For example, it could be argued that not only should the standard of p-value cutoffs be changed, but there needs to be a shift in how people think, from individual one-off testing to understanding studies as an accumulation of evidence. Shifting how people think about scientific questions is a daunting task and one that requires understanding of how people think and how they would be able to change that process.

The Need for Empirical Research

The picture just presented of problematic behaviors, their causes, and solutions is one of complexity and broadness. There are two types of dangers that can result in moving forward toward solutions to the problems of science. The first is disillusionment, giving up on any solutions because the road ahead is so convoluted. The second is to make assumptions that one solution or one behavior is important without first empirically testing those assumptions.

Empirical research provides the roadmap on how to fix the problems of science. It can help us answer important questions that will guide our responses to integrity issues: How widespread are the problems? Which causes lead to problems? What are the most effective solutions? What effects would some of these solutions have?

The remainder of this report aims to suggest ideas for empirical research on problems, causes, and solutions. Such empirical research will hopefully demystify and disentangle the tangled webs of causes and issues that cause problems, testing whether each aspect is important and what effect it has. It is the way forward to providing solutions and testing which ones work the best.

First, the report will explore research questions about specific problematic behaviors or issues in order to ascertain which ones are in need of solutions. From there, it will present research questions for causes of behaviors to see which ones are relevant for potential solutions. Finally, it will examine research questions for solutions, and present study designs that could be implemented right away.

Empirical Research Questions

Questionable Research Practices

In order to provide effective solutions, it is imperative to first determine what the issues are and how problematic they are. This section presents research questions on specific problematic behaviors in relation to scientific best practice and how prevalent they are. Causes or mediators of these behaviors and many others are explored in the next section.

Most of the research that has been conducted has centered on obviously problematic and widely discussed behaviors, often included under the umbrella term "questionable research practices" (QRPs), such as p-hacking and selective reporting. P-hacking entails selectively and strategically analyzing, selecting, or rounding data in order to produce statistically significant results. Selective reporting similarly involves a focus on statistically significant results, and involves only reporting variables, trials, or analyses that were statistically significant. These types of behaviors have found to be widespread among not only psychology (John et al., 2012) but other fields as well, such as the biosciences (Head et al., 2015).

The research thus far has found that researchers frequently engage in these QRPs that lead to massive problems for science by decreasing replicability and accuracy of scientific findings. Yet while it is clear that researchers take part in these behaviors, it is not clear how *willing* they are to do so.

On the one hand, it may be the case that researchers choose to engage in QRPs and are very willing to do so. It could be that incentives, whether related to employment or status, for dishonesty are so high that researchers are tremendously willing to engage in these behaviors. On the other hand, there are some reasons why researchers may not be willing at all to do so. First, to the extent that the value of science is tied to its objectivity and accuracy, there are dangerous risks for scientists who cut corners by engaging in these behaviors. Scientists who are caught for p-hacking or selective reporting, then, may take a stronger hit professionally and in the public eye than they would in a profession that is not seen as one that should be objective and accurate. It might follow that scientists would not be particularly willing to engage in these behaviors knowing the massive consequences for getting caught. Nor is it likely that people who have chosen to go into science take immense joy in taking shortcuts to produce a certain outcome, given the emphasis even early on in the educational system on the "objective" scientific method (Mellado, 1997).

Thus, an important question to consider when exploring QRPs is not only whether researchers engage in them, but also how willingly they do so. The answer to this question points to the extent of the problem at hand. If researchers frequently p-hack or selectively report and they are not very willing to do so, the next steps might be determining what causes these behaviors, and then providing solutions based on those causes. Yet if it turns out that researchers frequently p-hack or selectively report and they are very willing to do so, it is not enough to find causes of the behaviors and a solution for each cause. It is instead necessary to explore why they are willing to engage in the behaviors, and the reason may not be simple. This may point to causes, solutions, and even more problems or issues that would not arise otherwise, and may be more difficult to fix.

> Empirical research questions: How *willing* are researchers to engage QRPs such as p-hacking and selective reporting? Does this differ by field? Does willingness change depending on situational factors (e.g., lower professional incentives)?

Incentives are another piece of the puzzle for QRPs. Much discussion has maligned incentives of the academic world that reward a high quantity of publications, which have a lower likelihood of being accepted into a journal with nonsignificant results (Dwan et al., 2013). But it is not yet clear how important or impactful professional incentives are to researchers. It might be that incentives greatly impact researchers' behavior. On the other hand, it could be that professional incentives pale in comparison to other factors, such as personal incentives like status or appearing knowledgeable and capable. Before examining to what extent incentives cause problematic behavior, which the next section will explore, it is important to first establish that incentives are important in general.

> Empirical research questions: How important are professional incentives to researchers? How important are they compared to other types of incentives?

QRPs might also arise from a different issue. Some argue that researchers do not understand p-values very well. Researchers see p-values as entirely objective, which might lead to inappropriate and incorrect decisions about how to calculate p-values and which ones to use.

> Empirical research questions: How well do researchers understand p-values? In a given imaginary scenario in which none of their incentives are at play, how correct are researchers at identifying the correct p-value and justifying their choice? (e.g., one-tailed vs. two-tailed)? How frequent is inaccurate use of p-values, such as incorrect rounding?

In addition to obviously problematic behavior such as p-hacking and selective reporting, understanding the prevalence of intentional behavior that is not, at face value, as problematic is essential as well to be able to fully understand and outline best practices in science. There is not much systematic evidence about how common these kinds of behaviors are. Such behaviors or tendencies include collecting more data in order to find an effect, stopping data collection earlier than planned because significant results were found, researchers' political bias affecting the questions they ask and how stringently they check the findings, overgeneralizing results, and splitting the data into subgroups in order to find larger or significant effects.

> Empirical research questions: How prevalent is collecting more data after the fact in order to find an effect or different results? How prevalent is stopping data collection earlier than planned because significant results were found? Do researchers have political biases that make them want to find some findings more than others? Do those political biases, if they exist, affect the question they choose to research? Do those political biases, if they exist, make them more careful or less careful in conducting research? How prevalent is overgeneralizing results? How prevalent is splitting the data into subgroups in order to find larger effects?

In addition, errors of other kinds occur, but it is not yet clear how widespread they are. Both unintentional errors and intentional problematic behaviors can sometimes lead to the same outcome, such as non-replicability, so it is important to determine to what extent errors and intentional behaviors occur. One example of such errors is when even well-intentioned researchers who are trying to carry out a protocol misinterpret it when replicating a previous study. This may lead to replications not working or interventions not working on a large scale, if many different people are expected to carry out the same procedure, or at least have the same and correct understanding of the material.

> Empirical research questions: How often does unintended misinterpretation of study protocol occur? How many intended, compared to unintended, errors or misinterpretations are there?

Another error is when researchers assume that one failed replication means that the effect does not exist, even if the evidence is in actuality mixed with one success and one failure. This may introduce inaccuracies in the literature and exclude information that may be important for the literature to contain, preventing future studies from being able to correctly distinguish whether the effect occurs and under what conditions it does.

> Empirical research questions: Do scientists tend to assume after one failed replication that the effect has been proven wrong, when in reality the evidence is more indeterminate?

Other errors that contribute to inaccuracy in the collection of scientific knowledge include interpretation and citation errors. For instance, studies that are flawed or inaccurate may be cited by researchers who are not aware of the inaccuracies, or who are parroting other literature reviews on the same topic.

> Empirical research questions: How often are studies that are inaccurate or flawed cited? On a given topic, what percentage of cited studies are inaccurate or flawed?

Such lack of knowledge about which studies are inaccurate, and why, might disproportionately affect researchers or students from institutions that do not have a prominent role in the field or considerable resources, such as library resources. Resources might also include cultural knowledge, such as information passed between people about some study that has been retracted or is flawed, which some researchers from other places cannot access. This may make the inaccuracies in science especially prominent in work that is done outside the scope of the best research universities.

> Empirical research questions: Do those outside of the best research universities cite inaccurate or flawed studies more? Does this lead to further inaccurate citations?

Additionally, interpretation errors may occur on the part of the media. Sometimes a researcher might find an effect, but only in subgroups and not overall. The media, for a variety of reasons, might tell the wrong story about the study, generalizing it from happening only within subgroups to happening overall for everyone. Or sometimes the media might generalize scientific findings from a sample that included only certain types of people to the general population. These are errors that increase the inaccuracy of knowledge about the specific scientific field and its findings.

> Empirical research questions: How common is this? How often are studies described inaccurately by the media? Does that impact people's knowledge of science, perceptions of science, and trust in science?

Finally, it is necessary to do investigations of how prevalent problematic issues, rather than behaviors, are. For example, the "decline effect" describes the tendency for effect sizes to shrink over time with each study. The decline effect has been documented in various fields, but is still not well understood. Still missing are very systematic, extensive, cross-field meta-analyses of effect sizes to try to classify what kinds of effects get smaller and what don't.

> Empirical research questions: Which kinds of effects decline? Which kinds of effects don't decline? How prevalent are decline effects in each field? Are they smaller in some fields than others?

A more extensive look at problematic behaviors and issues follows in the next section as we explore causes of behaviors or issues.

Causes of Problematic Behaviors and Issues

Many problematic behaviors and issues occur behind closed doors. As such, it is difficult, even impossible, to find out why researchers engage in certain behaviors by just examining the behaviors. Empirical research can unearth the underlying causes behind issues, avoiding the inaccurate and even costly way of making faulty assumptions about why things happen and ending up with ineffective solutions.

Professional Incentives

Incentives are widely believed to cause, or at least increase, QRPs. There are powerful professional incentives to publish papers. Citation counts or measures such as the h-index and the number of publications are commonly used criteria for hiring, promotion, and tenure decisions within academia, despite the drawbacks of using such criteria (Fanelli, 2010; Reinstein et al., 2011). Competition for positions has increased in recent years, while the number of available academic jobs has not (Weir, 2011).

These professional incentives might make researchers aim to publish as many papers as possible, especially ones seen as novel. While such incentives spur academic output and ultimately scientific progress, they can interact with certain tendencies of the academic environment to foster, over time, more and more QRPs and problematic behavior. One tendency is for journals to accept more papers with significant effects or results than not, along with the widespread perception that papers with null effects will not be accepted. In addition, innovative and groundbreaking work is commonly aimed at being, at least within social psychology and other social science fields, counterintuitive and unexpected in relation to past theoretical work or common sense.

Thus, there is not only the incentive to engage in QRPs, but also an environment that encourages this behavior, both for those who want to engage in it and those who feel like they do not have a choice but to try. Researchers who have spent many years in graduate school may feel the pressure of limited job options and increased competition. Within another environment, the solution researchers consider might be to work harder, or to expand their professional network. Within academia, however, where citation counts and publication counts reign, they may instead realize the only option will be to get more papers published, any way that that is possible. When honest attempts to run studies yield null findings, researchers who feel that journals will not accept the paper may round some numbers or leave out certain variables or conditions to keep only significant results. Or, many honest attempts later, a researcher may finally find a significant effect and submit this counter-intuitive, "wow" paper to a journal, even if the effect is solely due to chance.

> Empirical research questions: Does the desire to publish a lot of papers increase the likelihood of engaging in QRPs? That is, if researchers were told that citation counts and the number of publications would not factor as much into decision-making as other factors, would they be less likely to engage in QRPs? If researchers were told that counterintuitive and surprising papers were not as important as thorough, "unsurprising" papers, would they be less likely to engage in QRPs? Is there a greater chance of p-hacking for "wow" papers that involve only a single study, compared to papers that contain multiple studies/replications?

Professional incentives to publish lots of papers may be rising, but there is no similar rise in incentives to be honest or transparent. Researchers are not especially rewarded for being transparent, and may in some circumstances even be punished for, for instance, going beyond word limits, or weakening a paper's perceived value. Researchers might avoid engaging in QRPs if there were a higher incentive to be transparent.

> Empirical research question: Does increasing the incentives to be transparent decrease the likelihood of engaging in QRPs?

There is most likely variation within researchers as to how susceptible they are to professional incentives. It is not clear merely from examining outcomes and incentives (e.g., professional incentives increase the likelihood of QRPs) which of two possible motivations people had while engaging in the problematic behavior. The first is gaming the system, no matter what it is or how difficult it is to do things honestly. The second is shaped by pressure from editors, advisors, reviewers, and oneself, only engaging in QRPs because there is no other way. This distinction is important because while the two groups share professional incentives, the first group may not be willing to be transparent or honest, while the second would.

Empirical research questions: What percentage of people would engage in QRPs regardless of external pressure? What percentage of people would be less willing to engage in QRPs if external pressure were lower or if there were another way to their goal (e.g., a guaranteed job offer)?

Some argue that it is not incentives, but cultural factors, that matter. Researchers learn implicit knowledge of what the field does or is supposed to do, as well as explicit knowledge of how to do certain tasks. This means not only that researchers might imitate and go along with their colleagues or advisors who engage in QRPs but also that researchers may be constrained to certain traditional techniques or methods, rather than trying newer and sounder methods.

Empirical research questions: How related are knowledge of what people in the field are "supposed" to do and what researchers actually do? Would telling people that others are using sounder methods increase willingness to use them as well? Would telling people that others are being honest and transparent increase willingness to be honest or transparent? Would telling people that others are engaging in QRPs increase willingness to also engage in QRPs? Do researchers with a stronger sense of the culture of the field, institution, or lab group produce less reproducible findings or more inaccurate methods or conclusions?

The impact of incentives to cut corners and of subsequent QRPs could be minimized by complete transparency, in which researchers reveal aspects of their research process, such as data, code, variables, all hypotheses tested, and all studies run. With transparency, researchers who engage in QRPs may be caught, and it can be determined whether non-replicability is due to errors in analysis or the file drawer problem.

While there have been initiatives to increase transparency, such as the creation of the Open Science Framework website, and encouraging researchers to publicly post their data, complete transparency is nevertheless absent from or has a minor role in much of academic work. There are several potential reasons, related to different kinds of incentives, as to why this may be.

One reason is that many academic journals are not encouraging or requiring transparency. Journals may not be willing to change their policies to require more transparency, such as more detailed writeups of every step of the analysis process, because they feel that people will submit to other journals instead. This incentive to publish the best submissions, then, makes journals less willing to encourage transparency, and researchers thus do not feel they need to take steps to do so.

> Empirical research questions: Would people submit to other journals if the journal they want to submit to institutes transparency policies? Are journals that have formidable rivals in other journals less willing to require or encourage transparency? If journals encourage, but do not require, transparency, do researchers start to consider taking steps toward transparency? If journals require transparency, do researchers follow suit? Does a greater signal from top journals increase the willingness of researchers to be transparent? What is the threshold of transparency requirements/encouragement for changing the intended journal? What is the limit at which researchers would move to another journal?

Another reason relates to incentives for researchers. Researchers have incentive to publish many papers as quickly as they can, and may fear that taking transparency measures, such as writing long and detailed preregistration documents, takes up too much precious time that could be devoted to new studies. Yet it might also be that transparency saves researchers' time. Transparency might speed up different kinds of processes, such as quickly figuring out what studies or analyses they have already done, immediately finding data or relevant code, running analyses within seconds, or thinking of new steps based on already-thought-out hypotheses.

> Empirical research questions: Does framing transparency as an incentive for researchers in terms of saving time increase their willingness to be transparent? And how does this compare to the impact of a more general incentive, such as improving the state of science in general, on willingness to be transparent?

Bias

Researchers are not free from bias. One bias that may plague researchers might stem from a deep investment in the way a research question turns out. This could be due to attacks from other researchers on the "other side" or the researcher's own political leaning. For instance, researchers could be motivated to protect their research when it is criticized, and thus be more susceptible to confirmation bias or bypassing analysis errors. Or, researchers might desire a certain outcome that aligns with their beliefs, making them less objective and more willing to engage in QRPs in order to reach a certain conclusion. On the other hand, having interest in the research question might lead to better-quality research than indifference toward the research. When researchers deeply care about the research, they might give greater attention and care into finding errors and choosing appropriate techniques and methods.

> Empirical research questions: Does caring about the research question lead to better or worse science (as measured, perhaps, by replicability)? Does caring about the research question increase or decrease willingness to engage in QRPs? Does perceived antagonism to a theory make people more defensive about their theory or research? Does perceived antagonism increase willingness to engage in QRPs? If people are given a goal in conducting research (e.g., addressing skepticism about it vs. understanding what is going on in the world), does that affect interpretation, analysis, and findings? Does that goal affect their willingness to engage in QRPs?

Criticism might not always a defensive response. Disagreeing in a civil way may increase the quality of science by finding errors while also avoiding triggering a strong defensive, and possibly biased, response from the researcher. Harsh, and perhaps even personal, criticism, however, might provoke defensive and biased reactions.

> Empirical research questions: Does disagreeing in a civil, polite manner decrease bias and willingness to engage in QRPs and increase replicability? Does disagreeing overly harshly increase bias, increase willingness to engage in QRPs, and decrease replicability?

If criticism is good for science, while bias is bad, the amount of political diversity within a field might decrease the amount of bias in scientific work while increasing criticism of it. It might be argued that political diversity improves the quality of science in making it, overall, less biased and more replicable. It could also be that political diversity creates more criticism, which might make work clearer, more evidence-based, less problematic, and more accurate.

Empirical research questions: Does diversity in political opinions lead to more replicable research? Does the criticism resulting from political diversity improve science? Does it make criticized work more evidence-based or replicable, or does it make researchers more entrenched in their own biases?

One bias that may plague researchers is the motivation to appear like a knowledgeable expert in a certain area. Appearing extremely knowledgeable might entail seeming to clearly understand the effect or results. This may mean engaging in behaviors such as throwing away moderators that do not work or contribute to confusion surrounding the effect.

Empirical research question: Does the desire to appear like a knowledgeable expert lead to fewer reported variables, moderators, and/or conditions in papers, compared to those who do not have this desire?

Another very similar type of motivation is having a simple narrative about the effect or research agenda. News articles or TED talks are much flashier when they proclaim that "parents like the middle child more than the first-born child," compared to "it seems that middle-aged, Norwegian parents like their middle child more than their first-born child sometimes, although they like the first-born child more other times." It could be that when researchers desire a simple narrative to encapsulate their research, they are more likely to engage in QRPs like selective reporting, and report interpretations of their findings that are overly simplistic.

Empirical research question: Does the desire to have a simple narrative increase bias and QRPs or cause researchers to present results as simpler or cleaner than they really are?

Lack of Accurate Knowledge
It is also important to understand what other types of factors increase the inaccuracy of science.

One factor is the lack of clear understanding about the decline effect and the resulting non-reproducibility of scientific work. It is not clear why the decline effect, which describes the decrease in effect size over time with each replication, occurs. It could be due to QRPs or simply heterogeneity. There is a lot of heterogeneity of different environments and participants between replications. This is especially the case with interventions, in which one intervention that was studied at one place at one time is carried out in many locations with different people running the study or participating in it. Perhaps this heterogeneity, which is probably not well understood for many effects, ultimately is responsible for the decreasing effect size across sites or labs.

> Empirical research questions: How much of the decline effect is due to flawed scientific behaviors (QRPs), and how much is due to heterogeneity? How much does heterogeneity explain decline effects?

It could be the case that the decline effect, or even non-reproducibility in general, occurs because the researchers who are drawn to doing replications are not at the skill level of the researchers who are producing original research. Perhaps they do not have the skillset or technical ability to properly carry about replications, and failures to replicate are due to unintentional researcher error.

> Empirical research question: Are researchers who are interested in doing direct replications lower-quality researchers (as measured in different ways, such as knowledge of research or ratings by experts of the quality of research papers)?

We also must consider inaccuracy of knowledge *about* science. Social psychology textbooks commonly present the field inaccurately. The most widely used social psychology textbooks often mention flawed studies and present effects as big and general, failing to mention moderators or complexity or messiness. In classrooms, instructors may similarly explain the state of research in a simpler, and thus perhaps inaccurate, way for two reasons. First is a fear that students will lose interest in the field after being taught about moderators or complexities, compared to simple and overgeneralized summaries. The second reason is not wanting to delve into the complexities of the research due to lack of knowledge on how best to convey that information. When the state of research is one of messiness and complexity, students without proper knowledge of the field will not be able to contribute in a meaningful way to future research or may carry inaccurate information about the science of the field with them to other industries.

Empirical research questions: Do instructors fear that students will lose interest in the field after being taught about complexities in the research? Are instructors unwilling to delve into those complexities? Do student perceptions of how compelling the field is change when students are taught more explicitly about moderators in research? What increases interest in the field more: simple narratives or nuanced narratives about research? What makes students more inclined to pursue research in the field? What makes them learn more knowledge about the field?

Proposed Solutions

Ioannidis (2014) called for rigorous, systematic empirical research to be done on potential solutions and interventions in order to inform decisions with evidence rather than conventions or "inertia," as is currently the case. Research is especially vital because solutions that may seem to make sense at first glance may have unintended and negative consequences, or no effect at all. For instance, rewards for openly sharing data and code may lead to situations in which the most conscientious and careful researchers, the only ones who were willing to share such material, are attacked by "reanalyzers who hunt for errors, no matter how negligible these errors are" (Ioannidis, 2015).

This section serves to heed his call, to encourage research on solutions that have not been examined in the literature yet, and to consider the complexities of each proposed solution and what its effects could be. Thus, the proposed research questions are not limited to how well the solution at hand would work, but also whether it might have unanticipated effects that need to be considered by decision makers.

Transparency

One widely proposed solution to problems of QRPs and non-reproducibility is that of transparency, or publicly revealing at least some, if not all, aspects of one's research process. The broad term of transparency includes such concepts as openly sharing data and the code used in analysis as well as pre-registration plans, in which researchers submit, in writing and prior to running a study, a document that lays out the hypotheses, variables, and analysis strategies that will be used in the study.

The hope is that with more transparency, researchers will be more careful, making fewer errors and committing fewer QRPs. The result, then, will be research that is more accurate and more replicable. Yet this assumption has not been empirically tested, though it is an imperative piece of information in order to decide whether transparency is a viable solution.

> Empirical research questions: Does transparency produce better research (e.g., more replicable and reliable)? Is there less evidence of QRPs (e.g., p-hacking) in more transparent research? Is more transparent research judged to be of higher quality than research that is not? Are researchers more honest with transparency compared to without transparency?

Preregistration plans have been the most widely discussed and analyzed transparency measures. Preregistration purportedly provides several advantages in certain situations but is not a perfect solution for all types of studies (see Coffman & Niederle, 2015; Olken, 2015).

> Empirical research question: Does preregistration decrease QRPs, increase disclosures that would otherwise not be disclosed, and produce more replicable and reliable research?

Preregistration might also be valuable for other secondary reasons. Having all the data and code available in a preregistration system saves time, as researchers do not have to hunt through code and their memories to recall what they did previously. In addition, researchers have higher confidence that their results are accurate and not due to error or fraud. Also, all studies that were run are registered, so researchers are less likely to forget that they had previously run ultimately inconclusive studies a long time ago to investigate the same effect.

> Empirical research questions: Does preregistration save researchers' time? Does preregistration lead to a longer or shorter research process (e.g., from conception of the study to publication)? Does hearing that preregistering saves time make researchers more willing to try it? Does preregistering decrease misremembering or forgetting about past inconclusive or shelved studies? Does preregistering lead to higher willingness to write up results, whether they are statistically significant or not?

Despite the advantages of preregistration, researchers warn of a potential danger: that having to register hypotheses and analyses in advance will restrain researchers from taking creative risks in their research. While such warnings have been speculative (e.g., Coffman & Niederle, 2015; Gelman, 2013), no study has empirically tested whether this assumption is true or not.

> Empirical research question: Does transparency (e.g., preregistration) decrease creativity (perhaps measured by self and other ratings on creativity, amount of risk taken, and complexity of research question)?

The effectiveness of transparency measures other than preregistration has also not yet been examined in the literature. Some transparency measures beyond preregistration that can be tested include (1) the requirement of a 21-word statement in which researchers vow that they are reporting all data and manipulations and measures, as well as (2) openly sharing data and coding materials. Such measures might make researchers more honest and disclose more of the information they might otherwise not have reported in their papers. However, it might also not have that intended effect. For instance, researchers may not be truthful in their 21-word statement, in which case the statement would have no or very little effect in increasing transparency and the accuracy of scientific work. Or researchers may edit their datasets and code to reflect only the final analyses after initial variables were removed or excluded.

> Empirical research questions: Does requiring a 21-word statement decrease QRPs, increase replicability, and increase disclosure? How truthful are authors in their 21-word statements? Does requiring openly sharing data and coding materials decrease QRPs, increase replicability, and increase disclosure?

Even if transparency is encouraged, it is not necessarily the case that researchers will embrace it. Transparency demands time and energy from researchers that they may not be willing to devote to it without incentives to do so. One potential incentive is a badge or reward for preregistering or for increasing transparency, such as by making the data available. This may work by increasing researchers' willingness to preregister and overcoming the initial barrier of entry. Perhaps, after trying it, researchers will be willing to embrace preregistration from then on. On the other hand, it is possible that the badge method would not work well because its success is contingent on people reading the paper, seeing the badge, and valuing it. If consumers do not notice the badge or value it, its ability to increase preregistration and transparency is hampered.

Empirical research questions: How willing are researchers to preregister studies? How willing are researchers to preregister studies if given an incentive (e.g., a reward or badge)? How effective are badges or rewards in increasing transparency? How much do people notice a badge? How much do they value it? What are the moderators at play in the effect of badges on willingness to preregister?

Another possible incentive is a financial one. Open Science Framework's Preregistration Challenge offered $1,000 to researchers who publish a study that was preregistered on the site. Such incentives might encourage preregistration. On the other hand, it might be that those who are interested in a financial incentive are those who are more susceptible to incentives in the first place. In addition, the prize requires the paper to be published. It could be, then, that in their desire for their paper to be published, researchers engage in QRPs that are not detectable via preregistration, such as rounding decimal points incorrectly to reach the cutoff point for statistical significance.

Empirical research questions: Does the prospect of an incentive with inherent value, such as a financial incentive, make researchers more likely to preregister? How does this kind of incentive affect willingness to be transparent? How does it affect the quality of the science? Does it decrease or increase QRPs?

A different type of incentive is a goal-oriented one. Rather than providing researchers with a financial incentive, perhaps a more impactful incentive would be shifting researchers' perspective from one of personal gain to one of using science to improve the quality of others' lives and to better the world. Perhaps an intervention activating this incentive would make people more careful and honest in their work, engaging in fewer QRPs and being more transparent.

Empirical research questions: Does activating this incentive/goal in researchers make them less willing to engage in QRPs? Does it make them more careful and honest in their scientific work? Does it increase transparency? Does priming an achievement goal lead researchers to be more willing to engage in QRPs compared to priming researchers with a generosity goal?

Even if individually incentivized, researchers still may not be willing to devote the time and resources that transparency requires. They may forgo the additional incentive in order to save on the costs of preregistration, for instance, and the end result may be most researchers ignoring transparency and only a few researchers embracing it. Thus, a shift in culture may be required, at a level higher than the individual researcher. In order for this change to occur, journal editors of top journals may need to be involved. If journal editors require transparency, other journal editors and researchers and reviewers may follow suit.

Empirical research question: Do transparency requirements or encouragements from journal editors make people more willing to be transparent?

Most journals do not have explicit policies for accessing data and transparency. As a result, even a researcher who wants to check another researcher's data and code will not know where to go to find such information. This researcher may not even be able to obtain the dataset if journals do not require authors to submit it and the authors do not want to reveal it. This could decrease transparency and increase QRPs. Similarly, in many universities, there is no office or staff member that is easily identifiable for addressing concerns of scientific integrity. This may keep questionable behavior from being reported. Perhaps having explicit policies, and a structured system such that researchers know exactly where to go to obtain data and measures, or to report questionable behavior, will keep researchers accountable.

Empirical research questions: If a journal has explicit policies or the journal has an organizational structure that enables researchers to obtain data or code from other researchers, do transparency and disclosure increase? Do QRPs decrease? If people knew where to go within a university to report scientific integrity violations, would they be more willing to report one? If people were told about an office that could take action on scientific integrity, would people be less willing to engage in QRPs?

Other steps journals can take that indirectly increase transparency involve a shift in perceptions of the circumstances for which researchers will receive rewards in the form of accepted publications. Some proposed solutions include allowing people to publish null results, messy results, and replications, and allowing for results-blind peer review. Results-blind peer review would enable reviewers to evaluate the study before observing the outcomes of the research, focusing instead on the quality of the question, its importance, and the quality and implementation of the research design, rather than the results. If journals made these changes, people might not be as incentivized to engage in QRPs or hide variables and analyses in order to find significant results.

> Empirical research questions: Does the perception that null results, messy results, and replications can be published decrease QRPs, increase replicability, and increase disclosure? Does results-blind peer review decrease QRPs, increase replicability, and increase disclosure?

Another change journals can make is to split the results section of the standard paper format into "findings" and "exploration" sections. Researchers may feel obligated to report speculation and results about which they are not confident as "results" to follow the standard research paper format. As a result, they may be more prone to making stronger claims than the evidence would warrant. Creating an "exploration" section within the results section—that is, not in the discussion section—may make people more forthcoming about which findings they are confident in and which ones are more speculative or need more data.

> Empirical research questions: Does splitting the results section this way make people more honest? Does it make them report more findings as speculation than they would otherwise? Does the language the researchers use change when using this new format (e.g., is their language more hesitant about weaker findings than when using the traditional format)?

The general scientific culture is important as well. Stigmatization of retractions may decrease transparency by motivating researchers to keep any mistakes, even unintentional ones, hidden. Taking steps to change that culture, by encouraging researchers to take pride in retractions or in being open and transparent, might help to increase transparency.

Empirical research question: Would an intervention to decrease stigmatization of retractions and admitting mistakes increase transparency and honesty?

Transparency could be the key to decreasing QRPs, fraud, and errors, which would all lead to more accurate and more replicable science. This section has explored transparency with these major goals in mind. However, transparency could provide advantages even beyond these. If researchers embraced transparency, that could affect perceptions of science and of scientists. People might take science more seriously, and be less likely to discount it.

Empirical research questions: Does enacting transparency affect public perceptions of science (and of scientists)? With greater transparency, do people draw different conclusions about scientific findings than they would with less transparency? With greater transparency, do people take science more seriously and are they less likely to discount it? What kinds of transparency are more convincing to laypeople than others?

Providing More Accurate Information

While QRPs and intentional problematic behaviors are essential to consider, much of the inaccuracy and non-reproducibility of science in recent years could also be largely due to lack of accurate knowledge or unintentional errors. For instance, 73.5% of English-language research paper retractions in a period of 10 years were due to error (Steen, 2010) rather than misconduct. Targeting intentional behaviors alone may not be enough to keep science as accurate and reproducible as possible.

According to a conference attendee who has served as an journal editor, researchers lack a surprisingly large amount of fundamental knowledge. Some of the knowledge includes why some analytical strategies can be problematic or inaccurate. This means that reviewers might also not be aware of this information, increasing errors in research if the research gets published, as well as non-replicability if other researchers try to replicate the original study using the correct analytical strategy. Creating a publicly available list of common errors or tips endorsed by top journals in each field might increase this fundamental knowledge and decrease the errors in research analysis.

SCIENCE REFORM 27

Empirical research questions: Do people who read a list of common errors and tips commit fewer errors in their research? Do they have more accurate knowledge after reading the list? Would people read this list if it were available?

One example of scientific information that people lack could be causing both intentional and unintentional QRPs such as fishing for significant effects. There is confusion, even among seasoned scholars, over when subgroup analysis is acceptable, such as to examine heterogeneity and moderators, and when it crosses the line into fishing in order to find significant effects. If this were made clearer to all researchers, these types of QRPs might diminish.

Empirical research question: Would an intervention in which researchers learn and think more about this topic with experienced researchers decrease fishing QRPs?

Other industries avoid these issues by requiring recertification every so often as old methods become outdated and improved by newer methods. This ensures that practitioners possess the knowledge they need. The absence of required recertification within academia makes it imperative for researchers to stay up to date on methods and research, which they may not be doing. This could lead to inaccuracies in methods, analysis, and interpretation.

Empirical research questions: In other fields, does recertification decrease errors? Does it increase knowledge of new methods? Would the process of recertification decrease errors, increase knowledge, and produce more replicable research?

Inaccurate knowledge about published research studies is also common. Many journals do not have a section for comments from other researchers or do not publish short critiques. It is thus difficult for researchers, particularly those who do not know the field or literature very well, to be able to tell if a paper has issues, such as if it has misused statistics. In the extreme case, researchers are not aware that the study they are trying to replicate or after which to model their own research was retracted. The retraction process is extremely slow (Trikalinos et al., 2008), and retracted papers are cited often even if it is clear that they have been retracted, which is not always the case (Budd et al., 1999). Even if researchers know which papers have been retracted and avoid citing them, they still might not be aware of the flaws in each paper even after it has been published. They may not know, for instance, that the methodology used in the paper is one that is not appropriate for the research question at hand and that using the correct methodology might lead to entirely different results.

The first of two solutions that have been proposed to address these issues suggests providing a clear and publicly accessible online comment section attached to every journal article. There, researchers can point out flaws in the study in a way that would be easily seen by others. This would reduce inaccuracy in science by reducing the number of flawed studies that would otherwise be used for background, evidence, or replication attempts. But such a system might be abused if, for instance, someone who did not like a certain researcher wrote negative comments that could ultimately steer others to incorrectly discount the study as flawed.

> Empirical research questions: Do people who see a clear, easily accessible online comment section attached to a journal article gain more accurate knowledge about the paper than those who do not see a comment section? Would people incorporate information from the comment section in their judgments about the paper? Would people cite the study less than if the comments were not there? Would people replicate it or incorporate it in their study less than if there were no comments? If given the opportunity to comment, would people who do not like a certain researcher or study write negative comments for even high-quality articles? Would a comment section increase replicability? Would a comment section decrease inaccurate citations and inaccurate knowledge about the field?

Another solution is post-publication peer review. Suggestions for this process include collecting and flagging studies that are considered to be of very good quality, and marking studies that are of subpar quality. Reviews would be conducted by qualified reviewers and not the general public. Reviews would not be concerned with how interesting the research is or how large the effects were, but about the quality of the research process described in the study. Other researchers may then have a guide to which studies are well done and which ones are deeply flawed. Only studies that are done well might then spread and provide the basis for future studies. Of course, this may have negative consequences, in limiting the scope of cited and utilized research to only a few studies. If reviews are unconsciously biased depending on the reputation of the author, the papers that are elevated in a field may only be those written by the most famous researchers, not the ones of the best quality.

> Empirical research questions: Do post-publication peer-review judgments affect people's judgments? Does post-publication peer review make people more knowledgeable about what good research is? Does post-publication peer review increase replicability? Are post-publication peer-review judgments biased depending on the reputation of the researcher(s)? Does post-publication peer review flag only the most famous scholars' research as good?

Other types of inaccurate knowledge about research also are common. As mentioned in previous sections, many psychological studies are often reported in textbook in a simplified manner, which makes students misunderstand the research and its implications. One solution might be to, in textbooks or in instruction, provide more detail about fewer studies. This would allow students to have a better understanding of the current state of the research in the field, although it could also confuse them or make them less interested in pursuing research.

> Empirical research questions: Does providing more detail about fewer studies and refraining from inaccurately overgeneralizing effects increase the accuracy of knowledge about the research? Does this confuse students? Does this make them less interested in pursuing the field or research?

Another issue is that textbooks present some areas of research in psychology as united, rather than as areas in which the answers are not very clear or resolved and fervently debated. This may create inaccurate assumptions and knowledge about the research field. Three different solutions may be effective. First, rather than general textbooks, students can instead read academic books focused on one specific area, such as attitudes. These books will most likely be more accurate and go through controversies and unanswered questions in detail. Second, instructors could also break an area into sub-areas to prevent students from assuming that even one area is entirely united. Third, the classic psychology studies that have been inaccurately overgeneralized or presented could be framed as part of a developmental period, paving the way for future studies. That can lead to more accurate summaries of later or current research that corrected those flawed studies.

> Empirical research questions: How does having students read standard textbooks versus these kinds of topical books affect perceptions of psychology, retention, and accuracy of knowledge about research in the field? Does framing research in that way increase retention, compared to how the material is taught now? Will it make interest in the field higher?

Correcting Known Errors
The solutions we have mentioned so far focus on correcting or adding to the knowledge people have about research. Non-reproducibility is also caused by unintentional errors, even for people who possess significant knowledge about research and methods. Examining these errors may particularly help to understand a form of non-reproducibility: the failure of small interventions to have an effect when scaled up in size.

One error that researchers commit is using a very small and underpowered study in initial interventions that may make an effect look real due to error. When the study is scaled up with more participants and enough power, the effect then disappears. Sufficiently powering the original study would prevent these apparent but false effects from inclusion in larger-scale replication attempts, decreasing non-reproducibility.

> Empirical research question: If a larger sample is used for initial studies, are there fewer failed replications when studies are scaled up?

In addition, there are often issues with the intervention or treatment such that the people carrying out the protocol interpret it differently than the researchers intended. This would mean that the intervention is changed, which would also change effects and perhaps even make them disappear. Requiring training supervised by the researcher who designed the treatment in which small pilot studies are run may prevent these issues. In addition, in the policy world, professional research firms are paid to do on-site evaluations to ensure that procedures and protocols are followed correctly. People are also paid to follow all procedures and detail each step in spreadsheets. Applying this method to academic research may be another viable solution.

Empirical research questions: Does this type of training lead to successful or replicable interventions? Does this third-party evaluation system improve accuracy and replicability? Does this third-party evaluation system catch errors?

Changing Cultures and Ways of Thinking
A discussion of solutions would be incomplete without delving into the complicated culture of the academic world and the perspectives that researchers hold in it. Solutions that target culture and perspective may be more difficult to enact, but have the potential to have the biggest impact on scientific practice.

One change that has been discussed is changing the way researchers think about research by shifting the use of and focus on p-values to looking instead at the accumulation of evidence for an effect. Researchers who use null hypothesis significance testing answer the binary question, "Is there a significant effect?" when examining the evidence for an effect, rather than looking at the collection of evidence in terms of how big the effect is. This could make researchers disregard studies that barely miss the p-value cutoff, p-hack in order to reach that cutoff, or take as truth a "one-off" study that passes the cutoff with an effect that is not actually real. An intervention in which researchers are taught to examine the accumulation of evidence and to use other metrics aside from p-values, such as effect sizes, confidence intervals, and Bayesian techniques, may curb these problems.

Empirical research questions: Does this type of intervention reduce focus on p-values? Does it reduce p-hacking? Does it lead to more accurate perceptions of the strength of an effect? Does it reduce the importance of one-off studies that may not contain real effects on people's perceptions of the research? Is research that uses Bayesian techniques rather than p-values more replicable?

Changing the culture in order to fit this style of thinking may be beneficial. Creating a culture in which researchers wait until they have accumulated a lot of evidence, and thus put out fewer but stronger papers, may reduce non-reproducibility because only effects that were found multiple times, not just once by chance, would be submitted for publication. An intervention in which researchers are told that fewer and more conclusive papers are more valued than papers in which a surprising effect is found once may reduce the file drawer problem, as well as QRPs such as selective reporting and p-hacking.

> Empirical research questions: Would this intervention reduce non-replicability? Would this intervention reduce the file drawer problem? Would this intervention reduce selective reporting? Would it reduce p-hacking? Would it increase confidence in results and in science?

This type of solution cannot be suggested without mentioning incentives. If the current incentive structure values as many publications as possible, and journals and media are more excited about counterintuitive and one-study ("wow") papers, researchers might not want to stray from their current strategy of aiming for "wow" papers. If it is not possible to overhaul the entire incentive structure, perhaps at the very least, actions that improve scientific practice can be further incentivized.

For example, incentivizing replication work may restrain the power that striving for the "wow" paper has on engaging in QRPs. Adding a section to CVs that lists replications and creating a simple counting system in which replications count as publications would make it easier for decision makers to use information other than citation counts in their decisions. This professional incentive may increase the number of replications that are done. This would uncover effects that do not replicate and potentially the QRPs and errors underlying the false effects.

> Empirical research questions: Would this new CV section and counting system decrease the number of people interested in striving for "wow" papers? Would they increase interest in conducting replications? Would they decrease non-replicability? Would they decrease the frequency of QRPs?

Another change that can be made to CVs is to provide more space for the discussion of various skills or accomplishments or even publications. For example, a graduate student might describe the way her creative teaching techniques revolutionized the way communication was taught at her university. This way, decision makers have a bountiful amount of information and are not restricted to numbers such as citation counts. This, in turn, would decrease the professional incentive to rack up as many publications as possible, which might lead to fewer QRPs and more carefully conducted research.

Empirical research questions: Would this new type of CV decrease non-reproducibility? Would it reduce QRPs? Would decision makers use this information in their decisions?

Investigating These Research Questions

A number of empirical research questions have been presented so far, some very broad and wide in scope and others more specific. To aid in the development of next research steps, this section will present a few possible study designs and examples that will illustrate how the research questions we have proposed can be developed into research studies that can be implemented.

The Field Experiment

Rather than being confined to the laboratory and to university student participants, a field experiment could examine the behavior of researchers as they do research. For instance, imagine you would like to test the effects of preregistration on the quality of science. You could randomly assign researchers to either preregister all of their studies or not to preregister any of their studies. Yoked pairs that are similar in terms of quality of research (perhaps rated by independent experts) can be compared when studies are completed in terms of the quality of the science that is produced, its replicability, and the number of papers that are submitted for publication.

The Observational Study

Sometimes there is not a variable to be manipulated or a treatment to be implemented, in which case an observational study can help to answer questions concerning, for instance, frequency and amount. Suppose you want to see how much would be left in the file drawer, or how many studies are abandoned or how many variables or studies are discontinued, after preregistration. You could pay researchers to put everything they do on a preregistration site such as Open Science Framework, and determine how many studies are started and how many end up being finished. This would allow you to determine how much would be in the file drawer if researchers were to adopt preregistration.

The Simulation

Equipped with the necessary resources, a natural experiment in which you create a world can be extremely illuminating because you would know all ground truths. For instance, in order to determine when and why p-hacking or other QRPs occur, you could create an experimental world in which smaller experiments will be simulated. Graduate students would do experiments in this simulated world and analyze the data. P-hacking and other QRPs can be observed and tracked as they occur within this environment, all while knowing the real truth value.

The Nonexperimental Cross-Sectional Comparison and/or Time Series Analysis

Rather than doing a costly experiment, you could do cross-sectional comparisons or time series analyses to see if a solution app whether preregistration procedures instituted by journals have certain effects on the journal (e.g., quality of results, number of submissions, impact factor). You could measure the impact of preregistration procedures instituted by journals on certain outcomes by comparing these outcomes on journals of similar quality, some that do not have any preregistration requirements and some that do. Or you could do a time series analysis to examine these outcomes for the same journals before and after they implement transparency guidelines.

Conclusion

Widespread concern about scientific methodology presents an opportunity for meta-research on how the process of scientific inquiry works, and thus on the behavior of researchers. Our goal here has been to identify potentially useful directions for such research addressing potentially problematic practices, the causes of such behaviors, and potential solutions. We look forward to seeing empirical research along these lines and others as well, in the service of maximizing the efficiency of scientific inquiry and the validity of scientific conclusions.

References

Budd, J. M., Sievert, M., Schultz, T. R., & Scoville, C. (1999). Effects of article retraction on citation and practice in medicine. *Bulletin of the Medical Library Association*, 87(4), 437.

Coffman, L. C., & Niederle, M. (2015). Pre-analysis plans have limited upside especially where replications are feasible. *Journal of Economic Perspectives*, 29(3), 81–98.

Dwan, K., Gamble, C., Williamson, P. R., & Kirkham, J. J. (2013). Systematic review of the empirical evidence of study publication bias and outcome reporting bias—an updated review. *PloS One*, 8(7), e66844.

Fanelli, D. (2010). Do pressures to publish increase scientists' bias? An empirical support from US states data. *PloS One*, 5(4), e10271.

Gelman, A. (2013). Preregistration of studies and mock reports. *Political Analysis*, 21(1), 40–41.

Head, M. L., Holman, L., Lanfear, R., Kahn, A. T., & Jennions, M. D. (2015). The extent and consequences of p-hacking in science. *PLoS Biology*, 13(3), e1002106.

Ioannidis, J. P. (2014). How to make more published research true. *PLoS Medicine*, 11(10), e1001747.

Ioannidis, J. P. (2015). Anticipating consequences of sharing raw data and code and of awarding badges for sharing. *Journal of Clinical Epidemiology*, 70, P258–P260.

John, L. K., Loewenstein, G., & Prelec, D. (2012). Measuring the prevalence of questionable research practices with incentives for truth telling. *Psychological Science*, 23(5), 524–532.

Levelt, W. J., Drenth, P. J. D., & Noort, E. (2012). Flawed science: The fraudulent research practices of social psychologist Diederik Stapel. http://www.tilburguniversity.edu/upload/3ff904d7-547b-40ae-85fe-bea38e05a34a_Final%20report%20Flawed%20Science.pdf

Mellado, V. (1997). Preservice teachers' classroom practice and their conceptions of the nature of science. *Science & Education*, 6(4), 331–354.

Olken, B. (2015). Promises and perils of pre-analysis plans. *Journal of Economic Perspectives*, 29(3), 61–80.

Open Science Collaboration. (2015). Estimating the reproducibility of psychological science. *Science*, 349(6251). https://www.science.org/doi/10.1126/science.aac4716

Reinstein, A., Hasselback, J. R., Riley, M. E., & Sinason, D. H. (2011). Pitfalls of using citation indices for making academic accounting promotion, tenure, teaching load, and merit pay decisions. *Issues in Accounting Education*, 26(1), 99–131.

Steen, R. G. (2011). Retractions in the scientific literature: Is the incidence of research fraud increasing? *Journal of Medical Ethics*, 37(4), 249–253.

Trikalinos, N. A., Evangelou, E., & Ioannidis, J. P. (2008). Falsified papers in high-impact journals were slow to retract and indistinguishable from nonfraudulent papers. *Journal of Clinical Epidemiology*, 61(5), 464–470.

Weir, K. (2011). The new academic job market. *GradPsych Magazine, American Psychological Association*. http://www.apa.org/gradpsych/2011/09/job-market.aspx

2
Improving Research Transparency in the Social Sciences
Registration, Preregistration, and Multiple Testing Adjustments

Garret Christensen and Edward Miguel[*]

Introduction

Openness and transparency have long been considered key pillars of the scientific ethos (Merton, 1973). Yet there is growing awareness that current research practices often deviate from this ideal, and can sometimes produce misleading bodies of evidence (Miguel et al., 2014). As we survey in this chapter, there is growing evidence documenting the prevalence of publication bias in economics and other scientific fields, as well as specification searching. Though peer review and robustness checks aim to reduce these problems, they appear unable to solve the problem entirely. While some of these issues have been widely discussed within economics for some time (DeLong & Lang, 1992; Dewald et al., 1986; Leamer, 1983), there has been a notable recent flurry of activity documenting these problems, and also generating new ideas for how to address them.

The goal of this chapter is to survey this emerging literature on research transparency and reproducibility, and synthesize the insights emerging in economics as well as from other fields—awareness of these issues has also recently come to the fore in political science (Gerber et al., 2001), psychology (Franco et al., 2016; Open Science Collaboration, 2015; Simmons et al., 2011), sociology (Gerber & Malhotra, 2008b), across the social sciences

---

[*] A similar paper with some related material was published as Christensen and Miguel (2018).

(Franco et al., 2014), finance (Harvey et al., 2016), and other research disciplines as well, including medicine (Ioannidis, 2005). We also discuss productive avenues for future work.

With the vastly greater computing power of recent decades and the ability to run a nearly infinite number of regressions (Sala-i-Martin, 1997), there is renewed concern that null-hypothesis statistical testing is subject to both conscious and unconscious manipulation. At the same time, technological progress has also facilitated various new statistical tools and potential solutions, including improved tests for publication bias, new ways to test the robustness of multiple estimates, and registration and preregistration of studies. Yet, as we discuss here, the progress to date is partial, with some journals and fields in the social sciences adopting new practices to promote transparency and reproducibility and many others not (yet) doing so.[1]

The rest of the paper is organized as follows. The first section focuses on documenting the problems, focusing on publication bias specification searching. The second section focuses on possible solutions to these issues: improved analytical methods, study registration, and pre-analysis plans. The final section discusses future directions for research as well as possible approaches to change norms and practices.

Evidence on Problems with the Current Body of Research

Multiple problems have been identified within the body of published research results in the social sciences. We focus on two that have come under greater focus in the recent push for transparency: publication bias and specification searching. Before describing them, it is useful to frame some key issues with a simple model.

---

[1] In addition to methodological concepts we discuss here, journals have been improving, requiring data (Bernanke, 2004; Wilson, 2012; Wilson, 2010), adopting guidelines such as the Transparency and Openness Promotion (TOP) Guidelines (McNutt, 2016; Nosek et al., 2015), and reviewing and publishing papers based on design rather than results (Chambers, 2013; Findley et al., 2016; Foster et al., 2018; Foster et al., 2019). Organizations such as the Center for Open Science (http://cos.io) and the Berkeley Initiative for Transparency in the Social Sciences (http://bitss.org) have also formed to educate and facilitate adoption. We discuss these in more detail in Christensen et al. (2019).

Publication Bias

Publication bias arises if certain types of statistical results are more likely to be published than other results, conditional on the research design and data used. This is usually thought to be most relevant in the case of studies that fail to reject the null hypothesis, which are thought to generate less support for publication among referees and journal editors.[2] If the research community is unable to track the complete body of statistical tests that have been run, including those that fail to reject the null (and thus are less likely to be published), then we cannot determine the true proportion of tests in a literature that reject the null. Thus it is critically important to understand how many tests have been run. The term "file drawer problem" was coined decades ago (Rosenthal, 1979) to describe this problem of results that are missing from a body of research evidence. The issue was a concern even earlier; see, for example, Sterling (1959), which warned of "embarrassing and unanticipated results" from type I errors if not significant results went unpublished.

Important recent research by Franco et al. (2014, 2016) affirms the importance of this issue in practice in contemporary social science research. They document that a large share of empirical analyses in the social sciences are never published or even written up, and the likelihood that a finding is shared with the broader research community falls sharply for "null" findings—that is, those that are not statistically significant (Franco et al., 2014).

Cleverly, the authors are able to look inside the file drawer through their access to the universe of studies that passed peer review and were included in a nationally representative social science survey, namely the National Science Foundation (NSF)-funded Time-Sharing Experiments in the Social Sciences, or TESS.[3] TESS funded studies across research fields, including in economics (e.g., Allcott & Taubinsky, 2015; Walsh et al., 2009) as well as political science, sociology, and other fields. Franco and colleagues tracked nearly all of the original studies over time, keeping track of the nature of the empirical results as well as the ultimate publication of the study, across the dozens of studies that participated in the original project.

They find a striking empirical pattern: Studies where the main hypothesis tested yielded null results are 40 percentage points less likely to be published

---

[2] Note that in a general sense "publication bias" could refer to the bias inherent in research publications from fads, topic timeliness, author status, political activism, or numerous other sources, but we mostly refer to the nonpublication of statistical null findings.

[3] See http://tessexperiments.org.

in a journal than those with a strongly statistically significant result, and a full 60 percentage points less likely to be written up in any form. This finding has potentially severe implications for our understanding of findings in whole bodies of social science research, if "zeros" are never seen by other scholars, even in working-paper form. It implies that the positive predictive value (PPV) of research is likely to be lower than it would be otherwise, and also has negative implications for the validity of meta-analyses, if null results are not known to the scholars attempting to draw broader conclusions about a body of evidence. The same TESS database yielded 32 psychology studies that the authors further analyzed, concluding that 40% of studies did not fully report all experimental conditions, and reported effects were twice as large as those unreported (Franco et al., 2016).

Consistent with these findings, other recent analyses have documented how widespread publication bias appears to be in economics research. Brodeur et al. (2016) collected a large sample of test statistics from papers in three top journals that publish largely empirical results (*American Economic Review*, *Quarterly Journal of Economics*, and *Journal of Political Economy*) from 2005 to 2011. They propose a method to differentiate between the journal's selection of papers with statistically stronger results and inflation of significance levels by the authors themselves. They begin by pointing out that a distribution of z-statistics under the null hypothesis would have a monotonically decreasing probability density. Next, if journals prefer results with stronger significance levels, this selection could explain an increasing density, at least on part of the distribution. However, Brodeur et al. hypothesize that observing a local minimum density before a local maximum is unlikely if only this selection process by journals is present. They argue that a local minimum is consistent with the additional presence of inflation of significance levels by the authors.

Brodeur et al. (2016) document a rather disturbing two-humped density function of test statistics, with a relative dearth of reported p-values just above the standard 0.05 level (i.e., below a t-statistic of 1.96) cutoff for statistical significance, and greater density just below 0.05 (i.e., above 1.96 for t-statistics). This is a strong indication that some combination of author bias and publication bias is fairly common. Using a variety of possible underlying distributions of test statistics, and estimating how selection would affect these distributions, they estimate the residual ("the valley and the echoing bump") and conclude that between 10% and 20% of marginally significant empirical results in these journals are likely to be unreliable. They also document that the proportion of misreporting appears to be lower in articles without "eye-catchers" (such as asterisks in tables that denote statistical significance), as well as in papers written by more senior authors, including those with tenured authors.

A similar pattern strongly suggestive of publication bias also appears in other social science fields, including political science, sociology, psychology, as well as in clinical medical research. Gerber and Malhotra (2008b) have used the caliper test, which compares the frequency of test statistics just above and below the key statistical significance cutoff, which is similar in spirit to a regression discontinuity design. Specifically, they compare the number of z-scores lying in the interval $[1.96 - X\%, 1.96]$ to the number in $[1.96, 1.96 + X\%]$, where X is the size of the caliper, and they examine these differences at 5%, 10%, 15%, and 20% critical values.[4]

These caliper tests are used to examine reported empirical results in leading sociology journals (*American Sociological Review*, *American Journal of Sociology*, and *Sociological Quarterly*) and reject the hypothesis of no publication bias at the 1-in-10-million level (Gerber & Malhotra, 2008b). Data from two leading political science journals (*American Political Science Review* and *American Journal of Political Science*) reject the hypothesis of no publication bias at the 1-in-32-billion level (Gerber & Malhotra, 2008a).

Psychologists have recently developed a related tool called the "p-curve," describing the density of reported p-values in a literature, that again takes advantage of the fact that if the null hypothesis were true (i.e., no effect), p-values should be uniformly distributed between 0 and 1 (Simonsohn et al., 2014a). Intuitively, under the null of no effect, a p-value less than 0.08 should occur 8% of the time, a p-value less than 0.07 occurs 7% of the time, etc., meaning a p-value between 0.07 and 0.08, or between any other 0.01-wide interval, should occur 1% of the time. In the case of true non-zero effects, the distribution of p-values should be right-skewed (with a decreasing density), with more low values (0.01) than higher values (0.04) (Hung et al., 1997).[5] In contrast, in bodies of empirical literature suffering from publication bias, or

---

[4] Note that when constructing z-scores from regression coefficients and standard errors, rounding may lead to an artificially large number of round or even integer z-scores. Brodeur et al. (2016) reconstruct original estimates by randomly redrawing numbers from a uniform interval (i.e., a standard error of 0.02 could actually be anything in the interval [0.015, 0.025]). This does not alter results significantly.

[5] Unlike economics journals, which often use asterisks or other notation to separately indicate p-values (0,.01), [0.01 <.05), and [.05,.1), psychology journals often indicate only whether a p-value is less than 0.05, and this is the standard used throughout (Simonsohn et al., 2014a).

"p-hacking" in their terminology, in which researchers evaluate significance as they collect data and only report results with statistically significant effects, the distribution of p-values would be left-skewed (assuming that researchers stop searching across specifications or collecting data once the desired level of significance is achieved).

To test whether a p-curve is right- or left-skewed, one can construct what the authors call a "pp-value," or p-value of the p-value—the probability of observing a significant p-value at least as extreme if the null were true—and then aggregate the pp-values in a literature with Fisher's method and test for skew with a χ^2 test. The authors also suggest a test of comparing whether a p-curve is flatter than the curve that would result if studies were (somewhat arbitrarily) powered at 33%, and interpret a p-curve that is significantly flatter or left-skewed than this as lacking in evidentiary value. The p-curve can also potentially be used to correct effect size estimates in literatures suffering from publication bias; corrected estimates of the "choice overload" literature exhibit a change in direction from standard published estimates (Simonsohn et al., 2014b).[6]

Thanks to the existence of study registries and ethical review boards in clinical medical research, it is increasingly possible to survey nearly the universe of studies that have been undertaken, along the lines of Franco et al. (2014). Easterbrook et al. (1991) reviewed the universe of protocols submitted to the Central Oxford Research Ethics Committee, and both Kirsch et al. (2008) and Turner et al. (2008) employ the universe of tests of certain antidepressant drugs submitted to the U.S. Food and Drug Administration (FDA), and all found significantly higher publication rates when tests yield statistically significant results. Turner et al. found that 37 of 38 (97%) of trials with positive (i.e., statistically significant) results were published, while only 8 of 24 (33%) with null (or negative) results were published; for a meta-meta-analysis of the latter two studies, see Ioannidis (2008).

A simple model of publication bias described in McCrary et al. (2016) suggests that, under some relatively strong assumptions regarding the rate of nonpublication of statistically nonsignificant results, readers of research studies could potentially adjust their significance threshold to "undo" the distortion by using a more stringent t-test statistic of 3.02 (rather than 1.96) to infer statistical significance at 95% confidence. They note that approximately

---

[6] For an online implementation of the p-curve, see http://p-curve.com. Also see a discussion of the robustness of the test in Simonsohn et al. (2015a) and Ulrich & Miller (2015).

30% of published test statistics in the social sciences fall between these two cutoffs. It is also possible that this method would break down and result in a "t-ratio arms race" if all researchers were to use it, so it is mostly intended for illustrative purposes.

As an aside, it is also possible that publication bias could work *against* rejection of the null hypothesis in some cases. For instance, within economics in cases where there is a strong theoretical presumption among some scholars that the null hypothesis of no effect is likely to hold (e.g., in certain tests of market efficiency), the publication process could be biased by a preference among editors and referees for nonrejection of the null hypothesis of no effect. This complicates efforts to neatly characterize the nature of publication bias and may limit the application of the method in McCrary et al. (2016).

Taken together, a growing body of evidence indicates that publication bias is widespread in economics and many other scientific fields. Stepping back, these patterns do not appear to occur by chance, but are likely to indicate some combination of selective editor (and referee) decision-making, the file drawer problem alluded to above, and/or widespread specification searching (the focus of the next subsection), which is closely related to what the Ioannidis (2005) model calls author bias.

Specification Searching

While publication bias implies a distortion of a body of multiple research studies, bias is also possible within any given study. In the 1980s and 1990s, expanded access to computing power led to rising concerns that some researchers were carrying out growing numbers of analyses and selectively reporting econometric analysis that supported preconceived notions—or were seen as particularly interesting within the research community—and ignoring, whether consciously or not, other specifications that did not.

One the most widely cited articles from this period is Leamer's (1983) "Let's Take the Con Out of Econometrics," which discusses the promise of improved research design (namely, randomized trials) and argues that in observational research, researchers ought to transparently report the entire range of estimates that result from alternative analytical decisions. Leamer's illustrative application employs data from a student's research project, namely U.S. data from 44 states, to test for the existence of a deterrent effect of the death penalty on the murder rate. (These data are also used in McManus

[1985].) Leamer classifies variables in the data as either "important" or "doubtful" determinants of the murder rate, and then runs regressions with all possible combinations of the doubtful variables, producing a range of different estimates. Depending on which set of control variables, or covariates, were included (among state median income, unemployment, percent population nonwhite, percent population 15 to 24 years old, percent male, percent urban, percent of two-parent households, and several others), the main coefficient of interest—the number of murders estimated to be prevented by each execution—ranges widely on both sides of zero, from 29 lives saved to 12 lives lost. Of the five ways of classifying variables as important or doubtful that Leamer evaluated, three produced a range of estimates that included zero, suggesting that inference was quite fragile in this case.

Echoing some of Leamer's (1983) recommendations, a parallel approach to bolstering applied econometric inference focused on improved research design instead of sensitivity analysis. LaLonde (1986) applied widely used techniques from observational research to data from a randomized trial and showed that none of the methods reproduced the experimentally identified, and thus presumably closer to true, estimate.[7]

Since the 1980s, empirical research practices in economics have changed significantly, especially with regards to improvements in research design. Angrist and Pischke (2010) make the point that improved experimental and quasi-experimental research designs have made much econometric inference more credible. Leamer (2010), however, argues that researchers retain a significant degree of flexibility in how they choose to analyze data, and that this leeway could introduce bias into their results.

Related points have been made in other social science fields in recent years. In psychology, Simmons et al. (2011) "prove" that listening to the Beatles' song "When I'm Sixty-Four" made listeners a year and a half younger. The extent and ease of this "fishing" in analysis is also described in political science by Humphreys et al. (2013), who use simulations to show how a multiplicity of outcome measures and of heterogeneous treatment effects (subgroup analyses) can be used to generate a false positive, even with large sample sizes. In statistics, Gelman and Loken (2013) agree that "[a] dataset

---

[7] In a similar spirit, researchers have more recently called attention to the lack of robustness in some estimates from random-coefficient demand models, where problems with certain numerical maximization algorithms may produce misleading estimates (Knittel & Metaxoglou, 2011; Knittel & Metaxoglou, 2013). McCullough and Vinod (2003) contains a more general discussion of robustness and replication failures in nonlinear maximization methods.

can be analyzed in so many different ways (with the choices being not just what statistical test to perform but also decisions on what data to [include] or exclude, what measures to study, what interactions to consider, etc.), that very little information is provided by the statement that a study came up with a $p<.05$ result."

The greater use of extra robustness checks in applied economics is designed to limit the extent of specification search and is a shift in the direction proposed by Leamer (1983), but it is unclear how effective these changes are in reducing bias in practice. As noted earlier, the analysis of 641 articles from three top economics journals in recent years presented in Brodeur et al. (2016) still shows a disturbing two-humped distribution of p-values, with relatively few p-values between 0.10 and 0.25 and far more just below 0.05. Their analysis also explores the correlates behind this pattern, and finds that this apparent misallocation of p-values just below the accepted statistical significant level was less pronounced for articles written by tenured authors, and tentatively find it less pronounced among studies based on randomized controlled trials (suggesting that improved research design itself may partially constrain data mining), but they did not detect any differences in the pattern based on whether the authors had publicly posted the study's replication data in the journal's public archive.

One area of analytical flexibility that appears particularly important in practice is subgroup analysis. In many cases, there are multiple distinct interaction effects that could plausibly be justified by economic theory, and current datasets have a growing richness of potential covariates. Yet it is rare for applied economics studies to mention how many different interaction effects were tested, increasing the risk that only statistically significant false positives are reported.

While there are few systematic treatments of this issue in economics, there has been extensive discussion of this issue within medical research, where the use of non-prespecified subgroup analysis is strongly frowned upon. The FDA does not use subgroup analysis in its drug approval decisions (Maggioni et al., 2007). An oft-repeated, and humorous, case comes from a trial of aspirin and streptokinase use after heart attacks conducted in a large number of patients (N = 17,187). Aspirin and streptokinase were found to be beneficial, except for patients born under Libra and Gemini, for whom there was a harmful (but not statistically significant) effect (ISIS-2 Collaborative Group, 1988). The authors included the zodiac subgroup analysis because journal editors had suggested that 40 subgroups be analyzed, and the authors relented under the condition that they could include a few subgroups of their own choosing to demonstrate the unreliability of such analysis (Schulz & Grimes, 2005).

New Research Methods and Tools

This section discusses several new methods and tools that have emerged in social science research over the past two decades—and more forcefully over the past 10 years—to address the concerns we have just discussed. These approaches have in common a focus on greater transparency and openness in the research process. They include improved analytical methods regarding model uncertainty and multiple testing adjustments, and study registration and pre-analysis plans; we discuss each in turn.

Improved Analytical Methods: Model Uncertainty and Multiple Testing Adjustments

There have been a number of different responses within economics to the view that pervasive specification searching and publication bias was affecting the credibility of empirical literatures. As mentioned earlier, there has been a shift toward a greater focus on prospective research design in several fields of applied economics and political science work. Experimental (Duflo et al., 2007) and quasi-experimental (Angrist & Pischke, 2010) research designs arguably place more constraints on researchers relative to earlier empirical approaches, since there are natural ways to present data using these designs that researchers are typically compelled to present by colleagues in seminars and by journal referees and editors. Prospective experimental studies also tend to place greater emphasis on adequately powering an analysis statistically, which may help to reduce the likelihood of publishing only false positives (Duflo et al., 2007).

There is also suggestive evidence that the adoption of experimental and quasi-experimental empirical approaches is beginning to address some concerns about specification search and publication bias: Brodeur et al. (2016) present tentative evidence that the familiar spike in p-values just below the 0.05 level is less pronounced in randomized controlled trial studies than in studies utilizing nonexperimental methods. Yet improved research design alone may not solve several other key threats to the credibility of empirical social science research, including the possibility that null or "uninteresting" findings never become known within the research community.

Understanding Statistical Model Uncertainty

In addition to improvements in research design, Leamer (1983) argued for greater disclosure of the decisions made in analysis, in what became known as "extreme bounds analysis." Research along these lines has dealt with model uncertainty by employing combinations of multiple models and specifications, as well as comparisons between them. Leamer himself has continued to advance this agenda (see Leamer, 2016). We describe several related approaches here.

Specification Curve

Simonsohn et al. (2015b) propose a method, which they call the "specification curve," that is similar in spirit to Leamer's extreme bounds analysis, but they recommend researchers test the exhaustive combination of analytical decisions, not just decisions about which covariates to include in the model. If the full exhaustive set is too large to be practical, a random subset can be used. After plotting the effect size from each of the specifications, researchers can assess how much the estimated effect size varies, and which combinations of decisions lead to which outcomes. Using permutation tests (for treatment with random assignment) or bootstrapping (for treatment without random assignment), researchers can generate shuffled samples with no true effect by construction, and compare the specification curves from these placebo samples to the specification curve from the actual data. Many comparisons are possible, but the authors suggest comparing the median effect size, the share of results with the predicted sign, and the share of statistically significant results with the predicted sign. A key comparison, which is analogous to the traditional p-value, is the percent of the shuffled samples with as many or more extreme results.

The paper builds specification curves for two examples: Jung et al. (2014), which tested the effect of the gender of hurricane names on human fatalities, and Bertrand and Mullainathan (2004), which tested job application callback rates based on the likely ethnicity of applicant names included in job résumés. Jung et al. (2014) elicited four critical responses taking issue with the analytical decisions (Bakkensen & Larson, 2014; Christensen & Christensen, 2014; Maley, 2014; Malter, 2014). The specification curve shows that 46% of curves from permuted data show at least as large a median effect size as the original, 16% show at least as many results with the predicted sign, and 85% show at least as many significant results with the predicted sign. This indicates that the results are likely to have been generated by chance. The Bertrand and Mullainathan (2004) specification curve, on the other hand, shows that fewer than 0.2% of the permuted curves generate as large a median effect, 12.5% of permuted curves show at least as many results with the predicted sign, and less than 0.2% of permuted curves show at least as many significant results with the predicted sign, providing evidence that the results are very unlikely to have been generated by chance.

Improved Publication Bias Tests

There have been significant advances in the methodological literature on quantifying the extent of publication bias in a given body of literature. Early methods include the Rosenthal (1979) method (the "fail-safe N"), while Galbraith (1988) advocated for radial plots of log odds ratios, and Card and Krueger (1995) tested for relationships between study sample sizes and t-statistics.

Statisticians have developed methods to estimate effect sizes in meta-analyses that control for publication bias (Hedges, 1992; Hedges & Vevea, 1996). The tools most widely used by economists tend to be simpler, including the widely used funnel plot, which is a scatterplot of some measure of statistical precision (typically the inverse of the standard error), versus the estimated effect size. Estimates generated from smaller samples should usually form the wider base of an inverted funnel, which should be symmetric around more precise estimates in the absence of publication bias. The method is illustrated with several economics examples in Stanley and Doucouliagos (2010). In addition to scrutinizing the visual plot, a formal test of the symmetry of this plot can be conducted using data from multiple studies and regressing the relevant t-statistics on inverse standard errors:

(eqn. 4) $$t_i = \frac{Estimated\ effect_i}{SE_i} = \beta_0 + \beta_1 \left(\frac{1}{SE_i}\right) + v_i.$$

The resulting t-test on β_0, referred to as the funnel asymmetry test (FAT) (Stanley, 2008), captures the correlation between estimated effect size and precision, and thus tests for publication bias.

Using the FAT, Doucouliagos and Stanley (2009) find evidence of publication bias in the Card and Krueger (1995) sample of minimum wage studies ($\beta_0 \neq 0$), consistent with their own interpretation of the published literature at that time. β_1 here can also be interpreted as the true effect (called the precision effect test, PET) free of publication bias, and Doucouliagos and Stanley (2009) find no evidence of a true effect of the minimum wage on unemployment. The authors also conduct the FAT-PET tests with 49 additional more recent studies in this literature and find the same results: evidence of significant publication bias and no evidence of an effect of the minimum wage on unemployment. Additional meta-analysis methods, including this "FAT-PET" approach, are summarized in Stanley & Doucouliagos (2012), while significant debate surrounding the validity, or falsifiability, of this and other meta-analysis techniques can be found in Vosgerau et al. (2019).

Multiple Testing Corrections
Other applied econometricians have recently called for increasing the use of multiple testing corrections in order to generate more meaningful inference in study settings with many research hypotheses (Anderson, 2008; Fink et al., 2014). The practice of correcting for multiple tests is already widespread in certain scientific fields (e.g., genetics) but has yet to become the norm in economics and other social sciences. Simply put, since we know that p-values fall below traditional significance thresholds (e.g., 0.05) purely by chance a certain proportion of the time, it makes sense to report adjusted p-values that account for the fact that we are running multiple tests, since this makes it more likely that at least one of our test statistics has a significant p-value simply by chance.

There are several multiple testing approaches, some of which are used and explained by Anderson (2008)—namely, reporting index tests, controlling the family-wise error rate (FWER), and controlling the false discovery rate (FDR). These are each discussed in turn below.

Reporting Index Tests
One option for scholars in cases where there are multiple related outcome measures is to forgo reporting the outcomes of numerous tests, and instead standardize the related outcomes and combine them into a smaller number of indices, sometimes referred to as a mean effect. This can be implemented for a family of related outcomes by making all signs agree (i.e., allowing

positive values to denote beneficial outcomes), demeaning and dividing by the control-group standard deviation, and constructing a weighted average (possibly using the inverse of the covariance matrix to weight each standardized outcome). This new index can be used as a single outcome in a regression model and evaluated with a standard t-test. Kling et al. (2007) implement an early index test in the "Moving to Opportunity" field experiment using methods developed in biomedicine by O'Brien (1984).

This method addresses some concerns regarding the multiplicity of statistical tests by simply reducing the number of tests. A potential drawback is that the index may combine outcomes that are only weakly related and may obscure impacts on specific outcomes that are of interest to particular scholars, although note that these specific outcomes could also be separately reported for completeness.

Controlling the FWER

The FWER is the probability that at least one true null hypothesis in a group is rejected (a type I error, or false positive). This approach is considered most useful when the "damage" from incorrectly claiming that *any* null hypothesis is false is high. There are several ways to implement this approach, with the simplest method being the Bonferroni correction of simply multiplying every original p-value by the number of tests carried out (Bland & Altman, 1995), although this is extremely conservative, and improved methods have been developed.

Holm's sequential method involves ordering p-values by class and multiplying the lower p-values by higher discount factors (Holm, 1979, p. 1). A related and more efficient recent method is the free step-down resampling method, developed by Westfall and Young (1993), which when implemented by Anderson (2008) implies that several highly cited experimental preschool interventions (namely, the Abecedarian, Perry, and Early Training Project studies) exhibit few positive long-run impacts for males.

Another recent method improves on Holm by incorporating the dependent structure of multiple tests. Lee and Shaikh (2014) apply it to reevaluate the Mexican PROGRESA conditional cash transfer program and find that overall program impacts remain positive and significant but are statistically significant for fewer subgroups (e.g., by gender, education) when controlling for multiple testing. List et al. (2016) propose a method of controlling the FWER for three common situations in experimental economics, namely testing multiple outcomes, testing for heterogeneous treatment effects in multiple subgroups, and testing with multiple treatment conditions.[8]

Controlling the FDR

In situations where a single type I error is not considered very costly, researchers may be willing to use a somewhat less conservative method than the FWER approach, and trade off some incorrect hypothesis rejections in exchange for greater statistical power. This is made possible by controlling the FDR, or the percentage of rejections that are type I errors. Benjamini and Hochberg (1995) detail a simple algorithm to control this rate at a chosen level under the assumption that the p-values from the multiple tests are independent, though the same method was later shown to also be valid under weaker assumptions (Benjamini & Yekutieli, 2001). Benjamini et al. (2006) describe a two-step procedure with greater statistical power, while Romano et al. (2008) propose the first methods to incorporate information about the dependence structure of the test statistics.

Multiple hypothesis testing adjustments have recently been used in finance (Harvey et al., 2016) to reevaluate 316 factors from 313 different papers that explain the cross-section of expected stock returns. The authors employ the Bonferroni, Holm (1979), and Benjamini et al. (2006) methods to account for multiple testing, and conclude that t-statistics greater than 3.0, and possibly as high as 3.9, should be used instead of the standard 1.96, to actually conclude that a factor explains stock returns with 95% confidence. Index tests and both the FWER and FDR multiple testing corrections are also employed in Casey et al. (2012) to estimate the impacts of a community-driven development program in Sierra Leone using a dataset with hundreds of potentially relevant outcome variables.

Study Registration

A leading proposed solution to the problem of publication bias is the registration of empirical studies in a public registry. This would ideally be a centralized database of all attempts to conduct research on a certain question, irrespective of the nature of the results, and such that even null (not

---

[8] Most methods are meant only to deal with the first and/or second of these cases. Statistical code to implement the adjustments in List et al. (2016) in Stata and MATLAB is available at: https://github.com/seidelj/mht.

statistically significant) findings are not lost to the research community. Top medical journals have adopted a clear standard of publishing only medical trials that are registered (De Angelis et al., 2004). The largest clinical trial registry is clinicaltrials.gov, which helped to inspire the most high-profile study registry within economics, the American Economic Association Randomized Controlled Trial Registry (Katz et al., 2013), which was launched in May 2013.[9]

While recent research in medicine finds that the clinical trial registry has not eliminated all underreporting of null results or other forms of publication bias and specification searching (Laine et al., 2007; Mathieu et al., 2009), they do allow the research community to quantify the extent of these problems and over time may help to constrain inappropriate practices. It also helps scholars locate studies that are delayed in publication, or are never published, helping to fill in gaps in the literature and thus resolving some of the problems identified in Franco et al. (2014).

Though it is too soon after the adoption of the AEA's trial registry to measure its impact on research practices and the robustness of empirical results, it is worth noting that the registry is already being used by many empirical researchers: since its inception in 2013, over 2,600 studies conducted in over 100 countries have been registered, and the pace of registrations continues to rise rapidly. Figure 2.1, Panel A, presents the total number of registrations over time in the AEA registry (through May 2019), and Panel B shows the number of new registrations per month. A review of the projects currently included in the registry suggests that there are a particularly large number of development economics studies, which is perhaps not surprising given the widespread use of field experimental methods in contemporary development economics.

In addition to the AEA registry, several other social science registries have recently been created, including the International Initiative for Impact Evaluation's (3ie) Registry for International Development Impact Evaluations (RIDIE, http://ridie.3ieimpact.org), launched in September 2013 (Dahl Rasmussen et al., 2011), and the Experiments in Governance and Politics (EGAP) registry (http://egap.org/content/registration), also created in 2013. The Center for Open Science's Open Science Framework (OSF, http://osf.io) accommodates the registration of essentially any study or research document by allowing users to create a frozen time-stamped

---

[9] The registry can be found online at: https://www.socialscienceregistry.org/.

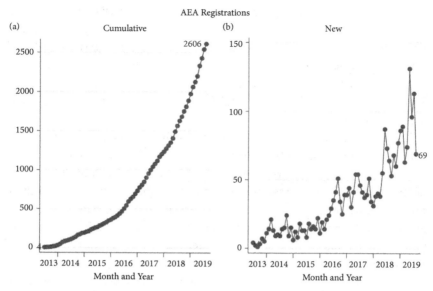

Figure 2.1. Studies in the AEA trial registry, May 2013 to May 2019. Figure shows the cumulative (Panel A) and new (Panel B) trial registrations in the American Economic Association Trial Registry (http://socialscienceregistry.org).
Figure available in public domain: http://dx.doi.org/10.7910/DVN/FUO7FC.

web URL with associated digital object identifier (DOI) for any materials uploaded to OSF. Several popular data storage options (including Dropbox, Dataverse, and GitHub) can also be synced with the OSF and its storage, creating a flexible way for researchers to register their research and materials. As of October 2016, over 7,300 public registrations have been created on OSF since the service launched in 2013.

Pre-Analysis Plans

In addition to serving as a useful way to search for research findings on a particular topic, most supporters of study registration also promote the preregistration of studies, including pre-analysis plans (PAPs) that can be posted and time stamped even before analysis data are collected or otherwise available (Miguel et al., 2014). Registration is now the norm in medical research for randomized trials, and registrations often include (or link to) prospective statistical analysis plans as part of the project protocol. Official guidance from the FDA's Center for Drug Evaluation and Research (CDER) from 1998 describes what should be included in a statistical analysis plan, and discusses eight broad categories: prespecification of the analysis; analysis sets; missing values and outliers; data transformation; estimation, confidence intervals, and hypothesis testing; adjustment of significance and confidence levels; subgroups, interactions, and covariates; and integrity of data and computer software validity (U.S. Food and Drug Administration, n.d.).

While there were scattered early cases of pre-analysis plans being used in economics, most notably by Neumark (2001), the quantity of published papers employing prespecified analysis has grown rapidly in the past few years, mirroring the rise of studies posted on the AEA registry.

There is ongoing discussion of what one should include in a PAP; detailed discussions include Glennerster and Takavarasha (2013), David McKenzie's World Bank Research Group blog post,[10] and a template for PAPs by Ganimian (2014). Ganimian's template may be particularly useful to researchers themselves when developing their own PAPs, and instructors may find it useful in their courses, and additional templates can be found on the OSF.

Building on, and modifying, the FDA's 1998 checklist with insights from these other recent treatments of PAPs, there appears to be a growing consensus that PAPs in the social sciences should consider discussing at least the following list of 10 issues:

1. Study design
2. Study sample
3. Outcome measures
4. Mean effects family groupings
5. Multiple hypothesis testing adjustments
6. Subgroup analyses
7. Direction of effect for one-tailed tests
8. Statistical specification and method
9. Structural model
10. Time stamp for verification

---

[10] http://blogs.worldbank.org/impactevaluations/a-pre-analysis-plan-checklist

PAPs are relatively new to the social sciences, and this list is likely to evolve in the coming years as researchers explore the potential, and possible limitations, of this new tool.

For those concerned about the possibility of "scooping" of new research designs and questions based upon a publicly posted PAP or project description, several of the social science registries allow temporary embargoing of project details. For instance, the AEA registry allows an embargo until a specific date or project completion. At the time of writing, the OSF allows a 4-year embargo until the information is made public.[11]

Examples of PAPs

Recent examples of economics papers based on experiments with PAPs include Casey et al. (2012) and Finkelstein et al. (2012), among others. Casey et al. (2012) discuss evidence from a large-scale field experiment on community-driven development projects in Sierra Leone. The project, called GoBifo, was intended to make local institutions in postwar Sierra Leone more democratic and egalitarian. GoBifo funds were spent on a variety of local public goods infrastructure (e.g., community centers, schools, latrines, roads), agriculture, and business training projects, and were closely monitored to limit leakage. The analysis finds significant short-run benefits in terms of the "hardware" aspects of infrastructure and economic wellbeing: The latrines were indeed built. However, a larger goal of the project, reshaping local institutions, making them more egalitarian, increasing trust, improving local collective action, and strengthening community groups, which the researchers call the "software effects," largely failed. There are a large number of plausible outcome measures along these dimensions, hundreds in total, which the authors analyze using a mean effects index approach for nine different families of outcomes (with multiple testing adjustments). The null hypothesis of no impact cannot be rejected at 95% confidence for any of the nine families of outcomes.

Yet Casey et al. (2012) go on to show that, given the large numbers of outcomes in their dataset, and the multiplicity of ways to define outcome measures, finding some statistically significant results would have been relatively easy. In fact, the paper includes an example of how, if they had had the latitude to define outcomes without a PAP, as has been standard practice

---

[11] See https://help.osf.io/hc/en-us/articles/360019930893-Register-Your-Project. Accessed August 2, 2019.

in most empirical economics studies (and in other social science fields), the authors could have reported either statistically significant and positive effects, or significantly negative effects, depending on the nature of the "cherry-picking" of results. We reproduce their results here as Table 2.1, where Panel A presents the statistically significant positive impacts identified in the GoBifo data and Panel B highlights negative effects. This finding

Table 2.1 Erroneous Interpretations Under "Cherry-Picking"

Outcome variable	Mean in control group	Treatment effect	Standard error
Panel A: GoBifo "weakened institutions"			
Attended meeting to decide what to do with the tarp	0.81	−0.04+	(0.02)
Everybody had equal say in deciding how to use the tarp	0.51	−0.11+	(0.06)
Community used the tarp (verified by physical assessment)	0.90	−0.08+	(0.04)
Community can show research team the tarp	0.84	−0.12*	(0.05)
Respondent would like to be a member of the VDC	0.36	−0.04*	(0.02)
Respondent voted in the local government election (2008)	0.85	−0.04*	(0.02)
Panel B: GoBifo "strengthened institutions"			
Community teachers have been trained	0.47	0.12+	(0.07)
Respondent is a member of a women's group	0.24	0.06**	(0.02)
Someone took minutes at the most recent community meeting	0.30	0.14*	(0.06)
Building materials stored in a public place when not in use	0.13	0.25*	(0.10)
Chiefdom official did not have the most influence over tarpaulin use	0.54	0.06*	(0.03)
Respondent agrees with "Responsible young people can be good leaders"	0.76	0.04*	(0.02)
Correctly able to name the year of the next general elections	0.19	0.04*	(0.02)

Reproduced from Casey et al., 2012, Table VI.
(i) significance levels (per comparison p-value) indicated by + $p < 0.10$, * $p < 0.05$, ** $p < 0.01$; (ii) robust standard errors; (iii) treatment effects estimated on follow-up data; and iv) includes fixed effects for the district council wards (the unit of stratification) and the two balancing variables from the randomization (total households and distance to road) as controls.

prompts us to ask the question: How many empirical social science papers with statistically significant results are, unbeknownst to us, really just some version of either Panel A or Panel B?

Finkelstein et al. (2012) study the politically charged question of the impacts of health insurance expansion, using the case of Oregon's Medicaid program, called Oregon Health Plan (OHP). In 2008, Oregon determined it could afford to enroll 10,000 additional adults, and it opted to do so by random lottery. Most of the analyses in the impact evaluation were laid out in a detailed PAP, which was publicly posted on the National Bureau of Economic Research's website in 2010, before the researchers had access to the data. This is important because, as in Casey et al. (2012), the researchers tested a large number of outcomes: hospital admissions through the emergency room (ER) and not through the ER; hospital days; procedures; financial strain (bankruptcy, judgments, liens, delinquency, medical debt, and non-medical debt, measured by credit report data); self-reported health from survey data; and so on. When running such a large number of tests, the researchers again could have discovered some "significant" effects simply by chance. The combination of the PAP and multiple hypothesis testing adjustments gives us more confidence in the main results of the study: that recipients did not improve significantly in terms of physical health measurements, but they were more likely to have health insurance, had better self-reported health outcomes, utilized ERs more, and had better detection and management of diabetes.

Additional studies that have resulted from the experiment have also employed PAPs, and they show that health insurance increased ER use (Taubman et al., 2014), had no effect on measured physical health outcomes after 2 years, but did increase health care use and diabetes management, as well as leading to lower rates of depression and financial strain (Baicker et al., 2013). The health care expansion had no significant effect on employment or earnings (Baicker et al., 2014).

Other prominent early examples of economics studies that have employed PAPs include poverty-targeting programs in Indonesia, an evaluation of the TOMS shoe company donation program, and a job training program in Turkey, among many others (Alatas et al., 2012; Hirshleifer et al., 2015; Olken et al., 2012; Wydick et al., 2014). The PAP tool is also spreading to other social sciences beyond economics. For instance, in psychology, a prespecified replication of an earlier paper that had found a link between female conception risk and racial prejudice failed to find a similar effect (Hawkins et al., 2015). In political science, the Election Research Preacceptance Competition ran a competition for work with PAPs based on the 2016 American National Election Studies data; eligible papers were required to register their analysis plan prior to the public release of the data.[12]

One issue that arises for studies that did register a PAP is the question of characterizing the extent to which the analysis conforms to the original plan, or if it deviates in important ways from the plan. To appreciate these differences, scholars will need to compare the analysis to the plan, a step that could be seen as adding to the burden of journal editors and referees. Even if the analysis does conform exactly to the PAP, there is still the possibility that authors are consciously or unconsciously emphasizing a subset of the prespecified analyses in the final study. Berge et al. (2015) develop an approach to comparing the distribution of p-values in the paper's main tables versus those in the PAP in order to quantify the extent of possibly selective reporting between the plan and the paper.

The Finkelstein et al (2012) study is a model of transparency regarding the presentation of results. To the authors' credit, all analyses presented in the published paper that were not prespecified are clearly labeled as such; in fact, the exact phrase "This analysis was not prespecified" appears in the paper six times. Tables in the main text and appendix that report analyses that were not prespecified are labeled with a "^" character to set them apart and are clearly labeled as such.

Strengths, Limitations, and Other Issues Regarding PAPs

There remain many questions about whether, when, and how PAPs could and should be used in social science research, with open debates about how useful they are in different subfields of the discipline. Olken (2015), for example, highlights both their "promises and perils." On the positive side, PAPs bind the hands of researchers and greatly limit specification searching, allowing them to take full advantage of the power of their statistical tests (even making one-sided tests reasonable).

A further advantage of the use of PAPs is that they are likely to help shield researchers from pressures to affirm the policy agenda of donors and policymakers, in cases where they have a vested interest in the outcome, or

---

[12] See https://www.erpc2016.com/.

when research focuses on politically controversial topics (such as health care reform). This is especially the case if researchers and their institutional partners can agree on the PAP, as a sort of evaluation contract.

On the negative side, PAPs are often complex and take valuable time to write. Scientific breakthroughs often come at unexpected times and places, often as a result of exploratory analysis, and the time spent writing PAPs may thus mean less time to spend on less structured data exploration.

Coffman and Niederle (2015) argue that there is limited upside from PAPs when replication (in conjunction with hypothesis registries) is possible. In experimental and behavioral economics, where lab experiments utilize samples of locally recruited students and the costs of replicating an experiment are relatively low, they argue that replication could be a viable substitute for PAPs. Yet there does appear to be a growing consensus, endorsed by Coffman and Niederle, that PAPs can significantly increase the credibility of reporting and analysis in large-scale randomized trials that are expensive or difficult to repeat, or when a study that relies on a particular contextual factor makes it impossible to replicate. Berge et al. (2015), for instance, carry out a series of lab experiments timed to take place just before the 2013 Kenya elections. Replication of this lab research is clearly impossible due to the unique context, and thus use of a PAP is valuable.

Olken (2015) as well as Coffman and Niederle (2015) discuss another potential way to address publication bias and specification search: results-blind review. Scholars in psychology have championed this method; studies that are submitted to such review are often referred to as "registered reports" in that discipline. Authors write a detailed study protocol and PAP and, before the experiment is actually run and data are collected, submit the plan to a journal. Journals review the plan for the quality of the design and the scientific value of the research question, and may choose to give "in-principle acceptance." This can be thought of as a kind of revise and resubmit that is contingent on the data being collected and analyzed as planned. If the author follows through on the proposed design, and the data are of sufficiently high quality (with sufficiently low sample attrition rates in a longitudinal study, etc.), the results are to be published regardless of whether they are statistically significant, and whether they conform to the expectations of the editor or referees, or to the conventional wisdom in the discipline.

Several psychology journals currently have begun using results-blind review, either regularly or in special issues (Chambers, 2013; Chambers et al.,

2014; Nosek & Lakens, 2014).[13] An issue of *Comparative Political Studies* was the first to feature results-blind review in political science (Ansell & Samuels, 2016; Findley et al., 2016), and it included both experimental and observational research studies. The *Journal of Development Economics* announced that it would pilot acceptance of these articles (Foster et al., 2018) and later fully adopted the practice (Foster et al., 2019). The rise in experimental studies and PAPs in economics, as evidenced by the rapid growth of the AEA registry, is likely to facilitate the wider acceptance of this approach.

Observational Studies

An important open question is how widely the approach of study registration and hypothesis prespecification could be usefully applied in nonprospective and nonexperimental studies. This issue has been extensively discussed in recent years within medical research but consensus has not yet been reached in that community. It actually appears that some of the most prestigious medical research journals, which typically publish randomized trials, are even more in favor of the registration of observational studies than the editors of journals that publish primarily in nonexperimental research (Dal-Ré et al., 2014; Epidemiology Editors, 2010; Lancet, 2010; Loder et al., 2010).

A major logical concern with the preregistration of nonprospective observational studies using preexisting data is that there is often no credible way to verify that preregistration took place before analysis was completed, which is different than the case of prospective studies in which the data have not yet been collected or accessed. In our view, proponents of the preregistration of observational work have not formulated a convincing response to this obvious concern.

The only economics study of which we are aware that has used a PAP on nonexperimental data was Neumark (2001). Based on conversations with David Levine, Alan Krueger appears to have suggested to Levine, who was the editor of the *Industrial Relations* journal at the time, that multiple researchers could analyze the employment effects of an upcoming change in the federal minimum wage with prespecified research designs, in a bid to eliminate "author effect," and that this could create a productive "adversarial collaboration" between authors with starkly different prior views on the likely

---

[13] A list of journals that have adopted registered reports is available at: https://osf.io/8mpji/wiki/home/.

impacts of the policy change (Levine, 2001). (The concept of adversarial collaboration—two sets of researchers with opposing theories coming together and agreeing on a way to test hypotheses before observing the data—is often associated with Daniel Kahneman; see, for example, Bateman et al. (2005).

The U.S. federal minimum wage increased in October 1996 and September 1997. Although Krueger ultimately decided not to participate, Neumark submitted a prespecified research design consisting of the exact estimating equations, variable definitions, and subgroups that would be used to analyze the effect of the minimum wage on the unemployment of younger workers using October, November, and December Current Population Survey (CPS) data from 1995 through 1998. This detailed plan was submitted to journal editors and reviewers prior to the end of May 1997. The October 1996 data started to become available at the end of May 1997, and Neumark assures readers he had not looked at any published data at the state level prior to submitting his analysis plan.

The verifiable "time stamp" of the federal government's release of data indeed makes this approach possible, but the situation also benefits from the depth and intensity of the minimum wage debate prior to this study. Neumark had an extensive literature to draw upon when choosing specific regression functional forms and subgroup analyses. He tests two definitions of the minimum wage, the ratio of the minimum wage to the average wage (common in Neumark's previous work) as well as the fraction of workers who benefit from the newly raised minimum wage (used in David Card's earlier work; Card, 1992a; Card, 1992b), and tests both models with and without controls for the employment rate of higher-skilled prime-age adults (as recommended by Deere et al., 1995). The results mostly fail to reject the null hypothesis of no effect of the minimum wage increase: Only 18 of the 80 specifications result in statistically significant decreases in employment (at the 90% confidence level), with estimated elasticities ranging from −0.14 to −0.3 for the significant estimates and others closer to zero.

A more recent study bases its analysis on Neumark's exact prespecified tests to estimate the effect of minimum wages in Canada and found larger unemployment effects, but the authors had access to the data before estimating their models and did not have an agreement with the journal, so the value of this "prespecification" is perhaps less clear (Campolieti et al., 2006). In political science, a prespecified observational analysis measured the effect of the immigration stances of Republican representatives on their 2010 election outcomes (Monogan, 2013).

It is difficult to see how researchers could reach Neumark's level of prespecified detail with a research question with which they were not already intimately familiar. It seems more likely that in a case where the researchers were less knowledgeable they might either prespecify with an inadequate level of detail or choose an inappropriate specification; this risk makes it important that researchers should not be punished for deviating from their PAP in cases where the plan omits important details or contains errors, as argued in Casey et al (2012).

It seems likely to us that the majority of observational empirical work in economics will continue largely as is for the foreseeable future. However, for important, intensely debated, and well-defined questions, it would be desirable in our view for more prospective observational research to be conducted in a prespecified fashion, following the example in Neumark (2001). Although prespecification will not always be possible, the fact that large amounts of government data are released to the public on regular schedules, and that many policy changes are known to occur well in advance (such as in the case of the anticipated federal minimum wage changes discussed earlier, with similar arguments for future elections), will make it possible for the verifiable prespecification of research analysis to be carried out in many settings.

Future Directions and Conclusion

The rising interest in transparency and reproducibility in the social sciences reflects broader global trends regarding these issues, both among academics and beyond. As such, we argue that "this time" really may be different than earlier bursts of interest in research transparency within economics (such as the surge of interest in the mid-1980s following Leamer's 1983 article) that later lost momentum and mostly died down.

The increased institutionalization of new practices—including through the new AEA randomized controlled trial registry, which has rapidly attracted hundreds of studies, many employing PAPs, something unheard of in economics until a few years ago—is evidence that new norms are emerging. The rise in the use of PAPs has been particularly rapid in certain subfields, especially development economics, pushed forward by policy changes promoting PAPs in the Jameel Poverty Action Lab, Innovations for Poverty Action, and the Center for Effective Global Action. Interest in PAPs, and more broadly in issues of research transparency and openness, appears to be particularly high among Ph.D. students and younger faculty (at least anecdotally), suggesting that there may be a generational shift at work.

At the same time, we have highlighted many open questions. The role that PAPs and study registration could or should play in observational empirical research—which represents the vast majority of empirical social science work, even a couple of decades into the well-known shift toward experimental designs—as well as in structural econometric work, macroeconomics, economic theory, and other subfields in economics and other social sciences remains largely unexplored. There is also a question about the impact that the adoption of these new practices will ultimately have on the reliability of empirical social science research. Will the use of study registries and PAPs lead to improved research quality in a way that can be credibly measured and assessed? To this point, the presumption among advocates (including ourselves, admittedly) is that these changes will indeed lead to improvements, but rigorous evidence on these effects, using meta-analytic approaches or other methods, will be important in determining which practices are in fact most effective, and possibly in building further support for their adoption in the profession.

References

Alatas, V., Banerjee, A., Hanna, R., Olken, B. A., & Tobias, J. (2012). Targeting the poor: Evidence from a field experiment in Indonesia. *American Economic Review, 102*(4), 1206–1240. https://doi.org/10.1257/aer.102.4.1206

Allcott, H., & Taubinsky, D. (2015). Evaluating behaviorally motivated policy: Experimental evidence from the lightbulb market. *American Economic Review, 105*(8), 2501–2538. https://doi.org/10.1257/aer.20131564

Anderson, M. L. (2008). Multiple inference and gender differences in the effects of early intervention: A reevaluation of the Abecedarian, Perry Preschool, and Early Training projects. *Journal of the American Statistical Association, 103*(484), 1481–1495. https://doi.org/10.1198/016214508000000841

Angrist, J. D., & Pischke, J.-S. (2010). The credibility revolution in empirical economics: How better research design is taking the con out of econometrics. *Journal of Economic Perspectives, 24*(2), 3–30. https://doi.org/10.1257/jep.24.2.3

Ansell, B., & Samuels, D. (2016). Journal editors and "results-free" research: A cautionary note. *Comparative Political Studies, 49*(13), 1809–1815. https://doi.org/10.1177/0010414016669369

Baicker, K., Finkelstein, A., Song, J., & Taubman, S. (2014). The impact of Medicaid on labor market activity and program participation: Evidence from the Oregon health insurance experiment. *American Economic Review, 104*(5), 322–328. https://doi.org/10.1257/aer.104.5.322

Baicker, K., Taubman, S. L., Allen, H. L., Bernstein, M., Gruber, J. H., Newhouse, J. P., Schneider, E. C., Wright, B. J., Zaslavsky, A. M., & Finkelstein, A. N. (2013). The Oregon experiment—Effects of Medicaid on clinical outcomes. *New England Journal of Medicine*, *368*(18), 1713–1722. https://doi.org/10.1056/NEJMsa1212321

Bakkensen, L. A., & Larson, W. (2014). Population matters when modeling hurricane fatalities. *Proceedings of the National Academy of Sciences USA*, *111*(50), E5331–E5332. https://doi.org/10.1073/pnas.1417030111

Bateman, I., Kahneman, D., Munro, A., Starmer, C., & Sugden, R. (2005). Testing competing models of loss aversion: An adversarial collaboration. *Journal of Public Economics*, *89*(8), 1561–1580. https://doi.org/10.1016/j.jpubeco.2004.06.013

Benjamini, Y., & Hochberg, Y. (1995). Controlling the false discovery rate: A practical and powerful approach to multiple testing. *Journal of the Royal Statistical Society. Series B (Methodological)*, *57*(1), 289–300.

Benjamini, Y., Krieger, A. M., & Yekutieli, D. (2006). Adaptive linear step-up procedures that control the false discovery rate. *Biometrika*, *93*(3), 491–507. https://doi.org/10.1093/biomet/93.3.491

Benjamini, Y., & Yekutieli, D. (2001). The control of the false discovery rate in multiple testing under dependency. *Annals of Statistics*, *29*(4), 1165–1188.

Berge, L. I. O., Bjorvatn, K., Galle, S., Miguel, E., Posner, D. N., Tungodden, B., & Zhang, K. (2015). *How Strong Are Ethnic Preferences?* (Working Paper No. 21715). National Bureau of Economic Research. http://www.nber.org/papers/w21715

Bernanke, B. S. (2004). Editorial statement. *American Economic Review*, *94*(1), 404–404.

Bertrand, M., & Mullainathan, S. (2004). Are Emily and Greg more employable than Lakisha and Jamal? A field experiment on labor market discrimination. *American Economic Review*, *94*(4), 991–1013. https://doi.org/10.1257/0002828042002561

Bland, J. M., & Altman, D. G. (1995). Multiple significance tests: The Bonferroni method. *BMJ: British Medical Journal*, *310*(6973), 170.

Brodeur, A., Le, M., Sangnier, M., & Zylberberg, Y. (2016). Star Wars: The empirics strike back. *American Economic Journal: Applied Economics*, *8*(1), 1–32.

Campolieti, M., Gunderson, M., & Riddell, C. (2006). Minimum wage impacts from a prespecified research design: Canada 1981–1997. *Industrial Relations: A Journal of Economy and Society*, *45*(2), 195–216. https://doi.org/10.1111/j.1468-232X.2006.00424.x

Card, D. (1992a). Do minimum wages reduce employment? A case study of California, 1987–89. *Industrial & Labor Relations Review*, *46*(1), 38–54. https://doi.org/10.1177/001979399204600104

Card, D. (1992b). Using regional variation in wages to measure the effects of the federal minimum wage. *Industrial & Labor Relations Review*, *46*(1), 22–37. https://doi.org/10.1177/001979399204600103

Card, D., & Krueger, A. B. (1995). Time-series minimum-wage studies: A meta-analysis. *American Economic Review*, *85*(2), 238–243.

Casey, K., Glennerster, R., & Miguel, E. (2012). Reshaping institutions: Evidence on aid impacts using a preanalysis plan. *Quarterly Journal of Economics*, *127*(4), 1755–1812. https://doi.org/10.1093/qje/qje027

Chambers, C. (2013). Registered reports: A new publishing initiative at Cortex. *Cortex*, *49*, 609–610. http://dx.doi.org/10.1016/j.cortex.2012.12.016

Chambers, C. D., Feredoes, E., D. Muthukumaraswamy, S., & J. Etchells, P. (2014). Instead of "playing the game" it is time to change the rules: Registered reports at AIMS Neuroscience and beyond. *AIMS Environmental Science, 1*(1), 4–17. https://doi.org/10.3934/Neuroscience.2014.1.4

Christensen, B., & Christensen, S. (2014). Are female hurricanes really deadlier than male hurricanes? *Proceedings of the National Academy of Sciences USA, 111*(34), E3497–E3498. https://doi.org/10.1073/pnas.1410910111

Christensen, G., Freese, J., & Miguel, E. (2019). *Transparent and Reproducible Social Science Research: How to Do Open Science.* https://www.ucpress.edu/book/9780520296954/transparent-and-reproducible-social-science-research

Christensen, G., & Miguel, E. (2018). Transparency, reproducibility, and the credibility of economics research. *Journal of Economic Literature, 56*(3), 920–980. https://doi.org/10.1257/jel.20171350

Coffman, L. C., & Niederle, M. (2015). Pre-analysis plans have limited upside, especially where replications are feasible. *Journal of Economic Perspectives, 29*(3), 81–98.

Dahl Rasmussen, O., Malchow-Møller, N., & Barnebeck Andersen, T. (2011). Walking the talk: The need for a trial registry for development interventions. *Journal of Development Effectiveness, 3*(4), 502–519. https://doi.org/10.1080/19439342.2011.605160

Dal-Ré, R., Ioannidis, J. P., Bracken, M. B., Buffler, P. A., Chan, A.-W., Franco, E. L., La Vecchia, C., & Weiderpass, E. (2014). Making prospective registration of observational research a reality. *Science Translational Medicine, 6*(224), 224cm1. https://doi.org/10.1126/scitranslmed.3007513

De Angelis, C., Drazen, J. M., Frizelle, F. A., Haug, C., Hoey, J., Horton, R., Kotzin, S., Laine, C., Marusic, A., Overbeke, A. J. P. M., Schroeder, T. V., & Sox, H. C. (2004). Clinical trial registration: A statement from the International Committee of Medical Journal Editors. *New England Journal of Medicine, 351*(12), 1250–1251. https://doi.org/10.1056/NEJMe048225

Deere, D., Murphy, K. M., & Welch, F. (1995). Employment and the 1990-1991 minimum-wage hike. *American Economic Review, 85*(2), 232–237.

DeLong, J. B., & Lang, K. (1992). Are all economic hypotheses false? *Journal of Political Economy, 100*(6), 1257–1272.

Dewald, W. G., Thursby, J. G., & Anderson, R. G. (1986). Replication in empirical economics: The Journal of Money, Credit and Banking project. *American Economic Review, 76*(4), 587–603.

Doucouliagos, H., & Stanley, T. D. (2009). Publication selection bias in minimum-wage research? A meta-regression analysis. *British Journal of Industrial Relations, 47*(2), 406–428. https://doi.org/10.1111/j.1467-8543.2009.00723.x

Duflo, E., Glennerster, R., & Kremer, M. (2007). Chapter 61: Using randomization in development economics research: A toolkit. In T. P. Schultz and J. A. Strauss (Eds.), *Handbook of Development Economics* (Vol. 4, pp. 3895–3962). Elsevier. http://www.sciencedirect.com/science/article/pii/S1573447107040612

Easterbrook, P. J., Gopalan, R., Berlin, J. A., & Matthews, D. R. (1991). Publication bias in clinical research. *Lancet, 337*(8746), 867–872. https://doi.org/10.1016/0140-6736(91)90201-Y

Epidemiology Editors. (2010). The registration of observational studies—When metaphors go bad. *Epidemiology, 21*(5), 607–609. https://doi.org/10.1097/EDE.0b013e3181eafbcf

Findley, M., Jensen, N. M., Malesky, E. J., & Pepinsky, T. B. (2016). Can results free review reduce publication bias? The results and implications of a pilot study. *Comparative Political Studies*, *49*(13), 1667–1703.

Fink, G., McConnell, M., & Vollmer, S. (2014). Testing for heterogeneous treatment effects in experimental data: False discovery risks and correction procedures. *Journal of Development Effectiveness*, *6*(1), 44–57. https://doi.org/10.1080/19439342.2013.875054

Finkelstein, A., Taubman, S., Wright, B., Bernstein, M., Gruber, J., Newhouse, J. P., Allen, H., & Baicker, K. (2012). The Oregon health insurance experiment: Evidence from the first year. *Quarterly Journal of Economics*, *127*(3), 1057–1106. https://doi.org/10.1093/qje/qjs020

Foster, A., Karlan, D., & Miguel, E. (2018, March 9). Registered reports: Piloting a pre-results review process at the *Journal of Development Economics*. https://blogs.worldbank.org/impactevaluations/registered-reports-piloting-pre-results-review-process-journal-development-economics

Foster, A., Karlan, D., Miguel, E., & Bogdanoski, A. (2019, July 15). Pre-results review at the *Journal of Development Economics*: Lessons learned so far. https://blogs.worldbank.org/impactevaluations/pre-results-review-journal-development-economics-lessons-learned-so-far

Franco, A., Malhotra, N., & Simonovits, G. (2014). Publication bias in the social sciences: Unlocking the file drawer. *Science*, *345*(6203), 1502–1505. https://doi.org/10.1126/science.1255484

Franco, A., Malhotra, N., & Simonovits, G. (2016). Underreporting in psychology experiments: Evidence from a study registry. *Social Psychological and Personality Science*, *7*(1), 8–12. https://doi.org/10.1177/1948550615598377

Galbraith, R. F. (1988). A note on graphical presentation of estimated odds ratios from several clinical trials. *Statistics in Medicine*, *7*(8), 889–894. https://doi.org/10.1002/sim.4780070807

Ganimian, A. (2014). *Pre-analysis plan template*. https://osf.io/exyb8/

Gelman, A., & Loken, E. (2013). *The garden of forking paths: Why multiple comparisons can be a problem, even when there is no "fishing expedition" or "p-hacking" and the research hypothesis was posited ahead of time*. http://www.stat.columbia.edu/~gelman/research/unpublished/p_hacking.pdf

Gerber, A., & Malhotra, N. (2008a). Do statistical reporting standards affect what is published? Publication bias in two leading political science journals. *Quarterly Journal of Political Science*, *3*(3), 313–326. https://doi.org/10.1561/100.00008024

Gerber, A., & Malhotra, N. (2008b). Publication bias in empirical sociological research: Do arbitrary significance levels distort published results? *Sociological Methods & Research*, *37*(1), 3–30. https://doi.org/10.1177/0049124108318973

Gerber, A. S., Green, D. P., & Nickerson, D. (2001). Testing for publication bias in political science. *Political Analysis*, *9*(4), 385–392.

Glennerster, R., & Takavarasha, K. (2013). *Running Randomized Evaluations: A Practical Guide*. Princeton University Press.

Harvey, C. R., Liu, Y., & Zhu, H. (2016). . . . and the cross-section of expected returns. *Review of Financial Studies*, *29*(1), 5–68. https://doi.org/10.1093/rfs/hhv059

Hawkins, C. B., Fitzgerald, C. E., & Nosek, B. A. (2015). In search of an association between conception risk and prejudice. *Psychological Science*, *26*(2), 249–252. https://doi.org/10.1177/0956797614553121

Hedges, L. V. (1992). Modeling publication selection effects in meta-analysis. *Statistical Science, 7*(2), 246–255.

Hedges, L. V., & Vevea, J. L. (1996). Estimating effect size under publication bias: Small sample properties and robustness of a random effects selection model. *Journal of Educational and Behavioral Statistics, 21*(4), 299–332. https://doi.org/10.3102/10769986021004299

Hirshleifer, S., McKenzie, D., Almeida, R., & Ridao-Cano, C. (2016). The impact of vocational training for the unemployed: Experimental evidence from Turkey. *Economic Journal, 126*(597), 2115–2146. https://doi.org/10.1111/ecoj.12211

Holm, S. (1979). A simple sequentially rejective multiple test procedure. *Scandinavian Journal of Statistics, 6*(2), 65–70.

Humphreys, M., Sierra, R. S. de la, & Windt, P. van der. (2013). Fishing, commitment, and communication: A proposal for comprehensive nonbinding research registration. *Political Analysis, 21*(1), 1–20. https://doi.org/10.1093/pan/mps021

Hung, H. M. J., O'Neill, R. T., Bauer, P., & Kohne, K. (1997). The behavior of the p-value when the alternative hypothesis is true. *Biometrics, 53*(1), 11–22. https://doi.org/10.2307/2533093

Ioannidis, J. P. (2008). Effectiveness of antidepressants: An evidence myth constructed from a thousand randomized trials? *Philosophy, Ethics, and Humanities in Medicine, 3*(1), 14. https://doi.org/10.1186/1747-5341-3-14

Ioannidis, J. P. A. (2005). Why most published research findings are false. *PLoS Medicine, 2*(8), e124. https://doi.org/10.1371/journal.pmed.0020124

ISIS-2 Collaborative Group. (1988). Randomised trial of intravenous streptokinase, oral aspirin, both, or neither among 17,187 cases of suspected acute myocardial infarction: ISIS-2. *Lancet, 332*(8607), 349–360. https://doi.org/10.1016/S0140-6736(88)92833-4

Jung, K., Shavitt, S., Viswanathan, M., & Hilbe, J. M. (2014). Female hurricanes are deadlier than male hurricanes. *Proceedings of the National Academy of Sciences USA, 111*(24), 8782–8787. https://doi.org/10.1073/pnas.1402786111

Katz, L., Duflo, E., Goldberg, P., & Thomas, D. (2013, November 18). *AEA e-mail announcement.* https://web.archive.org/web/20131128040053/http:/www.aeaweb.org:80/announcements/20131118_rct_email.php

Kirsch, I., Deacon, B. J., Huedo-Medina, T. B., Scoboria, A., Moore, T. J., & Johnson, B. T. (2008). Initial severity and antidepressant benefits: A meta-analysis of data submitted to the Food and Drug Administration. *PLoS Medicine, 5*(2), e45. https://doi.org/10.1371/journal.pmed.0050045

Kling, J. R., Liebman, J. B., & Katz, L. F. (2007). Experimental analysis of neighborhood effects. *Econometrica, 75*(1), 83–119. https://doi.org/10.1111/j.1468-0262.2007.00733.x

Knittel, C. R., & Metaxoglou, K. (2011). Challenges in merger simulation analysis. *American Economic Review, 101*(3), 56–59.

Knittel, C. R., & Metaxoglou, K. (2013). Estimation of random-coefficient demand models: Two empiricists' perspective. *Review of Economics and Statistics, 96*(1), 34–59. https://doi.org/10.1162/REST_a_00394

Laine, C., Horton, R., DeAngelis, C. D., Drazen, J. M., Frizelle, F. A., Godlee, F., Haug, C., Hébert, P. C., Kotzin, S., Marusic, A., Sahni, P., & Schroeder, T. V. (2007). Clinical trial registration—Looking back and moving ahead. *New England Journal of Medicine, 356*(26), 2734–2736. https://doi.org/10.1056/NEJMe078110

LaLonde, R. J. (1986). Evaluating the econometric evaluations of training programs with experimental data. *American Economic Review, 76*(4), 604–620.

Lancet. (2010). Should protocols for observational research be registered? *Lancet*, *375*(9712), 348. https://doi.org/10.1016/S0140-6736(10)60148-1

Leamer, E. E. (1983). Let's take the con out of econometrics. *American Economic Review*, *73*(1), 31–43.

Leamer, E. E. (2010). Tantalus on the road to asymptopia. *Journal of Economic Perspectives*, *24*(2), 31–46. https://doi.org/10.1257/jep.24.2.31

Leamer, E. E. (2016). S-values: Conventional context-minimal measures of the sturdiness of regression coefficients. *Journal of Econometrics*, *193*(1), 147–161. https://doi.org/10.1016/j.jeconom.2015.10.013

Lee, S., & Shaikh, A. M. (2014). Multiple testing and heterogeneous treatment effects: Re-evaluating the effect of PROGRESA on school enrollment. *Journal of Applied Econometrics*, *29*(4), 612–626. https://doi.org/10.1002/jae.2327

Levine, D. I. (2001). Editor's introduction to "The unemployment effects of minimum wages: Evidence from a prespecified research design." *Industrial Relations: A Journal of Economy and Society*, *40*(2), 161–162. https://doi.org/10.1111/0019-8676.00204

List, J. A., Shaikh, A. M., & Xu, Y. (2016). *Multiple Hypothesis Testing in Experimental Economics* (Working Paper No. 21875). National Bureau of Economic Research. http://www.nber.org/papers/w21875

Loder, E., Groves, T., & MacAuley, D. (2010). Registration of observational studies: The next step towards research transparency. *BMJ: British Medical Journal*, *340*, c950. https://doi.org/10.1136/bmj.c950

Maggioni, A. P., Darne, B., Atar, D., Abadie, E., Pitt, B., & Zannad, F. (2007). FDA and CPMP rulings on subgroup analyses. *Cardiology*, *107*(2), 97–102. https://doi.org/10.1159/000094508

Maley, S. (2014). Statistics show no evidence of gender bias in the public's hurricane preparedness. *Proceedings of the National Academy of Sciences USA*, *111*(37), E3834. https://doi.org/10.1073/pnas.1413079111

Malter, D. (2014). Female hurricanes are not deadlier than male hurricanes. *Proceedings of the National Academy of Sciences USA*, *111*(34), E3496. https://doi.org/10.1073/pnas.1411428111

Mathieu, S., Boutron, I., Moher, D., Altman, D. G., & Ravaud, P. (2009). Comparison of registered and published primary outcomes in randomized controlled trials. *Journal of the American Medical Association*, *302*(9), 977–984. https://doi.org/10.1001/jama.2009.1242

McCrary, J., Christensen, G., & Fanelli, D. (2016). Conservative Tests under Satisficing Models of Publication Bias. *PLoS ONE*, *11*(2), e0149590. https://doi.org/10.1371/journal.pone.0149590

McCullough, B. D., & Vinod, H. D. (2003). Verifying the solution from a nonlinear solver: A case study. *American Economic Review*, *93*(3), 873–892.

McManus, W. S. (1985). Estimates of the deterrent effect of capital punishment: The importance of the researcher's prior beliefs. *Journal of Political Economy*, *93*(2), 417–425.

McNutt, M. (2016). Taking up TOP. *Science*, *352*(6290), 1147–1147. https://doi.org/10.1126/science.aag2359

Merton, R. K. (1973). *The Sociology of Science: Theoretical and Empirical Investigations*. University of Chicago Press.

Miguel, E., Camerer, C., Casey, K., Cohen, J., Esterling, K. M., Gerber, A., . . . Laan, M. V. der. (2014). Promoting transparency in social science research. *Science*, *343*(6166), 30–31. https://doi.org/10.1126/science.1245317

Monogan, J. E. (2013). A case for registering studies of political outcomes: An application in the 2010 House elections. *Political Analysis, 21*(1), 21–37. https://doi.org/10.1093/pan/mps022

Neumark, D. (2001). The employment effects of minimum wages: Evidence from a prespecified research design. *Industrial Relations: A Journal of Economy and Society, 40*(1), 121–144. https://doi.org/10.1111/0019-8676.00199

Nosek, B. A., Alter, G., Banks, G. C., Borsboom, D., Bowman, S. D., Breckler, S. J., ... Yarkoni, T. (2015). Promoting an open research culture. *Science, 348*(6242), 1422–1425. https://doi.org/10.1126/science.aab2374

Nosek, B. A., & Lakens, D. (2014). Registered reports. *Social Psychology, 45*(3), 137–141. https://doi.org/10.1027/1864-9335/a000192

O'Brien, P. C. (1984). Procedures for comparing samples with multiple endpoints. *Biometrics, 40*(4), 1079–1087. https://doi.org/10.2307/2531158

Olken, B. A. (2015). Promises and perils of pre-analysis plans. *Journal of Economic Perspectives, 29*(3), 61–80. https://doi.org/10.1257/jep.29.3.61

Olken, B. A., Onishi, J., & Wong, S. (2012). *Should Aid Reward Performance? Evidence from a Field Experiment on Health and Education in Indonesia* (Working Paper No. 17892). National Bureau of Economic Research. http://www.nber.org/papers/w17892

Open Science Collaboration. (2015). Estimating the reproducibility of psychological science. *Science, 349*(6251), aac4716. https://doi.org/10.1126/science.aac4716

Romano, J. P., Shaikh, A. M., & Wolf, M. (2008). Control of the false discovery rate under dependence using the bootstrap and subsampling. *TEST, 17*(3), 417. https://doi.org/10.1007/s11749-008-0126-6

Rosenthal, R. (1979). The file drawer problem and tolerance for null results. *Psychological Bulletin, 86*(3), 638–641. https://doi.org/10.1037/0033-2909.86.3.638

Sala-I-Martin, X. X. (1997). I just ran two million regressions. *American Economic Review, 87*(2), 178–183.

Schulz, K. F., & Grimes, D. A. (2005). Multiplicity in randomised trials II: Subgroup and interim analyses. *Lancet, 365*(9471), 1657–1661. https://doi.org/10.1016/S0140-6736(05)66516-6

Simmons, J. P., Nelson, L. D., & Simonsohn, U. (2011). False-positive psychology undisclosed flexibility in data collection and analysis allows presenting anything as significant. *Psychological Science, 22*(11), 1359–1366. https://doi.org/10.1177/0956797611417632

Simonsohn, U., Nelson, L. D., & Simmons, J. P. (2014a). P-curve: A key to the file-drawer. *Journal of Experimental Psychology: General, 143*(2), 534–547. https://doi.org/10.1037/a0033242

Simonsohn, U., Nelson, L. D., & Simmons, J. P. (2014b). P-curve and effect size correcting for publication bias using only significant results. *Perspectives on Psychological Science, 9*(6), 666–681. https://doi.org/10.1177/1745691614553988

Simonsohn, U., Simmons, J. P., & Nelson, L. D. (2015a). Better P-curves: Making P-curve analysis more robust to errors, fraud, and ambitious P-hacking, a Reply to Ulrich and Miller (2015). *Journal of Experimental Psychology: General, 144*(6), 1146–1152. https://doi.org/10.1037/xge0000104

Simonsohn, U., Simmons, J. P., & Nelson, L. D. (2015b). *Specification Curve: Descriptive and Inferential Statistics on All Reasonable Specifications* (SSRN Scholarly Paper No. ID 2694998). Social Science Research Network. http://papers.ssrn.com/abstract=2694998

Stanley, T. D. (2008). Meta-regression methods for detecting and estimating empirical effects in the presence of publication selection. *Oxford Bulletin of Economics and Statistics*, 70(1), 103–127. https://doi.org/10.1111/j.1468-0084.2007.00487.x

Stanley, T. D., & Doucouliagos, H. (2010). Picture this: A simple graph that reveals much ado about research. *Journal of Economic Surveys*, 24(1), 170–191. https://doi.org/10.1111/j.1467-6419.2009.00593.x

Stanley, T. D., & Doucouliagos, H. (2012). *Meta-regression Analysis in Economics and Business*. Routledge.

Sterling, T. D. (1959). Publication decisions and their possible effects on inferences drawn from tests of significance—or vice versa. *Journal of the American Statistical Association*, 54(285), 30–34. https://doi.org/10.1080/01621459.1959.10501497

Taubman, S. L., Allen, H. L., Wright, B. J., Baicker, K., & Finkelstein, A. N. (2014). Medicaid increases emergency-department use: Evidence from Oregon's health insurance experiment. *Science*, 343(6168), 263–268. https://doi.org/10.1126/science.1246183

Turner, E. H., Matthews, A. M., Linardatos, E., Tell, R. A., & Rosenthal, R. (2008). Selective publication of antidepressant trials and its influence on apparent efficacy. *New England Journal of Medicine*, 358(3), 252–260. https://doi.org/10.1056/NEJMsa065779

Ulrich, R., & Miller, J. (2015). P-hacking by post hoc selection with multiple opportunities: Detectability by skewness test? Comment on Simonsohn, Nelson, and Simmons (2014). *Journal of Experimental Psychology: General*, 144(6), 1137–1145. https://doi.org/10.1037/xge0000086

U.S. Food and Drug Administration. (n.d.). *E9 statistical principles for clinical trials*. http://www.fda.gov/downloads/drugs/guidancecomplianceregulatoryinformation/guidances/ucm073137.pdf

Vosgerau, J., Nelson, L. D., Simonsohn, U., & Simmons, J. P. (2019). *99% Impossible: A Valid, or Falsifiable, Internal Meta-Analysis* (SSRN Scholarly Paper No. ID 3271372). Social Science Research Network. https://papers.ssrn.com/abstract=3271372

Walsh, E., Dolfin, S., & DiNardo, J. (2009). Lies, damn lies, and pre-election polling. *American Economic Review*, 99(2), 316–322. https://doi.org/10.1257/aer.99.2.316

Westfall, P. H., & Young, S. S. (1993). *Resampling-Based Multiple Testing: Examples and Methods for P-Value Adjustment*. John Wiley & Sons.

Wilson, R. (2012). Note from the editor. *American Journal of Political Science*, 56(3), 519.

Wilson, R. K. (2010). Editorial. *American Journal of Political Science*, 54(4), 837–838.

Wydick, B., Katz, E., & Janet, B. (2014). Do in-kind transfers damage local markets? The case of TOMS shoe donations in El Salvador. *Journal of Development Effectiveness*, 6(3), 249–267. https://doi.org/10.1080/19439342.2014.919012

3
What Can We Do About Our (Untrustworthy) Literature?

Harold Pashler and Christine R. Harris

Many people look to the psychological literature for credible knowledge. The goals of these people are highly varied. For example, the thousands of college psychology instructors around the world must decide each semester what is known about their subject that merits presenting to students through lecture and reading. At the core, this is a judgment about credibility (as well as other things). If a large proportion of the work presented in a course is fallacious, it is hard to see how it can provide much value for its students, and it may well do harm. Content aside, any aspiration to promote "critical thinking" can hardly be served by presenting false findings unless the errors are exposed and discussed. In addition to instructors, a small but influential subgroup of academics toil to produce the constant stream of new books and articles that summarize each literature. Their work products include textbooks, review articles published in journals like *Psychological Bulletin*, *Annual Review* chapters, and so forth. These publications tend to be highly cited because of the great appetite that exists for credible summaries of research findings. Here, too, actual correctness is the key to whatever value these reviews have.

Looking out beyond the academic context, there are a vast numbers of practitioners around the world in different fields who seek to draw practical guidance from research about human psychology, or work to create new interventions or methods that might utilize scientific findings. For example, the Scottish educational system recently altered its teaching approach to embrace the notion of "Growth Mindset" based upon psychological research published by Dweck and colleagues. Unfortunately, the findings have not proven replicable (Li & Bates, 2017). Many of the most widely read books produced by psychologists are written with practitioners and the general public in mind. For example, several books tell advise teachers about what psychological research can tell us about the most effective strategies for teaching and instruction (e.g., Browen et al., 2014; Carey, 2015). All of these consumers of psychology require valid information from the psychology literature or else they are wasting their time and squandering limited resources.

The question posed in this chapter is a concrete one: How should these various groups deal with the fact that grave doubts are now emerging about the validity of our published literature? This emergence is strikingly rapid. Ten years ago, if someone had asked, "What are the best practices for dealing with uncertainties in the psychological literature?" it is our impression that the questioner would have received a few bits of caution accompanied by a lot of reassurance. "You can't believe everything you read," they probably would have been told. "Some results may not hold up to independent validation, but you'll be in good shape if you look for results that enjoy multiple lines of empirical support." They might have been told to keep their eyes open for "convergent validation" or "conceptual replication," evidence that supports a claim using different outcome variables and perhaps different types of experimental logic. Direct replications, or the absence thereof, would not have been the subject of much discussion (indeed, it could not have been, since direct replications were very scarce in the literature at that time.) Unfortunately, all of this reassurance now rings hollow, to put it mildly.

The Psychological Literature's Credibility Crisis

The so-called replicability crisis that has engulfed behavioral science emerged in about 2010. While the sense of crisis[1] has inevitably ebbed, the underlying erosion of credibility in the field has only grown since then, leaving in its wake a field full of doubt about what has been accomplished. An increasing number of scientists believe that a large proportion of the published results in the psychological literature are likely to be flat-out erroneous. "Erroneous" here does not mean "embodying incomplete theoretical insights or containing ideas that require further refinement." Rather, it means "containing flatly false empirical claims."

---

[1] Some have objected to the term "crisis" as presupposing that research practices had gotten worse over time. There is considerable evidence that they may have (see, for example, the multi-decadal decline in assessment of demand effects in psychological research documented by Klein et al., 2012, strongly suggestive of ever-increasing corner cutting by investigators), but pursuing that question would lead too far afield for the present chapter.

The first sounds heralding this crisis (or, as some would prefer, crisis of confidence) stemmed from some odd and seemingly disconnected events taking place around 2010. One was the Diederik Stapel case, the discovery of fraud on a massive scale being committed in a well-known Dutch social psychology lab (Carey, 2011). Another was the repeated failures in three or four cognitive psychology labs to confirm some of the best-known findings in the field of social cognition involving behavioral priming effects (Bower, 2012). A third was the publication in a prominent journal of findings purportedly confirming a form of paranormal perception incompatible with the laws of physics (Wagenmakers et al., 2011). Shortly afterward, Simmons et al. (2011) published a highly influential paper showing through simulation how data-analysis practices that were often seen as rather innocuous forms of corner cutting can easily cause completely spurious positive findings to reach conventional criteria of statistical significance. These practices are now widely referred to as "p-hacking," a term that encompasses a variety of ways of exploiting hidden flexibility in analytic strategy in order to obtain at least one significant result, such as testing different dependent variables and placing weight on positive results obtained with any one of these variables.

The present chapter focuses on the question: Is the lack of confidence well justified, and if so, how should the various groups that seek wisdom from the literature respond to this credibility crisis? While the "crisis" has spawned a great many (sometimes very insightful and useful) articles on the question of how research practices might be reformed in the future, the topic of the present chapter is something that has received far less discussion: What should we do with the literature we have, if we can't believe it as we have in the past?

We start by briefly reviewing some of the empirical evidence arising since about 2012 that explains why, for many, the idea of a severely corrupted literature has grown from a dark suspicion to something more like resigned acceptance. Then we consider various arguments about why the problem might not be so bad as it looks. Unfortunately, we shall see that those palliative efforts fall flat. Finally, we offer suggestions for steps the field can take to recover its credibility and confidence.

Recent Evidence of Widespread Published Error

As just noted, one of the earliest events that helped to herald the contemporary replicability crisis was the uncovering of the massive Dutch fraud case involving prominent social cognition researcher Diederik Stapel (Vogel, 2011). The case received a great deal of attention to the lurid misbehavior it revealed. But perhaps its most disturbing aspect was rather little remarked upon. While Stapel evidently published dozens and dozens of fraudulent papers claiming all kinds of interesting social cognition effects, the literature contained not a single published report of a failure to replicate any of these studies, not even (as far as we know) any descriptions of failures in conference posters. The credit for the public exposure of what was happening, and the retraction of more than 50 papers, rests solely with three young whistleblowers whose identities are not yet publicly known. In short, the "inherent" scrutiny that is supposed to be at the very core of the scientific enterprise was nowhere to be seen.

The most direct and empirical attempt to assess the reproducibility of psychological science as a whole was reported by the Open Science Collaboration (2015). This effort, unprecedented in size and scope, looked at research findings from a set of 100 papers published in 2008 in three different journals covering cognitive and social psychology. An attempt was made to replicate one study from each paper, and the effort was undertaken with careful attention to fidelity and statistical power, including looking to original authors for advice. The final results showed that only 36% of the replications reported a statistically significant effect confirming what was reported in the original studies. While the authors did not claim to have tried to reproduce a truly random sample of studies, the set that they concentrated upon came from a wide enough range of articles and involved articles published in sufficiently prestigious journals that onlookers generally conceded that the results are broadly informative about the state of the psychological literature.

Somewhat later, the journal *Social Psychology* published a special issue describing the results of a large number of preregistered replication attempts on social psychology findings judged important to the field. A thorough Bayesian analysis of the results was presented by Marsman et al. (2017), who concluded that only 3 out of 44 effect size measures were credibly shown to lie in a range not containing zero and having the same sign as the original effect. In short, the results of this less random sample of studies selected to be of interest to social psychologists was quite disastrous by any standard.

Looking back before the "crisis," Makel et al. (2012) reported that about 1% of psychology articles reported replications of prior research. The crisis itself appears to have changed that, however, and in the last 5 years, researchers have been emboldened to check out results in the literature at an unprecedented rate. It would certainly appear that, of the recent wave of direct replication attempts, many fewer than half have confirmed the original results they sought to reproduce, at least in the area of social psychology. Surveying the dismal landscape, LeBel et al. (2017) listed among the resounding failures: "ego-depletion, superiority-of-unconscious decision-making effect, Macbeth effect, power posing, mood on helping effect, money priming, cleanliness priming, elderly priming, achievement priming, professor priming, God/religious priming, font disfluency on math performance, color priming, mate priming, U.S. flag priming, heat priming, honesty priming, distance priming, embodiment of secrets, embodiment of warmth" (p. 257). They were able to find just a handful of recent successful replications, and note "unfortunately, however, such successful replications are much fewer relative to the hundreds of unsuccessful replications that have now been published" LeBel et al., 2017, p. 258).

In short, while we are certainly not in a position to say whether Ioannidis's sobering suggestion that most published results are false (Ioannidis, 2005) correctly describes behavioral science literature, we can be pretty sure that at least some areas of behavioral science have literatures whose credibility is, for all practical purposes, deeply undermined.

Are Replicability Concerns Overstated?

Quite a few psychologists have come forward to argue that concerns about replication are overstated. Their arguments take very diverse forms. Let us examine some of the better-known examples.

Statistics Minimize the Problematic

It is our impression that when the replicability crisis began, many psychologists were startled by the suggestion that type I errors could be very frequent, and their surprise revealed some basic statistical misunderstandings. In essence, their response was to say: "But we have collectively adopted an alpha level of 0.05, and that automatically ensures that we are keeping our type I errors down to 5% on average. So how could far more than 5% of our findings be unreal?" In fact, statisticians have been reminding scientists for decades that the alpha level does not impose a ceiling on the proportion of positive findings that could reflect type I errors—even assuming that all assumptions of conventional statistical testing are true. If power for detecting the sort of effect sizes that occur in the field is low and if only a modest fraction of the hypotheses being tested represent real effects, then type I errors can easily outnumber real effects *among the population of published positive findings* (Button et al., 2013). Alpha level merely puts a cap on the conditional probability of obtaining a difference where there is no difference—it does not put a cap on the probability that obtained differences are false alarms.

A more sophisticated form of statistical reassurance is the suggestion that we should never have expected replication to work every time by the criterion "new study shows a statistically significant difference in the same direction as the original" (Maxwell et al., 2015; Stanley & Spence, 2014). This argument would have considerable merit if the studies producing failure generally had only the same sample size as the original studies, but in most of the cases we have discussed, the failures are observed in studies with considerably larger sample sizes (we are avoiding the term "well powered" here because it is never clear what effect size should be assumed in making such a determination.) One can see crude indices that make the same point even more simply; for example, in the Open Science Collaboration replication of 100 studies, approximately 25% of these studies (powered to show significant differences in the "right direction" 90% of the time assuming the original effect size) produced effects in the wrong direction. In general, it is certainly true that the term "failure to replicate" can be construed in a number of interestingly different ways (see Simonsohn, 2015, for an insightful perspective), but it seems unlikely that complexities surrounding this definition can provide any innocuous explanation for the various (and continuing) stream of non-replications of well-known effects from the literature.

Problems Are Confined to Theoretically Uninteresting Claims?

A more intriguing response to the replicability crisis has been the claim that we should not worry too much about widespread failures to replicate because the findings that are failing rarely involve findings or ideas of any fundamental importance to the psychological discipline. Fiedler (2017), for example, says that a common research strategy in certain areas of psychology has been what he terms "sexy-hypothesis testing" and that such effects tend to draw more attention than they deserve. He points out that if this means testing hypotheses with a low a priori probability of being correct, it naturally reduces the positive predictive value of positive findings. At the end of the day, he seems to say, we should not get too worried if these sexy effects prove ephemeral. The implication is that within each field lies a more substantial body of ideas and results.

One problem with this response is that the judgment of theoretical depth is highly subjective. Consider the area that has probably become more notorious than any other for producing consistent failures whenever independent replication is attempted, namely social and behavioral priming (Bartlett, 2013). Here the "mere exposure" to concepts or ideas is said to have the effect of unconsciously increasing or decreasing a person's propensity to produce related judgments and behavior; a famous example is the claim that reading words related to the elderly makes people tend to walk more slowly for some time afterwards. Are these effects of any deep significance for psychological theory? Or are they mere parlor tricks, standing apart from some more serious corpus of social cognition thinking? Fiedler appears to hold the latter view, as do other psychologists we have spoken with. Nonetheless, Daniel Kahneman (2011) devoted an entire chapter of his career-summarizing book *Thinking Fast and Slow* to the topic of behavioral priming. In that chapter, he contended that these diverse priming phenomena verified (and showed the real-world importance of) some of the key theoretical ideas he developed in his book, starting with the distinction between two purportedly different cognitive systems (reflected in the title of his book). Aware that the results would be very surprising to many of his readers, Kahneman cautioned them that "Doubt is not an option!", noting the statistical significance of the results. (Recently, Kahneman seems to have changed his mind about this, saying he "placed too much faith in underpowered studies"; Retraction Watch, Feb. 20, 2017).

The point here goes far beyond the case of Kahneman and priming, however. The many findings that have failed in recent replication checks may be seen by some as mere "cute effects" devoid of theoretical import, but there are academic specialists working on such effects who attribute theoretical importance to them. For example, shortly before the avalanche of non-replication of behavioral priming effects, Loersch and Payne (2011) presented an "integrative model of the effects of primes on perception, behavior, and motivation" offering a complex scheme to explain the wide variety of priming effects (many of which figure into LeBel et al.'s list of discredited effects quoted earlier in the chapter). While specialists of this sort are often the most eager to defend the research and publication practices that underlie whatever literature in which they are immersed, in some sense they also may be the greatest victims of those practices. After all, no one would wish to become a specialist on an unreproducible effect (a stature akin to being a Bigfoot expert or an authority on the taxonomy of flying pigs). Anyone who creates complex theories that assume the reality of nonexistent effects has labored in immense futility. (Philosophers starting with Bacon have pointed out the crucial role that exploring false ideas plays in advancing knowledge, but they referred to analyzing and ruling out false ideas, not embracing and elaborating upon them.)

Still, Fiedler is undoubtedly correct on the purely statistical point that if researchers investigate hypotheses predicted by theories, rather than interesting conjectures devised on a purely intuitive basis, it might be the case that the effects they look for will have a higher prior likelihood. If so, this in turn can be expected to increase the positive predictive value for the findings that reach significance (i.e., the conditional probability of a real effect existing given that a significant difference occurs). However, if theoretical hunches are poor in quality, relying upon theory should instead lower the likelihood of differences observed being real. We are not aware of any basis whatever for choosing among these scenarios, so we see little consolation for the field in this analysis.

Overlooked Moderators

In the past 5 years, it would appear that the most commonly voiced defense of the validity of the psychological literature as a whole is the contention that failures to replicate may be occurring because the replication study differed from the original study in some crucial but unsuspected variable or detail. From this perspective, the failure to replicate does not indicate that the original finding was invalid (e.g., a type I error and/or due to p-hacking). It merely shows that the finding is narrower in its generalizability than had been suspected—being subject as it is to the influence of a hitherto unsuspected moderator variable. Indeed, this suggestion seems to be an essentially universal reaction by authors of papers that have not been successfully replicated: "You must have failed to duplicate some crucial feature of our study, possibly one that was never mentioned in the original article."

As one concrete example, take the failure by many teams of investigators (e.g., Klein et al., 2014; Rohrer et al., 2015) to confirm the claim that activating the concept of money changes political and social attitudes, as reported by Caruso et al. (2013). Responding to these failures, Schuler and Wänke (2016) noted that the original studies were performed using students at the University of Chicago. Perhaps, Schuler and Wanke reasoned, the use of University of Chicago students was crucial. After all, they argued, that particular university has historically been noted for its prominent free-market-oriented economics department, and perhaps this attracts students who have different affective associations relating to the concept of money than do other college students. (The plausibility of this analysis was reduced when Caruso himself subsequently—and very commendably—attempted unsuccessfully to replicate his own results using a larger sample of University of Chicago students as subjects; Caruso et al., 2017.)

To take another example, writing in *Science*, Ramirez and Beilock (2011) reported that when students spent 10 minutes writing about their feelings about math problems, this caused them to perform better on a "high-pressured" math exam. The reported effect was sizable, to say the least: Cohen's d = 2.48. A recent multisite replication failed to confirm this result, finding essentially zero effect. Responding to the replication failure, the original authors argued that the replication work may have created a lower degree of stress than the original study.

Several writers defending past practices in behavioral science have promoted this general line of thinking. According to Dijksterhuis et al. (2014), "Most psychological phenomena tend to have many moderators (including factors that cannot always be easily controlled in a lab)" (p. 202). Similarly, Stroebe and Strack (2014) said that replication failures frequently occur because "important moderators were not spelled out by a theory" (p. 66).

We lay out a very general difficulty for this point of view, which has not been discussed in the literature to our knowledge. While it is certainly logically possible that an effect requires some narrow set of conditions, it raises the question of how the original investigators managed to stumble upon this set of conditions. The more fragile an effect is (in the sense of requiring a relatively unusual constellation of choices for the relevant variables), the more difficult it would be to ever have gotten the effect in the first place.

One account might be that the original experimenters learned through trial and error what set of conditions is necessary to elicit an effect. This account seems especially implausible in most situations. If there are many different relevant variables, it would require an extensive program of research to identify the correct combination(s) and this could not be done without creating a very large file drawer of failed attempts. That enormous file drawer would of course be very hard to distinguish from the case where there was no real effect and a success here or there was a type I error. Indeed, to conclude otherwise, the original investigators would have to duplicate the result several times, to show that they could "elicit the effect at will."

We have never heard of any author of a study that couldn't be replicated claiming to be in that situation. Indeed, if investigators *were* in that situation and heard of a non-replication, it would make sense that they would respond with confidence to any word of non-replication. If they had truly identified a difficult-to-reproduce recipe for producing an effect and had good evidence of their ability to duplicate it at will, they should welcome the challenge to produce it again, starting in their own labs. The remarkable rarity of that response suggests that they generally have no such recipes. We have, however, seen cases of "peek-a-boo" moderators (Harris et al., 2013): moderators that specific authors sometimes include in their studies and sometimes omit. If an effect is contingent on a moderator, it makes little sense ever to omit it from analyses once its importance had been discovered. Yet the literature on supposed effects of menstrual cycle phases changing women's judgments and preferences is fraught with this. Discussion of moderators seems finally to have petered out: After years of contentious debate on whether women's preferences for men with masculine faces changed based on the phase of their menstrual cycle (e.g., DeBruine et al., 2010; Harris, 2011; Harris, 2012), the original authors of this work finally conducted their own study and basically withdrew their claims, saying, "Analyses showed no evidence that preferences for facial masculinity were related to changes in women's salivary steroid hormone levels" (abstract, Jones et al., 2017).

Another argument one could make in favor of moderators as the cause of failures to replicate would be to say that the original investigators have not identified the recipe through systematic trial-and-error learning, but rather have apprehended it intuitively and without any ability to articulate it. They know how to make it work, but do not know what variables are critical. This is an interesting idea but appears to discard most of the features of science as conventionally understood (with falsifiability being near the top of the list). It also concedes that a finding lacks generalizability, and therefore importance.

In evaluating proposals involving moderators, it would be very helpful to know something of the overall likelihood of large interactions. Some writers have suggested that behavioral science may be treacherous specifically in that human behavior is prone to powerful interactions. There is no doubt that powerful interactions are *possible* with human behavior; variables sometimes interact in highly replicable ways. On the other hand, that does not mean that that strong interactions are *common*. Looking at interactions in the literature is of course useless for addressing this question, due to publication bias.

Ryne Sherman and one of us recently looked at the entire population of unpublished interactions in five of the largest available behavioral science datasets containing experimental manipulations and ample demographic and other subject variables. We assessed the magnitude of interactions of all combinations of predictor and outcome variables. While it was common to find that a Variable B affected outcome Variable X to some degree, finding that Variable A moderated the effect of Variable B on outcome Variable X proved rare, to a degree that surprised us (Sherman & Pashler, under review). The conclusion would seem to be: While interactions certainly occur from time to time, one should not generally bet on them. Thus, when a direct replication attempt fails, one should seriously consider the possibility that the original result was wrong, rather than assuming that some unsuspected interaction has blocked the original effect from occurring (lacking concrete evidence for that possibility).

In line with this, the Many Labs study (Klein et al., 2014) showed that when multiple labs tried to replicate the same effects, some of the effects "worked" and some didn't. But variability in the magnitude of the observed effect across labs was not much in excess of what would have been expected just based on sampling error. That is, the data were roughly consistent with the assumption that the true effect sizes were the same in all the labs, despite the many inevitable subtle differences between subject populations, laboratory environment, and so forth. This again raises doubt about the general proposition that behavioral science data are inherently unstable or subject to an extraordinary degree of perturbation by unknown variables differing from one implementation of a study to another. Of course, many of the studies in Klein et al. (2014) were online studies with relatively impoverished contexts, and there may be other types of studies that are not so homogeneous in their effects.

How to Deal with the Problem

For the reasons we have described, it appears that we do indeed have a very large problem with the psychological literature. Customary methods of literature review cannot generally be relied upon to yield accurate information, due to the biases introduced by publication bias, biased data analysis (p-hacking), and, to a hopefully lesser degree, fraud. This means that an unknown, but likely high, proportion of the contents of the textbooks of at least some disciplines in our field are completely erroneous. (Again, we are not talking about incomplete understanding or imperfect theories; we are talking about simple claims of differences that cannot be relied upon because studies were so poorly executed—with the authors weaving flukes or the products of corrupt research practices together to make stories.) So if that is what we have, what do we do about it?

The replicability crisis has spawned a tremendous outpouring of ideas and arguments about how to improve science going forward. For example, reformers have advocated lowering the critical alpha level to 0.005 or lower (Benjamin et al., 2018); abandoning binary hypothesis testing and replacing it with graded confidence intervals (Cumming, 2014) or various Bayesian statistics; requiring authors to present multiple demonstrations of new effects; requiring or rewarding preregistered methods (Chambers, 2015); requiring investigators to provide raw data to reviewers (Morey et al, 2016); and many others. Unfortunately, these reforms, while intriguing and promising to various degrees, provide little guidance for interpreting the existing literature. Given raw data, one can re-analyze data in line with several of these reformist approaches, as has been done quite frequently in the past few years. However, if the key contaminating factor is publication bias, these methods cannot be expected to remove the biases. Even less can be done when one only has access to summary data.

Use Meta-Analysis to Uncorrupt Our Results?

Can meta-analysis provide techniques to extract estimates of underlying effect size from the literature in a way that corrects for publication bias? For decades, observant researchers have been aware of publication bias (Smart, 1964) and over almost as a long a period, meta-analysts have been looking for methods of counteracting it. If one assumes a simple and "clean" idea about what the publication bias process looks like, simulations suggest that it may be potentially possible to correct for it to some limited degree (McShane et al., 2016). However, difficulties arise when the literature has been corrupted in relatively complex and probabilistic fashion, as is sure to be the case with any real scientific literature.

One interesting recent attempt to develop a method of extracting ground-truth effect sizes from a literature subject to publication bias is the technique referred to as "p-curve" (Simonsohn et al., 2014). The technique is based on the relative number of significant results in different sub-ranges of the range of significant p-values. When an effect is real and power is reasonable, p-values at the lower end (e.g., $p < 0.01$) should occur more frequently than p-values closer to the alpha level (e.g., those lying in the range $0.04 < p < 0.05$). P-hacking, on the other hand, has been claimed to produce an excess of results just below 0.05. While there is some evidence that big portions of the psychological literature as a whole have an excess of results near 0.05 (cf., Krawczyk, 2015), it would be a mistake to assume that p-hacking always drags the p-value just across the 0.05 boundary. This may be true of iterative strategies of p-hacking (in which the data analyst modifies the analytic strategy [e.g., adding a covariate], does a new analysis, and retains the modification if and only if it "improves" the p-value). But it would not be true to the same degree of noniterative strategies, such as discarding the "worst" 10% of subjects (the ones contributing least to the obtaining of the desired effect) before doing any data analysis.

The field of parapsychology provides a rather interesting demonstration of the limits of meta-analytic correction for publication bias. Bem et al. (2015) reported a meta-analysis of 90 studies on the "anomalous prediction of the future." The authors found that "P-curve analysis, a recently introduced statistical technique, estimate[d] the true effect size of our database to be 0.20, virtually identical to the effect size of [Bem, 2011] original experiments (0.22) and the closely related 'presentiment' experiments (0.21)." For those who start with the premise that anomalous anticipation of the future is an effect that has a ground-truth effect size of exactly zero (and that publication bias is likely to contaminate this literature, despite rather impressive and undoubtedly sincere efforts to avoid that), this work is very illuminating. Given that premise, the fact that the p-curve method gives a bill of good health to paranormal phenomena directly implies that we cannot rely upon it to distinguish real effects from effects conjured up by some mixture of biased publication, biased data analysis, and fraud. (In our opinion, fraud should not be assumed to occur at any greater degree in parapsychology than it does in mainstream academic fields, especially since the incentives for producing impressive results in parapsychology are surely far smaller than those found in more mainstream academic fields.)

Speaking of fraud, however, the p-curve method is also likely to be highly distorted by even a small amount of fraud. It is interesting that at least one recent case of apparent fraud seemed to involve the manufacture of highly significant p-values, not marginal ones (Enserink, 2012).

Another interesting case for examining the effectiveness of meta-analysis and its correctives relates to the famous "ego depletion hypothesis" of Baumeister and colleagues. A "standard" meta-analysis by Hagger et al. (2010) appeared to show a rather large effect (d = 0.62). A later meta-analysis by Carter and McCullough (2014) explored the use of corrective methods such as PET-PEESE to remove publication bias. This dramatically reduced the evidence. A later paper by Carter et al. (2015) performed a much more exhaustive effort to dig up unpublished results. The need to conduct a serious search for the "gray literature" has been pointed out by meta-analysts (e.g., Conn et al., 2003), yet it is rarely put into practice. For example, Carter et al. (2015) reviewed conference proceedings from many meetings (including poster sessions) and appealed personally to investigators to dig up unpublished results. This further reduced the evidence for ego depletion phenomena. Since that time, new preregistered large-scale studies have failed to replicate the basic effects (e.g., Gomes & McCullough, 2015; Lurquin et al., 2016). The results suggest that ordinary meta-analysis is likely to suggest the existence of moderate effects in even the most corrupted literatures. Various corrective techniques may help, but one can hardly place great faith in their results. Moreover, the opportunity to dig up gray literature of older effects is obviously going to be rapidly declining with time, making the likelihood of that succeeding increasingly hopeless. (On a more optimistic note, however, with growing respect for open science practices, the situation might perhaps be altered in a favorable direction.)

Another recent paper reinforces the point that, as its authors put it in the title of their paper, "meta-analyses are no substitute for registered replications" (Van Elk et al., 2015). These authors conducted a PET-PEESE meta-analysis that suggested that effects in the literature on "religious priming" were entirely due to publication bias, whereas a Bayesian meta-analysis concluded that there was some small signal present among the bias and noise. How, they ask, can this tool rescue us from a literature corrupted by publication bias (and possibly worse) if the various means for implementing it do not agree?

The Benign Neglect Approach

One option for dealing with any problem is to ignore it and hope things might just get better. What's so wrong with trying it here? As a field, we could decide that we are tired of all the crisis talk, and we are just going to go on doing what we are now doing. We'll make do with the literature we have, act as if it has an authority that we know it lacks, and maybe some of us will try to make that literature increasingly better in the future. What is so wrong with that plan? It seems to us that the field is likely to pay two very different kinds of costs (and, indeed, that we have already begun to pay these costs).

Cost to Psychology's Reputation

The first cost is a reputational cost. A few years ago, we suggested that the educated public appears to be rapidly losing faith in psychological research (Pashler & de Ruiter, 2017). This trend appears to be accelerating. Recently, for example, *Vox* magazine carried a prominent article with the subtitle "The most famous psychological studies are often wrong, fraudulent, or outdated." It would be naive as well as condescending to think that the public (which pays the bills for much of the psychological research enterprise) is going to remain in the dark about the fact that large parts of our literature describe imaginary findings. It would be sad and ironic indeed if, just as psychologists are realizing that they need to collect data on a much larger scale than they have done in the past in order to get statistically reliable knowledge, they should find that they lack the resources even to do what they were doing before.

Erosion of the Open Nature of Science

When we have had occasion to discuss the topic of this chapter with cognitive psychologists, the response we have heard has almost always been something amounting to "Yes, it's a shame that social psychology is such a disaster.

But cognitive psychology is pretty much okay, isn't it? Things generally replicate there, I think." Some voice suspicions that developmental psychology or some other areas are also afflicted.

These reactions reflect a newly emerging state of affairs that we believe will cause many problems. But before getting to these problems, is there merit to the idea that some areas of behavioral science have untrustworthy literatures while others contain largely sound empirical findings? There is little doubt that a high proportion of the more well-publicized fraud cases and failures to replicate have arisen in social psychology. Are the problems of psychology largely far worse in that field? It is easy to see why certain fields might be in relatively better shape. For example, cognitive and perceptual studies most typically collect many repeated measures from each subject in each condition ("fully within-subject designs"). The two priming literatures—in social psychology and cognitive psychology—provide a rather dramatic example of this. For example, a fairly typical social priming study is that of Bargh et al. (1996) claiming that reading achievement-related words increased subjects' cognitive performance. Experiment 1 in that paper involved a between-subject design with about 40 subjects per condition, each subject working on three puzzles. By contrast, a typical recent study of lexical-decision priming in the cognitive literature (Yap et al., 2013) used a fully within-subject design and had 60 trials per participant per condition. This kind of method greatly enhances power and precision for the estimation of within-subject effects (as confirmed in realistic simulations by Rouder & Haaf, 2018, and Smith & Little, 2018).

Thus, it is not implausible that cognitive and perceptual research might be in better shape than other areas such as social psychology. But one does not have to look very hard to find worrisome areas within the cognitive sciences. In the field of cognitive neuroscience, brain imaging research appears to have produced great numbers of extremely small-n studies (due to the cost of the technology) with methods that offer extraordinary experimenter flexibility for selecting both regions of interest in the brain (Vul et al., 2009) and data-analysis methods (Carp, 2012). All of these factors will conspire to produce many imaginary effects, and the method is so complex that replication is a rarity and often fails when tried (Turner et al., 2018). Similar problems have started coming to light recently in other areas of cognitive neuroscience. For example, Luck and Gaspelin (2017) recently showed that "common and seemingly innocuous methods for quantifying and analyzing ERP effects can lead to very high rates of significant-but-bogus effects, with the likelihood of obtaining at least one such bogus effect exceeding 50% in many experiments" (p. 146). So there would seem to be little justification for assuming that cognitive science is broadly free of the most severe replicability problems.

The PRRR project produced a slightly higher replication success rate for cognitive psychology as compared to social psychology, but the difference was not enormous. Wilson and Wixted (2018) suggested that the differences might reflect the fact that cognitive psychologists study effects with a higher prior probability of being real than do social psychologists, although the results are open to other interpretations.

Moreover, even if it were the case that some fields of psychology have relatively more credible literatures than others, the idea that some behavioral scientists have secret knowledge about which areas are credible and which are not—and that they generally keep this knowledge to themselves—should not be seen as an acceptable state of affairs. The spirit of science is a publicly verifiable process whereby theory and data are improved through open dissemination and debate.

If it should be the case that some subset of experienced practitioners hold the private opinion that the published empirical findings in some areas of their own discipline lack all credibility, it is incumbent on them to share this knowledge with students and colleagues and to act upon it in shared university governance and promotion practices. Failing to do so probably even violates the academic integrity standards adopted by many universities and professional societies. Even more obvious, tolerating secret gaps in research quality across the discipline does a disservice to all the practitioners and students who approach the literature of psychology looking for guidance and wisdom. It also disguises the fact that some areas of study are more difficult than others, which can lead to greater incentives to cut corners in order to publish at the rate of the easier areas.

An Alternative Approach: Honest Conservative Labeling

We come now to suggest our favored approach, a proposal that one of us (together with J. P. de Ruiter) outlined in a briefer format elsewhere (Pashler & de Ruiter, 2017). We believe that many of the costs just described—reputational ruin for psychology, disservice to the public, and betrayal of scientific standards—can be countered much more easily and decisively than it might appear. Remarkably, we contend that the power to fix these problems is within the grasp of the community of scholars who produce reviews (including textbooks, review chapters, and so forth). In our view, what reviewers of literatures need to do is to incorporate *explicit and highly conservative labels* regarding the degree of confirmation that any given research finding has received. The top category—which we call Class 1—should not be applied unless a research finding has been confirmed in a direct and preregistered replication. Conceptual replications do not count here (unless preregistered as attempts to do as direct a replication as possible while making necessary updates/adjustments for *context*[2]). The fact that "everybody knows X is a real effect" must not count, either (as far as we can tell, "everybody knew" that Kamin blocking and behavioral priming and the ego depletion effect were robust effects, too.) A second category—Class 2—would be applied to findings that have been credibly reported in adequately powered research designs. A Class 3 rating would apply to merely suggestive findings that have been suggested in low-powered studies. Multiple diverse conceptual replications at the Class 3 level (a fair description of the literature covered by Kahneman in his now-famous chapter on behavioral priming) would be summarized as "a large literature composed of Class 3 findings." That is, they would not all add up to a Class 1 designation.

This "honest labeling" proposal admittedly has a few unappetizing consequences. Many of us—including the present authors—do suspect that there are large swaths of research within big parts of psychology where statistical power is good (usually because of general reliance upon repeated measures and within-subject designs) and most results will probably replicate. In these areas, we suspect, most of the findings reported probably stand up. Still, a field that means to take itself seriously needs to brand any result lacking in preregistered replication (including many of our own) as Class 2 (strongly suggested in the literature but not scientifically confirmed). All research that is based on single studies and/or low-powered designs we would call Class 3 evidence, or, to borrow a phrase from Harold Jeffreys's (1961) classic theory of probability, "worth no more than a bare mention."

The idea of classifying a single experiment that has reached conventional significance levels as a merely preliminary finding is actually in close accord with the preferences of English statistician Ronald A. Fisher himself.

---

[2] The authors are grateful to the editors of this volume for this suggestion. There are some studies whose materials are inherently time bound (e.g., in political psychology), and in these cases, literal duplication of the original materials would not be a sensible way to test the underlying hypothesis.

In his 1935 book *The Design of Experiments*, Fisher suggested people should view this test as entirely preliminary. He said: "It is usual and convenient for experimenters to take 5 per cent as a standard level of significance, in the sense that they are prepared to ignore all results which fail to reach this standard, and, by this means, to eliminate from further discussion the greater part of the fluctuations which chance causes have introduced into their experimental results" (p. 13).

Fisher added this interesting comment: "In relation to the test of significance, we may say that a phenomenon is *experimentally demonstrable* when we know how to conduct an experiment which will rarely fail to give us a statistically significant result" (our italics). The notion of experimentally demonstrable effect corresponds closely with what we propose for Class 1. This is of course exactly what all the troubled literatures are notably lacking in.

We believe that this disciplinary self-control would, if broadly adopted, have dramatic and generally desirable consequences. Results labeled as having only second- or even third-class empirical support will draw the attention of new researchers as worthy topics of investigation. We will surely discover that a great many of the results we believe to be already well established are indeed experimentally demonstrable. Far from being a waste of time, this will produce a great outpouring of good news: "Behavioral scientists actually do know something (after all)!" As robust results are confirmed, they can be cited in textbooks with confidence. But can any sensible person doubt that in doing so, we will also find that a good number of results that we thought we knew are not in fact true?

What we suggest is basically a complete cessation of what has become a very bad habit in academia: the constant overclaiming and overstating of what evidence really shows. The people best situated to stamp down on this bad practice, it seems to us, are those entrusted with performing literature reviews. The consequences of doing otherwise seem pretty clear: If we continue to pretend to know what we do not know, to have shown things that we have not shown, our field will continue to lose respect and resources, likely at an accelerating rate.

Acknowledgment

This work was supported by the National Science Foundation (Grant DRL-1631681 to R. Baraniuk, Rice University, Principal Investigator).

References

Bargh, J. A., Chen, M., & Burrows, L. (1996). Automaticity of social behavior: Direct effects of trait construct and stereotype activation on action. *Journal of Personality and Social Psychology, 71*(2), 230.

Bartlett, T. (2013, Jan. 30). The power of suggestion. *Chronicle of Higher Education.* www.chronicle.com/article/Power-of-Suggestion/136907/

Bem, D. J. (2011). Feeling the future: Experimental evidence for anomalous retroactive influences on cognition and affect. *Journal of Personality and Social Psychology, 100*(3), 407.

Bem, D., Tressoldi, P., Rabeyron, T., & Duggan, M. (2015). Feeling the future: A meta-analysis of 90 experiments on the anomalous anticipation of random future events. *F1000 Research, 4,* 1188.

Benjamin, D. J., Berger, J. O., Johannesson, M., Nosek, B. A., Wagenmakers, E. J., Berk, R., . . . Cesarini, D. (2018). Redefine statistical significance. *Nature Human Behaviour, 2*(1), 6.

Bower, B. (2012). The hot and cold of priming: Psychologists are divided on whether unnoticed cues can influence behavior. *Science News, 181*(10), 26–29.

Brown, P. C., Roediger III, H. L., & McDaniel, M. A. (2014). *Make It Stick.* Harvard University Press.

Button, K. S., Ioannidis, J. P., Mokrysz, C., Nosek, B. A., Flint, J., Robinson, E. S., & Munafò, M. R. (2013). Power failure: Why small sample size undermines the reliability of neuroscience. *Nature Reviews Neuroscience, 14*(5), 365.

Carey, B. (2011, November 2). Fraud case seen as a red flag for psychology research. *New York Times,* A3.

Carey, B. (2015). *How We Learn: The Surprising Truth About When, Where, and Why It Happens.* Random House Trade Paperbacks.

Carp, J. (2012). On the plurality of (methodological) worlds: Estimating the analytic flexibility of fMRI experiments. *Frontiers in Neuroscience, 6,* 149.

Carter, E. C., Kofler, L. M., Forster, D. E., & McCullough, M. E. (2015). A series of meta-analytic tests of the depletion effect: Self-control does not seem to rely on a limited resource. *Journal of Experimental Psychology: General, 144*(4), 796.

Carter, E. C., & McCullough, M. E. (2014). Publication bias and the limited strength model of self-control: Has the evidence for ego depletion been overestimated? *Frontiers in Psychology, 5,* 823.

Caruso, E. M., Shapira, O., & Landy, J. F. (2017). Show me the money: A systematic exploration of manipulations, moderators, and mechanisms of priming effects. *Psychological Science, 28*(8), 1148–1159.

Caruso, E. M., Vohs, K. D., Baxter, B., & Waytz, A. (2013). Mere exposure to money increases endorsement of free-market systems and social inequality. *Journal of Experimental Psychology: General, 142*(2), 301.

Chambers, C. D. (2015). Ten reasons why journals must review manuscripts before results are known. *Addiction, 110*(1), 10–11.

Conn, V. S., Valentine, J. C., Cooper, H. M., & Rantz, M. J. (2003). Grey literature in meta-analyses. *Nursing Research, 52*(4), 256–261.

Cumming, G. (2014). The new statistics: Why and how. *Psychological science, 25*(1), 7–29.

DeBruine, L. M., Jones, B. C., Frederick, D. A., Haselton, M. G., Penton-Voak, I. S., & Perrett, D. I. (2010). Evidence for menstrual cycle shifts in women's preferences for masculinity: A response to Harris (2011) "Menstrual Cycle and Facial Preferences Reconsidered." *Evolutionary Psychology, 8,* 768–775.

Dijksterhuis, A., Van Knippenberg, A., & Holland, R. W. (2014). Evaluating behavior priming research: Three observations and a recommendation. In D. C. Molden (Ed.), *Understanding* Priming Effects in Social Psychology (pp. 205–217; 205). Guilford Press.

Enserink, M. (2012, June 25). Rotterdam marketing psychologist resigns after university investigates his data. *Science.* https://www.science.org/content/article/rotterdam-marketing-psychologist-resigns-after-university-investigates-his-data

Fiedler, K. (2017). What constitutes strong psychological science? The (neglected) role of diagnosticity and a priori theorizing. *Perspectives on Psychological Science, 12*(1), 46–61.

Fisher, R. A. (1935). *The Design of Experiments.* Edinburgh: Oliver & Boyd.

Gomes, C. M., & McCullough, M. E. (2015). The effects of implicit religious primes on dictator game allocations: A preregistered replication experiment. *Journal of Experimental Psychology: General, 144*(6), e94.

Hagger, M. S., Wood, C., Stiff, C., & Chatzisarantis, N. L. D. (2010). Ego depletion and the strength model of self-control: A meta-analysis. *Psychological Bulletin, 136,* 495–525. doi:10.1037/a0019486

Harris, C. R. (2011). Face preferences and menstrual cycle reconsidered. *Sex Roles, 64,* 669–681.

Harris, C. R. (2013). Shifts in masculinity preferences across the menstrual cycle: Still not there. *Sex Roles, 69*(9–10), 507–515. doi:10.1007/s11199-012-0229-0

Harris, C. R., Chabot, A., & Mickes, L. (2013). Shifts in methodology and theory in menstrual cycle research on attraction. *Sex Roles, 69*(9–10), 525–535.

Ioannidis, J. P. (2005). Why most published research findings are false. *PLoS Medicine, 2,* e124.

Jeffreys, H. (1961). *Theory of Probability.* Clarendon Press.

Jones, B. C., Hahn, A. C., Fisher, C. I., Wang, H., Kandrik, M., Han, C., ... DeBruine, L. M. (2018). No compelling evidence that preferences for facial masculinity track changes in women's hormonal status. *Psychological Science, 29*(6), 996–1005.

Kahneman, D. (2011). *Thinking, Fast and Slow.* Farrar, Straus and Giroux.

Klein, O., Doyen, S., Leys, C., Magalhães de Saldanha da Gama, P. A., Miller, S., Questienne, L., & Cleeremans, A. (2012). Low hopes, high expectations: Expectancy effects and the replicability of behavioral experiments. *Perspectives on Psychological Science, 7*(6), 572–584.

Klein, R. A., Ratliff, K. A., Vianello, M., Adams Jr, R. B., Bahník, Š., Bernstein, M. J., ... Cemalcilar, Z. (2014). Investigating variation in replicability: A "many labs" replication project. *Social Psychology, 45*(3), 142.

Krawczyk, M. (2015). The search for significance: A few peculiarities in the distribution of P values in experimental psychology literature. *PloS One, 10*(6), e0127872.

LeBel, E. P., Berger, D., Campbell, L., & Loving, T. J. (2017). Falsifiability is not optional. *Journal of Personality and Social Psychology, 113,* 254–261. doi:10.1037/pspi0000106

Li, Y., & Bates, T. (2017). Does mindset affect children's ability, school achievement, or response to challenge? Three failures to replicate. Unpublished manuscript. https://osf.io/preprints/socarxiv/tsdwy/download

Loersch, C., & Payne, B. K. (2011). The situated inference model: An integrative account of the effects of primes on perception, behavior, and motivation. *Perspectives on Psychological Science, 6*(3), 234–252.

Luck, S. J., & Gaspelin, N. (2017). How to get statistically significant effects in any ERP experiment (and why you shouldn't). *Psychophysiology, 54*(1), 146–157.

Lurquin, J. H., Michaelson, L. E., Barker, J. E., Gustavson, D. E., Von Bastian, C. C., Carruth, N. P., & Miyake, A. (2016). No evidence of the ego-depletion effect across task characteristics and individual differences: A pre-registered study. *PloS One, 11*(2), e0147770.

Makel, M. C., Plucker, J. A., & Hegarty, B. (2012). Replications in psychology research: How often do they really occur? *Perspectives on Psychological Science, 7*(6), 537–542.

Marsman, M., Schönbrodt, F., Morey, R. D., Yao, Y., Gelman, A., & Wagenmakers, E.-J. (2017). A Bayesian bird's eye view of "Replications of Important Results in *Social Psychology*." *Royal Society Open Science, 4*, 160426

Maxwell, S. E., Lau, M. Y., & Howard, G. S. (2015). Is psychology suffering from a replication crisis? What does "failure to replicate" really mean? *American Psychologist, 70*, 487–498.

McShane, B. B., Böckenholt, U., & Hansen, K. T. (2016). Adjusting for publication bias in meta-analysis: An evaluation of selection methods and some cautionary notes. *Perspectives on Psychological Science, 11*(5), 730–749.

Morey, R. D., Chambers, C. D., Etchells, P. J., Harris, C. R., Hoekstra, R., Lakens, D., ... Vanpaemel, W. (2016). The Peer Reviewers' Openness Initiative: Incentivizing open research practices through peer review. *Royal Society Open Science, 3*(1), 150547.

Open Science Collaboration. (2015). Estimating the reproducibility of psychological science. *Science, 349*(6251), aac4716.

Pashler, H., & de Ruiter, J. P. (2017). Taking responsibility for our field's reputation. *APS Observer, 30*(7).

Ramirez, G., & Beilock, S. L. (2011). Writing about testing worries boosts exam performance in the classroom. *Science, 331*(6014), 211–213.

Retraction Watch (2017). https://retractionwatch.com/2017/02/20/placed-much-faith-underpowered-studies-nobel-prize-winner-admits-mistakes/

Rohrer, D., Pashler, H., & Harris, C. R. (2015). Do subtle reminders of money change people's political views? *Journal of Experimental Psychology: General, 144*(4), e73.

Rouder, J. N., & Haaf, J. M. (2018). Power, dominance, and constraint: A note on the appeal of different design traditions. *Advances in Methods and Practices in Psychological Science, 1*, 1–8.

Schuler, J., & Wänke, M. (2016). A fresh look on money priming: Feeling privileged or not makes a difference. *Social Psychological and Personality Science, 7*(4), 366–373.

Simmons, J. P., Nelson, L. D., & Simonsohn, U. (2011). False-positive psychology: Undisclosed flexibility in data collection and analysis allows presenting anything as significant. *Psychological Science, 22*, 1359–1366.

Simonsohn, U. (2015). Small telescopes: Detectability and the evaluation of replication results. *Psychological Science, 26*(5), 559–569.

Simonsohn, U., Nelson, L. D., & Simmons, J. P. (2014). P-curve: A key to the file-drawer. *Journal of Experimental Psychology: General, 143*(2), 534.

Smart, R. G. (1964). The importance of negative results in psychological research. *Canadian Psychologist/Psychologie Canadienne, 5*(4), 225.

Smith, P. L., & Little, D. R. (2018). Small is beautiful: In defense of the small-N design. *Psychonomic Bulletin & Review, 25*, 2083–2101.

Stanley, D. J., & Spence, J. R. (2014). Expectations for replications: Are yours realistic? *Perspectives on Psychological Science, 9*(3), 305–318.

Stroebe, W., & Strack, F. (2014). The alleged crisis and the illusion of exact replication. *Perspectives on Psychological Science, 9*(1), 59–71.

Turner, B. O., Paul, E. J., Miller, M. B., & Barbey, A. K. (2018). Small sample sizes reduce the replicability of task-based fMRI studies. *Communications Biology, 1*(1), 62

Van Elk, M., Matzke, D., Gronau, Q., Guang, M., Vandekerckhove, J., & Wagenmakers, E. J. (2015). Meta-analyses are no substitute for registered replications: A skeptical perspective on religious priming. *Frontiers in Psychology, 6,* 1365.

Vogel, G. (2011). Psychologist accused of fraud on "astonishing scale." *Science, 334*(6056), 579.

Vul, E., Harris, C., Winkielman, P., & Pashler, H. (2009). Puzzlingly high correlations in fMRI studies of emotion, personality, and social cognition. *Perspectives on Psychological Science, 4*(3), 274–290.

Wagenmakers, E.-J., Wetzels, R., Borsboom, D., & Van Der Maas, H. L. (2011). Why psychologists must change the way they analyze their data: The case of psi: Comment on Bem (2011). *Journal of Personality and Social Psychology, 100*(3), 426–432.

Wilson, B. M., & Wixted, J. T. (2018). The prior odds of testing a true effect in cognitive and social psychology. *Advances in Methods and Practices in Psychological Science, 1,* 1–12. https://doi.org/10.1177/2515245918767122

Yap, M. J., Balota, D. C., & Tan, S. E. (2013). Additive and interactive effects in semantic priming: Isolating lexical and decision processes in the lexical decision task. *Journal of Experimental Psychology: Learning, Memory and Cognition, 39,* 140–158.

4
Is Science in Crisis?

Daniele Fanelli

Crisis:
1) A time of intense difficulty or danger.
2) A time when a difficult or important decision must be made.
3) The turning point of a disease when an important change takes place, indicating either recovery or death.
Oxford Living Dictionaries (Oxford University Press, 2017)

Readers of this book may be concerned that science is in crisis, and for good reasons. Perhaps they have read articles decrying a fraud and retraction "epidemic" (e.g., Castillo, 2014), or followed conference reports discussing remedies to a reproducibility crisis (e.g., (Rhodes, 2016), or maybe they came across online news divulging evidence that science is totally broken (e.g., Marinus et al., 2014). These articles are mere examples of a rapidly expanding literature that, directly or indirectly, expounds the belief that contemporary science is less reliable than in the past because it is plagued by results that are fabricated, falsified, or biased and are consequently irreproducible, ultimately due to growing pressures to publish and other misaligned incentives that are perverting the ethos of scientists.

This belief constitutes what I will call the "crisis narrative" about science. It is a narrative, in the sense that it offers a compelling, plausible, and coherent account of the condition of modern research. The consistency and popularity of this narrative was well captured by results of a survey that the "News" section of the journal *Nature* conducted among its readers: 90% agreed that there is a "slight" or "significant" crisis, and between 40% and 70% agreed that selective reporting, fraud, and pressures to publish "always" or "often" contribute to making research irreproducible (Baker, 2016). The crisis narrative is still growing in popularity. Although "scientific crises" of various kinds have been discussed in the literature before, articles that implicitly or explicitly assume that there is a crisis of reproducibility and integrity have proliferated since 2014 (Fanelli, 2018).

The compelling nature of this narrative has arguably driven much-needed research on the possible problems of contemporary science and on ways to improve it—the very subject matter of this book. Up until 5 or 10 years ago, good meta-research data were extremely rare, and anecdotal evidence—including the uncovering of spectacular cases of scientific misconduct (e.g., Levelt et al., 2012), the publishing of highly perplexing research studies (e.g., LeBel & Peters, 2011), and the widespread personal observation, shared by the author of this chapter, that it would be extremely easy to get away with cheating in research—justified concerns for the possibility that modern research might indeed be in deep trouble. In such a condition of limited knowledge and reasonable suspicions, expounding a crisis narrative helped to attract much-needed research efforts and funding. By virtue of these efforts, the last few years have blessed us with a torrent of meta-research studies of increasing size and methodological sophistication.

Did the many empirical studies generated by the crisis narrative ultimately confirm its somber implications? This chapter will provide an overview recent empirical evidence concerning the main tenets of the crisis narrative—that is, that fabricated, falsified, biased, and irreproducible results are widespread and increasing, due to growing pressures to publish—and in light of such evidence it will suggest that this question has a general answer, which could always be given and never is.

How Many Scientists Engage in Scientific Misconduct and Questionable Research Practices?

Numerous surveys have asked scientists directly how often they had engaged in scientific misconduct, which in most documents is defined as data fabrication, data falsification, and plagiarism (henceforth, FFP). This literature is limited by its methodological heterogeneity: Surveys differ from one another in crucial methodological details, including how they worded their questions, delivered the survey, and measured the answers, which are known to affect survey results. Nonetheless, using meta-analytical methods, it was possible to extrapolate from this literature a percentage of respondents who denied ever engaging in misconduct, and therefore conclude that on average at least 1% to 2% of survey respondents declared that they had knowingly engaged in FFP at least once (Fanelli, 2009; Pupovac & Fanelli, 2015).

In addition to questions about FFP, surveys typically asked about questionable research practices (QRPs), a phrase used to indicate a heterogeneous class of behaviors that, even though not unequivocally unethical, might in many cases lead to problems, including the misrepresentation of research results. Typical examples of QRPs include dropping data points from an analysis or failing to publish negative results. Unfortunately, most surveys have used their own lists and definitions of QRPs, which impedes any meta-analytical summary of their results. Nonetheless, survey results are consistent in showing that the percentages of self-reported QRPs are generally much higher than FFP and inversely proportional to their perceived gravity (Fanelli, 2009).

Earlier surveys were mostly conducted in the United States and amongst biomedical researchers. More recent surveys have been conducted in other countries, including Iran (Khadem-Rezaiyan & Dadgarmoghaddam, 2017), Nigeria (Okonta & Rossouw, 2013), Hong Kong (Jordan & Gray, 2013), Croatia (Pupovac et al., 2017), Sweden (Hofmann et al., 2015), Norway (Hofmann et al., 2013), The Netherlands (Tijdink et al., 2014), Italy (Agnoli et al., 2017), Egypt, Lebanon, and Bahrain (Felaefel et al., 2017), and in specific disciplines, such as psychology (John et al., 2012), economics (Necker, 2014), and management (Hopp & Hoover, 2017), and have also used more accurate methodologies (e.g., incentives for truth telling; John et al., 2012).

These more recent surveys yield a picture that is generally consistent with earlier meta-analytical results. They suggest that there is a non-zero but typically small percentage (i.e., below 5%) of respondents who admit having engaged in FFP at least once and a much higher percentage who report engaging in questionable behaviors that may represent improper conduct. Surveys in developing countries appear to yield higher rates of reported misbehavior (e.g., Felaefel et al., 2017; Okonta & Rossouw, 2013), although methodological heterogeneity impedes accurate cross-survey comparisons.

How Many Papers Are Affected by Scientific Misconduct and QRPs?

It would be tempting to extrapolate survey data to make direct inferences about the prevalence of misconduct and bias in the scientific literature, but doing so would be quite improper, for several reasons. First, survey results are very sensitive to methodological choices, and this makes them hard to generalize. Second, since responding to survey questions is usually voluntary, survey results may not be representative of the population of scientists at large.

Third, even if survey results were methodologically robust and representative, the resulting admission rates would only inform us about how many scientists engaged in FFP or QRPs at least once; it would not inform us about the actual number of publications affected by these behaviors. The latter quantity may be substantially lower, according to a study on German psychologists. In this study, respondents were presented with a list of QRPs and were asked (1) whether they had ever engaged in each of the listed behaviors and (2) in what proportion of papers they had done so. Intriguingly, whereas responses to the first question were in reasonable agreement with the results of other surveys, answers to the second question suggested that the percentage of literature affected by misconduct and QRPs might be about five times lower than the corresponding self-reported behavior (Fiedler & Schwarz, 2016).

However, no matter how accurate we make it, an estimate of the number of publications affected by FFP and QRPs would not be sufficient to truly quantify the prevalence of these issues, because the *severity* of each instance of misbehavior would be unknown. This is particularly the case for QRPs, which by definition may or may not represent improper methodological choices. Dropping data points from an analysis, for example, might represent anything from a perfectly sound methodological choice to an egregious act of misrepresentation of results (Fanelli, 2019a). For another example, the practice generally defined as HARKing (hypothesizing after the results are known), which is likely to be one of the most common QRPs in behavioral research (Fiedler & Schwarz, 2016), is not universally harmful as typically believed, because it comes in different forms, many of which are harmless or even beneficial (Rubin, 2017b).

Therefore, assessing the extent to which the scientific literature is actually suffering from the effects of misconduct and (improper) QRPs requires not just an estimate of the prevalence of these behaviors, but also a direct estimation of the *effects* that these practices have on representative samples of research publications. Unfortunately, this distinction is seldom made in the literature. In the text that follows, we will try to keep the two concepts separate, and we will first look at existing evidence on the prevalence of FFP and

QRPs in the literature, and then at evidence of their impact in terms of reproducibility and other possible problems.

Prevalence of Data Fabrication and Falsification

Estimating the prevalence of fabricated and falsified results in the literature is straightforward to do in principle, but difficult in practice. If in principle fabrication and falsification are relatively well-defined issues that are easy to detect, in practice the information necessary to detect them is rarely available in published studies. Most studies to date do not share their raw data and code (Iqbal et al., 2016; Kidwell et al., 2016; Naudet et al., 2018) and, even if they did, methods to assess their possible fraudulent nature would be too laborious and unreliable to yield large-scale conclusive results (e.g., Birajdar & Mankar, 2013; Hüllemann et al., 2017).

At the time of writing this chapter, only one study was able to credibly assess the prevalence of data fabrication in a large random sample of publications. This study focused on papers containing images of biological material or Southern blot gels, and looked for evidence of problematic duplications, manipulations, and copying and pasting of portions of images within the same publication. Out of over 20,000 papers published in 40 scientific journals from 1995 to 2004, 3.8% contained problematic figures, and about half of these suggested deliberate manipulation (Bik et al., 2016). This study further observed that problematic image duplications were relatively common in publications from a few developing countries, particularly China and India. A later re-analysis of this data that used a matched-control approach confirmed the latter finding and estimated that the odds of producing duplicated images for authors working in China and India were, respectively, about four times and five times the odds measured on authors in the United States (Fanelli et al., 2018).

Quite intriguingly, therefore, the best evidence available to date concerning the prevalence of data fabrication and falsification in the literature corroborates the picture suggested by surveys: It suggests that there is a small percentage (circa 1.8%, in this case) of studies being affected by some form of falsification or fabrication, and that the risk of misconduct might be higher in developing countries. However, despite its considerable sample sizes and methodological quality, this study has important limitations that impede us from making clear generalizations. On the one hand, the percentage of detected duplications is likely to be conservative, because not all duplications might have been detected, especially if they involved reusing portions of images taken from different publications. On the other hand, it is unknown how many of the detected image manipulations consisted of errors or benign embellishment of results, rather than deliberate misrepresentations. Furthermore, this study assessed a highly specific form of misconduct, which may not reflect the prevalence of other forms of fabrication and falsification.

Prevalence of P-hacking

Estimating the prevalence of QRPs is harder than for fabrication and falsification in principle, but easier in practice. It is harder in principle, because QRPs are by definition a heterogeneous category of behaviors that may or may not be legitimate. It is simpler in practice, because many data-related QRPs, if improper, will generate measurable biases in the distribution of published statistics. This is the case, in particular, for behaviors aimed at artificiously lowering the magnitude of p-values, a subcategory of QRPs collectively known as "p-hacking."

The most pernicious forms of p-hacking may be used by researchers whose results initially fall short of conventional thresholds of statistical significance (in particular, $p < 0.05$), and who "push" the p-value below that threshold by trying out multiple ad hoc practices, such as selectively excluding outliers, respecifying the model, reoperationalizing the outcome measures, selectively reporting p-values, and others (Hartgerink et al., 2016). If common in a research community, such practices will produce an excess of p-values right below the 0.05 threshold and a dearth right above it, producing a "bump" in the distribution of p-values.

Several studies have looked for the p-value bump in a variety of literatures, yielding contradictory results. Some studies failed to observe it (Jager & Leek, 2014; Krawczyk, 2015; Vermeulen et al., 2015), whereas others claimed to have found it (e.g., Ginsel et al., 2015; Leggett et al., 2013; Masicampo & Lalande, 2012). A positive findings was also reported by the broadest and most accurate study of this kind, which had extracted p-values from the literature of all scientific disciplines and studied their distribution using the "p-curve" method, in which the shape of the distribution of observed p-values is compared to the uniform distribution that would be expected if all p-values were derived from true null hypotheses. This study claimed that p-hacking was common (Head et al., 2015). However, it also suggested that the literatures of all disciplines had high evidential value and p-hacking had very modest effects on the conclusions of meta-analyses. This distinction cannot be emphasized enough: Finding *statistically* significant evidence of p-hacking is not the same as showing that p-hacking has a *substantively* significant impact of the literature. Somewhat ironically, however, the literature on p-hacking and other statistical issues in research appears to have overlooked this distinction.

In a further ironic twist, a later re-analysis suggested that all results just listed that had purportedly found the p-values bump were sensitive to methodological choices and/or were irreproducible (Hartgerink, 2017; Lakens, 2015a; Lakens, 2015b). Following these critiques, a large confirmatory p-curve analysis in psychology examined over 158,000 test results extracted from over 3,000 articles in eight high-impact journals and found no bump and therefore no evidence for p-hacking (Hartgerink et al., 2016). The only QRP for which this study found evidence was an improper rounding of p-values (e.g., presenting a $p = 0.055$ as $p < 0.05$). This is a relatively minor distortion, which was detectable at all solely because the test statistics underlying the incorrectly rounded p-values had been reported correctly. In other words, p-values had been rounded improperly, but the results and statistics had been presented correctly and with no bias.

In all fairness to the p-hacking literature, methodological criticisms and simulation studies have called into question the power of p-curve analyses to detect p-hacking in observational research (Bruns & Ioannidis, 2016) and/or in large heterogeneous samples of p-values taken from multiple fields and methodologies (Bishop & Thompson, 2016; Gelman & O'Rourke, 2014). This suggests that these negative results do not necessarily disprove the existence of p-hacking. However, they suggest that p-hacking may only be detectable within a sample of carefully collected p-values taken from a highly homogeneous literature. Claims that p-hacking is widespread in science or even in a specific discipline, therefore, are not supported by evidence. To any extent that such evidence exists, moreover, it falls short of suggesting that the impact of p-hacking is large.

Prevalence of Publication Bias

A second form of bias, which may result from QRPs, is publication bias, also known as the file drawer problem. This is the tendency for study results that report null or nonsignificant findings to remain unpublished and therefore to be laid to rest in scientists' metaphorical file drawers. Unlike p-hacking, the file drawer problem is well understood and has been described, measured, and studied for decades (Rosenthal, 1979; Song et al., 2010). The causes and general impact of this phenomenon, however, are not as well established as many researchers may think.

The culprits most commonly indicated for publication bias are journal editors and peer reviewers who allegedly are more likely to reject null and nonsignificant results. However, studies that tried to quantify the alleged biases of editors and peer reviewers have yielded contradictory results (Song et al., 2010), suggesting alternative explanations for publication bias (e.g., Senn, 2012). Indeed, publication bias is often generated by researchers themselves, who perceive their null results to be of lower interest or lower reliability and therefore not worth the effort to write up and publish. This is largely, for example, what was found by a recent study that "unlocked the file drawer" in a cohort of 221 studies in the social sciences: Whereas the vast majority of studies with strong or mixed results had been prepared for publication, 65% of null findings had not been written up. When asked about their reasons for not writing up null results, authors mentioned, besides the belief that such results would be less publishable, the perception that their methods were poor or flawed, and their desire to prioritize other projects (Franco et al., 2014).

Therefore, publication bias can often be ascribed to questionable choices made by authors themselves, who perceive their null results to be of lower quality and interest. Such choices are certainly questionable, but not necessarily wrong (they are QRPs in the literal sense), because in some cases a null finding might genuinely result from an error or a flawed methodology and should not be published. Indeed, all else being equal, there are in principle many more ways in which methodological errors in a study produce a false negative than a false positive. As an information-theory analysis suggests, the information value of null and negative results drops very rapidly as the number of uncontrolled experimental variables (e.g., experimental conditions, theoretical assumptions, alternative causal explanations) increases (Fanelli, 2019a).

The prevalence and impact of publication bias are a matter of debate, too. The theoretical reasons that make publication bias problematic are well understood: If only statistically significant findings are published, then smaller studies will tend to be published only when they produced large effects due to sampling error. This may create a literature that overestimates the magnitude of observed effects, and a meta-analysis based on this literature would yield biased estimates. The extent to which this bias occurs across research fields, however, is unknown. Studies on publication bias are numerous in biomedical research and increasingly in the behavioral sciences. However, such studies could, again somewhat ironically, suffer themselves from a publication bias (Dubben & Beck-Bornholdt, 2005), which suggests that the prevalence and importance of the file drawer effect in science could be overestimated.

My colleagues and I have assessed the prevalence of publication bias and other bias-related patterns in a representative sample of meta-analyses from all disciplines. Of particular interest for this discussion were two possible symptoms of publication bias in meta-analysis: (1) a small-study effect, in which studies with smaller sample sizes tend to report effects of larger magnitude, and (2) a gray-literature effect, in which study results that are smaller in magnitude tend to appear in secondary publication outlets, including conference abstracts, students' dissertation, and public repositories. We obtained surprisingly ambiguous results (Fanelli et al., 2017). Both small-study effects and gray-literature biases were measurable to statistically significant levels across the sample. However, only small-study effects were detected to substantively significant levels, whereas differences between gray and non-gray literature explained, at most, little over 1% of the variability of primary outcomes.

Moreover, the distribution of both these effects was very broad, heterogeneous, and overlapping with zero. This suggested that if on the one hand there are certainly research fields (defined by the primary literature in a meta-analysis) in which these effects are important, there are many other fields in which they are not observed at all, or even fields in which the opposite patterns are observed (i.e., larger studies and studies appearing in the gray literature report effect sizes of larger magnitude). Therefore, even though our results found statistically significant signals of the most common bias-related patterns, they fell short of conclusively showing pervasive publication bias in science.

Crucially, if smaller studies are designed differently from larger ones, a factor that our analyses could not control for, small-study effects in meta-analyses may result from phenomena that have little to do with publication bias, indeed with bias altogether. A recent study attempted to control for this confounding factor by measuring the strength of publication bias in homogeneous subsamples of primary studies taken from nearly 600 meta-analyses in psychology and medicine. In line with the evidence just reported, it concluded that publication bias was weak and that it caused, at most, less than 4% overestimation of effect sizes in meta-analyses (Van Aert et al., 2019).

How Many Published Research Findings Are False?

Ever since the publication of John Ioannidis's landmark essay (Ioannidis, 2005), researchers in all disciplines have been alerted to the fact that, even if misconduct and QRPs were completely absent from the literature, many published findings could be false. More accurately, they could be false positives (i.e., findings that reject the null hypothesis at conventional levels of statistical significance even though the null hypothesis is true). Also defined as type I errors, false positives are a physiological byproduct of the null-hypothesis significance testing (NHST) methodology, widely used in the biomedical and social sciences. P-hacking and publication bias (described earlier in the chapter) might increase the prevalence of type I errors, but these might be common in any field in which many of the hypotheses being tested are incorrect (i.e., many null hypotheses are true), statistical power is low (i.e., even when null hypotheses are false, many studies will fail to reject them), and the threshold for accepting a finding as significant is low (as in the widely accepted convention of $p < 0.05$).

Following these concerns, multiple studies have set out to measure the average statistical power in the literature and found it to be discouragingly low. Areas including neuroscience (Button et al., 2013), economics (Ioannidis et al., 2017), management research (Cashen & Geiger, 2004), gene–disease and environment–disease association studies (Dumas-Mallet et al., 2017), and cognitive neuroscience and psychology (Szucs & Ioannidis, 2016) have estimated statistical power well below the recommended 0.8 level. Such low statistical power suggests that the literature of these disciplines may abound with false negatives as well as false positives. However, it does not prove conclusively that this is the case, because estimates of power as well as of the prevalence of false negatives and false positives require strong and mostly untestable assumptions about the literature being examined, including assumptions about the average magnitude of true effect sizes, the average prevalence and strength of bias, and the average proportion of tested hypotheses that are correct.

For example, a study estimated that, in the recent psychological literature, the average statistical power to detect small, medium, and large effects (i.e., Cohen's d of 0.2, 0.5, and 0.8, respectively) was 0.12, 0.44, and 0.73 (Szucs & Ioannidis, 2016). Therefore, the statistical power of studies in this literature may be low or close to the recommended 0.8 level, depending on whether these studies are measuring effects that are small or large. Now, the true magnitude of effects being measured is unknown, and it can only be estimated from the literature itself, after making assumptions about how biased the literature actually is. If we assume no bias, calculations based on power suggest that the psychological literature in question would produce more than 50% of false-positive results only if less than 1 in 10 of the tested hypotheses were correct (Szucs & Ioannidis, 2016). If we assume an extremely high bias of 0.3, which entails that 30% of nonsignificant findings are reported as significant (although this approach to modeling bias has been criticized; see Goodman & Greenland, 2007), the majority of published findings would be false only if less than half of tested hypotheses were correct (Szucs & Ioannidis, 2016).

Therefore, even under the most pessimistic levels of bias, most published findings in psychology would be false only if most tested hypotheses were false to begin with. Whether this is truly the case it is anyone's guess, because we lack a methodology to estimate the level of theoretical strength of a field (Rubin, 2017a). However, several lines of reasoning suggest that the a priori chances of a tested hypothesis being correct are likely to vary widely across studies and research fields. This prior probability of formulating a correct hypothesis could be very low in studies that explore entirely new phenomena or phenomena of high complexity (i.e., that emerge from many interacting variables), and that do so with little prior evidence and using new and poorly understood methodologies. Studies in psychology and other social and biological disciplines might or might not be of this kind because if, on the one hand, many studies in these disciplines address phenomena of great complexity, on the other hand they usually build upon previous results, using established methods and deriving their predictions from supported theories and prior evidence (Moonesinghe et al., 2007). Denying the latter would amount to denying that psychology and other sciences ever make any real progress at all. Therefore, to any extent that a field does make cumulative progress, then most published research findings in that field might not be false positives after all.

It is also important to note that statistical power was typically not found to be uniformly low, but rather to vary substantially in magnitude across subfields or methodologies. Intriguingly, at least two independent studies observed that extremely low power was found among genetic association studies (Dumas-Mallet et al., 2017; Nord et al., 2017). For this and other reasons, this area closely matches the conditions that may make most published findings false (Stroebe, 2016). It perhaps not a coincidence, therefore, that genetic epidemiology was the source of inspiration for the original claim that most published research findings are false: High rates of false and irreproducible results have indeed been documented in this area (Hirschhorn et al., 2002; Ioannidis et al., 2001), and the very calculations that had suggested that most published research findings might be false were based on techniques used in high-throughput genetic analyses (Ioannidis, 2005).

Therefore, the field that generated the paradigmatic claim that most published research findings are false may be structurally predisposed to producing false claims. Other areas of science might certainly be in the same condition, but there is no strict theoretical reason to assume that this is the case. The extent to which the problems noted in genetic epidemiology affect the rest of science, and therefore the risk that most published research findings are false, is an empirical question that needs to be answered on a field-by-field basis, in line with what the essay itself had actually suggested (Ioannidis, 2005).

How Many Studies Are Irreproducible?

Concerns that the reproducibility of published results is too low are closely connected to the concerns for an excess of false positives just discussed. Indeed, both concerns may have been inspired by data from genetic association studies, in which early, promising results were frequently contradicted by subsequent findings (e.g., Ioannidis & Trikalinos, 2005). Anecdotal evidence from meta-analyses suggested that this might represent a general phenomenon in science, which was branded the "decline effect" (Schooler, 2011).

The decline effect does indeed appear to be a common phenomenon, but it is far from ubiquitous: Similarly to gray-literature biases (discussed earlier), when it was measured across a large representative sample of meta-analyses, the decline effect explained a very small portion of the variability of studies' outcomes, and it was broadly distributed, suggesting that it may affect significantly some fields of research and not affect many others at all (Fanelli et al., 2017). In other words, in some fields, early publications report promising strong effects that subsequent studies show to be of smaller or null magnitude, whereas in other fields this does not happen, and later studies either confirm earlier results or show them to be even larger than initially estimated.

Evidence of some decline effect is not necessarily indicative of a dysfunctional science, because a certain amount of irreproducibility ought to be expected in most research fields. When a study is repeated on a new sample, even if the original methodology is repeated exactly, differences between the old and new populations being sampled may lead to lower effect sizes measured in the new study (Gorroochurn et al., 2007). Furthermore, the inevitable presence of measurement error in the both the original and the replication study makes expectations to observe the same effect in the two studies largely unrealistic (Stanley & Spence, 2014).

As studies have accumulated, the unavoidable variability of effects measured across populations has emerged as a fundamental barrier to reproducibility (Gelman, 2015). Such differences between populations may not necessarily be random, but they appear to be so to us because of our own scientific ignorance. A well-known phenomenon in biology, for example, is that of "reaction norms," in which a measured effect is modulated by unknown environmental (contextual) factors. This may give rise to a "reproducibility paradox," in which the underlying effect is genuine and constant, but studies measuring it appear to be irreproducible in proportion to how precise they are (Voelkl & Wurbel, 2016).

Progress in studying and improving reproducibility may have been stifled by a lack of clarity about what aspect of reproducibility is being discussed. Most researchers concerned with a reproducibility crisis are interested in the reproducibility of results but are confronting at least three separate kinds of reproducibility: the reproducibility of methods, that of results, and that of inference (Goodman et al., 2016). Reproducing a study's methods is in principle always possible, and the reproducibility of methods can be improved by promoting transparency and better reporting. Applied to the same dataset, this reproducibility of methods should lead to the exact same result. When these methods are applied to a different population or dataset, however, results may not necessarily be identical. In particular, results are likely to diverge in fields that study highly complex phenomena and nondeterministic systems. Publication and research biases might increase the failure rate of this reproducibility of results, but such failures are expected to occur quite independently of any QRPs.

Furthermore, replicating a methodology exactly is impossible, because full information is unlikely to ever be available. Even when conducted with the help of the original authors and following its original description to the letter, the methodology of a replication attempt is bound to diverge from the original methodology in ways that escape the awareness of the researchers involved, because a multitude of unknown factors and "tacit" methodological choices are by definition overlooked. These methodological divergences may be random, but their impact is not: They are more likely to disrupt or cancel entirely the signal detected in the original study than they are to reinforce it. In other words, contrary to what most statistical analyses of reproducibility assume, the magnitude of effect sizes measured in a replication study should be expected to be lower than that originally reported (Fanelli, 2019a).

Therefore, the question to be asked is not whether irreproducible findings occur at all, but what rate of reproducibility ought to be considered unjustifiably and unacceptably low. Various lines of reasoning discussed in previous paragraphs suggest that the answer is highly field specific. Nonetheless, a plausible starting point may be to posit that a literature that reproduces less than 50% of the time might raise some concerns. A reproducibility of 50% corresponds to the average value that ought to be observed if, across fields of research or across different studies within a field, there is a balance between all possible degrees of reproducibility: from findings that are completely irreproducible under any condition to those that are instead reproduced exactly in all contexts. Hence, concerns for a reproducibility "crisis" would be justified if, as a first approximation, less than half of published studies were found to be reproducible.

Several remarkable studies have attempted to measure the reproducibility of studies in psychology and other disciplines. In most cases, their results suggested that reproducibility was above 50%. A "Many Labs" study selected 13 "classic and contemporary" effects from the psychological literature and had them replicated 36 times in different settings. It concluded that 11 (85%) were consistently replicated (Klein et al., 2014). A similar study, which recruited 25 laboratories and had each one of them replicate 10 different effects that had not yet been published, found that eight results (80%) were consistently replicated and two were not (Schweinsberg et al., 2016). Intriguingly, the two effects that were reported as not replicating were originally null effects, which the subsequent replications had found to be significant. This suggests that the only two "false" claims in the sample of 10 findings were false negatives, not false positives. It also entails that all 10 hypotheses tested were correct. Hence these findings contradict some of the assumptions underlying the claim that most published studies in psychology are false (Szucs & Ioannidis, 2017; see earlier discussion).

Outside the discipline of psychology, results are similarly positive. Successful replications were reported for at least 11 out of 18 laboratory experiments in behavioral economics (61%), although estimates based on the prediction intervals method, which gives a more accurate estimate of the likelihood to reproduce a finding, suggested an 89% replication rate (Camerer et al., 2016). The replicability of a sample of 21 social science experiments published in the journals *Nature* and *Science* was estimated to be between 57% and 67%, depending on the method of estimation (Camerer et al., 2018), and that of 40 behavioral studies in experimental philosophy between 70% and 78% (Cova et al., 2018). Results of the Reproducibility Initiative in Cancer Biology indicated that, at the time of writing this chapter, 9 out of 14 studies were fully or partially reproduced (64%), 2 results could not be interpreted clearly, and only 3 studies were deemed to be not reproduced (eLIFE, 2019).

Reproducibility rates below 50% were purportedly measured, at the time of writing, by only two studies. One, a Many Labs type of project, aimed at testing the subsistence of a "semester effect," by which results of psychological experiments on students change as the academic year progresses. As a side-product of this analysis, the study reported that only 3 out of 10 (33%) of the effects examined were replicated consistently, 2 of which with effect sizes significantly lower compared to the original reports (Ebersole et al., 2016). However, this study differed in many characteristics from the aforementioned Many Labs study. For example, this study recruited labs on a voluntary basis, without selecting them for their level of expertise. In the authors' own estimation, these differences made this study not a conclusive reproducibility test (Ebersole et al., 2016).

The other study that reportedly found low reproducibility is the Reproducibility Initiative in Psychology (RIP), arguably the most ambitious reproducibility study to date. It selected 100 studies from three prominent journals in psychology, and invited a consortium of laboratories to select one study and try to reproduce it, following, whenever possible, methodologies that had been approved by the authors of the original studies. The RIP was widely reported as suggesting disappointingly low reproducibility, circa 37%, but this was only according to some of the reproducibility criteria examined (in particular, how many replication studies rejected the null at the 0.05 level and how many studies were subjectively rated, by the replicators, as having replicated). Notably, however, the RIP had also reported that 47% of replication results were within the 95% confidence interval of the original finding, and that if original and replication were combined in a meta-analysis, 68% of resulting effects were still statistically significant. Notably, there is yet no consensus on which criterion ought to be followed, or indeed if completely different metrics of reproducibility ought to be used instead. Had the RIP employed prediction intervals, for example, which are relatively more realistic estimations of the likelihood to reproduce a finding, its estimate of reproducibility would have been 77% (Patil et al., 2016).

Therefore, to any extent that current evidence about reproducibility can be generalized, it does not suggest that most studies published in psychology and other fields are irreproducible, as the crisis narrative would suggest. Skeptical readers may once more deem the current estimations of reproducibility inconclusive, because they employ subtly different methods, because they are often limited by small samples, and because there is no consensus on how reproducibility ought to be defined and estimated. However, they would have to acknowledge that these studies offer the best evidence available. These studies were expressly designed to estimate reproducibility and in most cases they did not show dismally low levels of reproducibility, as they certainly could have.

Therefore, in light of all the evidence we have discussed, there appears to be little reason to conclude that misconduct, bias, or irreproducibility is pervasive in science. The case presented, I believe, goes beyond the mere absence of evidence of a crisis. Nonetheless, even if skeptical readers interpret all the evidence we have reviewed as merely inconclusive, they would still have to accept that the burden of proof rests on the claim that science is in crisis. Claiming otherwise would entail that science must be assumed to be in crisis in the absence of evidence and until irrefutable proof of the contrary is provided—which is a scientifically dubious position to take.

No one disputes that misconduct, bias, and QRPs are real phenomena that deserve attention. They are as old as science itself, and certainly much more can be done to tackle them today. However, given the manifest progress that science has allowed us to make on all fronts, surely the "null hypothesis" that meta-researchers ought to be testing is that the system—despite all its imperfections—is "not broken." Evidence collected so far does not compel us to reject this null.

However, it may still be the case that the problems we have discussed are increasing in prevalence and impact, and this in itself would justify concerns for a possible crisis in science. This is the question we move to next.

Are Fabricated, Falsified, Biased, and Irreproducible Results Increasing?

The fact that scientists today are concerned about a crisis cannot be taken as evidence that a crisis exists, because similar concerns have been expressed cyclically, if not continuously, throughout the history of science. In the discipline of psychology, for example, several crises have been debated and discussed in the 1980s, 1970s, and earlier (Faye, 2012; Giner-Sorolla, 2012). Concerns about the deleterious effects of a "publish or perish" academic culture were already published in the 1950s (Garfield, 1996; Siegel & Baveye, 2010). More than a century earlier, in 1830, the famous mathematician Charles Babbage published an essay on the "decline of science in England," in which he produced one of the first taxonomies of research misconduct and discussed the possible ill consequences of the professionalization of science (Babbage, 1830). Nearly two centuries before Babbage, right at the dawn of science itself, Robert Boyle dedicated two essays to the problem of false and irreproducible results, discussing it in much the same terms as it is discussed today (Bishop, 2015).

Historical evidence of past problems, of course, does not rule out the possibility that genuine crises may indeed have occurred in the past, nor does it entail that a crisis is not occurring today and therefore that modern concerns are not justified. Quite the contrary: It is evident that contemporary science is facing numerous radical transformations that could in theory threaten its integrity. However, as will be discussed, there is no unambiguous indication that problems with integrity and reproducibility are increasing, at least not in the terms postulated by the crisis narrative.

Scientific misconduct is widely believed to be rising, largely because in the last few decades there has been a rapid increase in the number of retractions of scientific publications, most of which are due to misconduct (Fang et al., 2012). However, the recent increase in retractions is almost entirely accounted for by the growing number of journals that have started issuing retractions (Fanelli, 2013). Not only did most scientific journals not retract articles in the past, they actually had no retraction policies. Indeed, many journals still lack such policies today. This fact was well documented by a study conducted in 2014, which found that only 65% of high-impact biomedical journals had a retraction policy; and this datum marked a substantial improvement from the 21% that had been recorded 10 years earlier on a similar sample of journals (Atlas, 2004; Resnik et al., 2015).

In addition to the diffusion of retraction policies in journals, the recent rise in retractions is most plausibly explained by the strengthening of national policies to investigate allegations of misconduct (whose development and effectiveness are empirically documented (Fanelli et al., 2015; Resnik et al., 2015) and the increased awareness and scrutiny that these structures have facilitated. The recent rise in retractions, therefore, is primarily, if not entirely, the symptom of positive innovations that should be celebrated, not decried as evidence of spreading dishonesty (Fanelli, 2013).

A second factor often cited in support of the belief that scientific misconduct may be increasing is the perception that pressures to publish have increased. In reality, it is unknown whether pressures to publish have literally increased, because "pressures" are subjective phenomena that would be difficult to measure and compare across studies or over time. However, it is certainly true that academic career advancement criteria in many countries have moved toward making greater use (and misuse) of bibliometric measures and indicators (Hicks et al., 2015), and it is therefore reasonable to hypothesize that scientists may be experiencing increasing pressures to meet demands imposed by these metrics, and thus engage in QRPs or FFP. However, several analyses have failed to show a direct connection between having high bibliometric scores and engaging in fraud or questionable practices. Researchers who publish more papers, more frequently, and in high-impact journals are equally or less likely to engage in misconduct (Fanelli et al., 2018), to have their papers retracted (Fanelli et al., 2015), and to publish biased effect sizes (Fanelli et al., 2017), and are more likely to issue corrections to their papers, the latter arguably being a manifestation of research integrity (Fanelli et al., 2015). Furthermore, there is actually no clear evidence that scientists are publishing at higher rates. An analysis of over 42,000 researchers who published throughout the 20th century in journals indexed by the Web of Science suggests that, while it is true that researchers have co-authored many more papers over time, their fractional (i.e., co-author-adjusted) publication output may have been higher in the 1950s than it is today (Fanelli & Larivière, 2016).

There is also no clear evidence that QRPs have increased. A few studies claimed to have observed that a bump in the distribution of p-values around the 0.05 threshold had grown over the years, which suggested that p-hacking was increasing. However, as noted in previous sections, re-analyses of these data have disconfirmed their results (Hartgerink et al., 2016; Lakens, 2015a). A large-scale computational analysis of statistical reporting errors in p-values found no evidence of an increase in such errors across eight major psychology journals between 1985 and 2013, which contradicts speculations that scientists might be increasingly "sloppy" in their work (Nuijten et al., 2016).

A few lines of evidence suggest that publication bias might have modestly increased in recent decades, but this evidence is inconclusive. The magnitude of small-study effects and decline effects has modestly increased, from 1984 to 2013, in a sample of meta-analyses taken from the behavioral and social sciences (Fanelli et al., 2017). However, this trend could reflect changes not in the publication practices of researchers, but rather in the methodology used by meta-analysts, who may be more likely to include gray literature and heterogeneous studies in their pooled estimates. Multiple independent studies found that the ratio of positive to negative results reported in the abstracts of publications has been increasing, which would suggest a possible rise in publication bias (de Winter & Dodou, 2015; Fanelli, 2012; Pautasso, 2010). However, these studies do not necessarily prove that publication bias is increasing. An alternative explanation could be that scientists are simply more likely to embed their negative results in longer studies that present multiple findings. This latter interpretation is supported by recent evidence that scientific papers are getting longer, denser with more information, and packed with more experimental results, at least in a few biomedical and psychological journals (Sherman et al., 1999; Vale, 2015).

Most of the temporal trends entailed by the crisis narrative, therefore, are not supported by evidence. However, other trends that are not contemplated by the crisis narrative might be a cause for concern. For example, evidence mentioned earlier that fractional productivity is not increasing and that scientific papers are not getting shorter suggests that the QRP known as "salami slicing" (fractioning results of a study into multiple smaller publications) is not spreading as many believe. What might be becoming more common, however, are questionable authorship practices in which authors "salami slice" not their papers but their collaborations (Fanelli, 2019b). Such hyper-collaborative practices would be questionable to the extent that authors "spread themselves thin" by contributing very little effort to many separate projects, artificiously inflating their publication lists. As another example, while there is no direct evidence to suggest that scientific misconduct is growing in scientifically active countries due to pressures to publish, several lines of evidence suggest that the risk of scientific misconduct may be higher in developing countries, particularly China and India. This suggests that the global prevalence of scientific misconduct might indeed be increasing, simply because these countries are contributing an increasing proportion of studies to the scientific literature. The average reproducibility of studies might also be declining, not because of rising misconduct or QRPs, but merely because scientific research may be tackling phenomena of increasing complexity, as some research suggests (Low-Décarie et al., 2014; Rodriguez-Esteban & Loging, 2013).

In Conclusion: Does Empirical Evidence Suggest That There Is a Crisis in Science?

As I have tried to emphasize throughout the chapter, many of the studies reviewed here suffer from limitations and may be interpreted as inconclusive by the skeptical reader. However, even if deemed inconclusive, this is the best evidence that we have and it does not suggest that we should reject the "null hypothesis" that most research fields in most disciplines across science are "not broken." This is not, of course, equivalent to saying all research fields are free from problems. Far from it. Indeed, I hope that this chapter succeeded in conveying the sense that a general answer to the question has already emerged from this broad and increasingly sophisticated literature. It is an answer that could have always been given, and never was. The answer is: "It depends." It depends, in particular, on what we mean by words like "crisis" and "science."

It Depends on What We Mean by "Crisis"

If by using the word "crisis" we mean that science is in the "critical stage of a disease" (an "epidemic" of false results, as some have put it), beyond which either death or recovery awaits, then the answer ought to be a resounding "no." To any extent that available evidence has spoken, it does not suggest that fabricated, falsified, biased, and irreproducible results are overwhelming the scientific literature, nor does the evidence suggest that these are increasing in prevalence. For this reason, I have argued elsewhere that the crisis narrative ought to be abandoned, because it is not only not supported empirically but also potentially and unfairly damaging to the reputation of science and the morale of researchers (Fanelli, 2018).

However, if by saying that science is in "crisis" we mean that science is in a critical period, because it is facing new challenges that require important decisions to be made, then the answer may be "yes." Contemporary science is certainly facing rapid and radical transformations, which mirror those occurring in many other human activities, largely because of the development of information and communication technologies. Scientists are enjoying an unprecedented capacity to work in large and global communities, to study phenomena of increasing subtlety and complexity, and to share their methods and results swiftly and completely. These developments are empowering the scientific community, but have their downsides in the form of new challenges that need to be addressed. As multiple studies suggest, for example, the quality and integrity of published research may not be homogeneous throughout the world, and developing countries may need to catch up; studies about complex phenomena are less likely to be reproducible; the development of ever more complicated and flexible computational tools may increase the probability that biases creep into published results; finally, the culture of sharing and democratization of expertise that is likely to characterize the younger generations of scientists is revolutionizing how research is conducted and communicated.

Therefore, if by "crisis" we mean "new challenges," then we may well say that science is facing a crisis. However, it is a crisis brought about by novelties that make science more powerful than ever, and this fact ought to be celebrated, not lamented. All present and future efforts to improve the integrity and reliability of research would find perfect justification under this "new challenges" narrative (Fanelli, 2018).

It Depends on What We Mean by "Science"

If by "science" we mean the entirety of the scientific literature or even the entire literature of a discipline like psychology or biomedicine, then there is no evidence of such a crisis in science. Studies that assessed large samples of literatures purported to represent one or more disciplines have not suggested that fabricated, falsified, biased, false, and irreproducible findings are in the majority or that their proportion is increasing.

However, there is ample evidence to suggest that there might be localized "crises" in specific fields of research. By "research field" I intend to indicate not a domain, like "social sciences," or a discipline, like "psychology," or a subdiscipline, like "social psychology," but a relatively narrow community of scientists and/or a literature that is addressing a well-defined research question. A "field" in this definition is represented by the literature captured by a review, and especially systematic reviews and meta-analyses. Large studies assessing statistical power, bias, and reproducibility have typically suggested that issues are heterogeneously distributed across methodologies and/or research topics. Furthermore, theoretical considerations suggest that the various issues that underlie concerns for a crisis are likely to depend on specific characteristics of the phenomena being studied, the methodologies used to study them, and the cultures of the scientific communities that are using those methodologies.

It is not a coincidence that virtually all of the meta-research studies mentioned in this chapter were affected by one of two possible limitations: Their samples were either (1) too narrow and specific to be generalizable or (2) too broad to yield accurate results. These may be insurmountable limitations of the meta-research program, indeed of any project that aims to study a phenomenon as complex as science. Science is a peculiar subject of investigation, because it is at once a unitary phenomenon and a highly diversified one. Science is unitary because, across fields, it consists in the same process: an organized and collective encoding of knowledge, in which patterns and regularities are uncovered and subsumed under theories of increasing generality (Fanelli, 2019a). In its practical manifestations, however, science is a highly diverse and dynamically evolving set of activities.

Fields of science are born, develop, and eventually die out around questions about empirical phenomena that vary widely in their frequency, relevance, regularity, and complexity. Methodologies that are developed to tackle this diversity of phenomena will consequently vary enormously in their accuracy, power, complexity, and reproducibility as well as in the kind of ethical and scientific challenges they may face. Theories to explain and predict such phenomena will develop at varying speed depending on the field. Consequently, the theoretical strength of hypotheses tested will vary across fields, and so will the levels of inferential reproducibility. Rather than trying to simplify the picture by drawing averages across disciplines or across all of science, meta-science should strive to explain, predict, and manage this diversity at an adequately fine-grained level (Fanelli, 2019a).

The literature on research integrity and meta-research reviewed in this chapter exemplifies perfectly the challenges of studying extremely complex phenomena: It has yielded contradictory findings, incorrect hypotheses, and irreproducible results. The fact that the risk of fabricated, falsified, biased, and irreproducible results depends on properties of research fields may be the most important lesson that a decade of meta-research has taught us. And we are still learning.

References

Agnoli, F., Wicherts, J. M., Veldkamp, C. L. S., Albiero, P., & Cubelli, R. (2017). Questionable research practices among Italian research psychologists. *PLoS One*, *12*(3), e0172792. https://doi.org/10.1371/journal.pone.0172792

Atlas, M. C. (2004). Retraction policies of high-impact biomedical journals. *Journal of the Medical Library Association*, *92*(2), 242–250. http://www.ncbi.nlm.nih.gov/pubmed/15098054%0Ahttp://www.pubmedcentral.nih.gov/articlerender.fcgi?artid=PMC385306

Babbage, C. (1830). Reflections on the decline of science in England and on some of its causes. In M. Campbell-Kelly (Ed.), *The Works of Charles Babbage*. Pickering.

Baker, M. (2016). Is there a reproducibility crisis? *Nature*, *533*(7604), 452–454.

Bik, E. M., Casadevall, A., & Fang, F. C. (2016). The prevalence of inappropriate image duplication in biomedical research publications. *Mbio*, *7*(3), e00809-16. https://doi.org/10.1128/mBio.00809-16

Birajdar, G. K., & Mankar, V. H. (2013). Digital image forgery detection using passive techniques: A survey. *Digital Investigation*, *10*(3), 226–245. https://doi.org/10.1016/j.diin.2013.04.007

Bishop, D. (2015). Publishing replication failures: Some lessons from history. http://deevybee.blogspot.co.uk/2015/07/publishing-replication-failures-some.html

Bishop, D. V. M., & Thompson, P. A. (2016). Problems in using p-curve analysis and text-mining to detect rate of p-hacking and evidential value. *PeerJ*, *4*, 16. https://doi.org/10.7717/peerj.1715

Bruns, S. B., & Ioannidis, J. P. A. (2016). P-curve and p-hacking in observational research. *PLoS One*, *11*(2), 13. https://doi.org/10.1371/journal.pone.0149144

Button, K. S., Ioannidis, J. P. A., Mokrysz, C., Nosek, B. A., Flint, J., Robinson, E. S. J., & Munafo, M. R. (2013). Power failure: Why small sample size undermines the reliability of neuroscience. *Nature Reviews Neuroscience*, *14*(5), 365–376. https://doi.org/10.1038/nrn3475

Camerer, C. F., Dreber, A., Forsell, E., Ho, T. H., Huber, J., Johannesson, M., . . . Wu, H. (2016). Evaluating replicability of laboratory experiments in economics. *Science*, *351*(6280), 1433–1436. https://doi.org/10.1126/science.aaf0918

Camerer, C. F., Dreber, A., Holzmeister, F., Ho, T.-H., Huber, J., Johannesson, M., . . . Wu, H. (2018). Evaluating the replicability of social science experiments in *Nature* and *Science* between 2010 and 2015. *Nature Human Behaviour*. https://doi.org/10.1038/s41562-018-0399-z

Cashen, L. H., & Geiger, S. W. (2004). Statistical power and the testing of null hypotheses: A review of contemporary management research and recommendations for future studies. *Organizational Research Methods*. https://doi.org/10.1177/1094428104263676

Castillo, M. (2014). The fraud and retraction epidemic. *American Journal of Neuroradiology*, 35(9), 1653–1654.

Cova, F., Strickland, B., Abatista, A., Allard, A., Andow, J., Attie, M., . . . Zhou, X. (2018). Estimating the reproducibility of experimental philosophy. *Review of Philosophy and Psychology*. https://doi.org/10.1007/s13164-018-0400-9

de Winter, J. C. F., & Dodou, D. (2015). A surge of p-values between 0.041 and 0.049 in recent decades (but negative results are increasing rapidly too). *PeerJ*, 3, e733. https://doi.org/10.7717/peerj.733

Dubben, H. H., & Beck-Bornholdt, H. P. (2005). Systematic review of publication bias in studies on publication bias. *British Medical Journal*, 331(7514), 433–434. https://doi.org/10.1136/bmj.38478.497164.F7

Dumas-Mallet, E., Button, K. S., Boraud, T., Gonon, F., & Munafo, M. R. (2017). Low statistical power in biomedical science: A review of three human research domains. *Royal Society Open Science*, 4(2), 11. https://doi.org/10.1098/rsos.160254

Ebersole, C. R., Atherton, O. E., Belanger, A. L., Skulborstad, H. M., Allen, J. M., Banks, J. B., . . . Nosek, B. A. (2016). Many Labs 3: Evaluating participant pool quality across the academic semester via replication. *Journal of Experimental Social Psychology*, 67, 68–82. https://doi.org/10.1016/j.jesp.2015.10.012

eLIFE. (2019). Reproducibility Project: Cancer Biology. https://elifesciences.org/collections/9b1e83d1/reproducibility-project-cancer-biology

Fanelli, D. (2009). How many scientists fabricate and falsify research? A systematic review and meta-analysis of survey data. *PLoS One*. https://doi.org/10.1371/journal.pone.0005738

Fanelli, D. (2012). Negative results are disappearing from most disciplines and countries. *Scientometrics*, 90(3), 891–904. https://doi.org/10.1007/DOI 10.1007/s11192-011-0494-7

Fanelli, D. (2013). Why growing retractions are (mostly) a good sign. *PLoS Medicine*, 10(12), 1–6. https://doi.org/10.1371/journal.pmed.1001563

Fanelli, D. (2018). Is science really facing a reproducibility crisis, and do we need it to? *Proceedings of the National Academy of Sciences USA*, 115(11), 2628–2631. https://doi.org/doi.org/10.1073/pnas.1708272114

Fanelli, D. (2019a). A theory and methodology to quantify knowledge. *Royal Society Open Science*, 6(4). https://doi.org/10.1098/rsos.181055

Fanelli, D. (2019b). Pressures to publish: What effects do we see? In M. Biagioli & A. Lippman (Eds.), *Beyond Publish or Perish: Metrics and the New Ecologies of Academic Misconduct*. MIT Press.

Fanelli, D., Costas, R., Fang, F. C., Casadevall, A., & Bik, E. M. (2018). Testing hypotheses on risk factors for scientific misconduct via matched-control analysis of papers containing problematic image duplications. *Science and Engineering Ethics*, in press. https://doi.org/10.1007/s11948-018-0023-7

Fanelli, D., Costas, R., & Ioannidis, J. P. A. (2017). Meta-assessment of bias in science. *Proceedings of the National Academy of Sciences USA*, 114(14), 3714–3719. https://doi.org/10.1073/pnas.1618569114

Fanelli, D., Costas, R., & Larivière, V. (2015). Misconduct policies, academic culture and career stage, not gender or pressures to publish, affect scientific integrity. *PLoS One, 10*(6), e0127556. https://doi.org/10.1371/journal.pone.0127556

Fanelli, D., & Larivière, V. (2016). Researchers' individual publication rate has not increased in a century. *PLoS One, 11*(3), e0149504. https://doi.org/10.1371/journal.pone.0149504

Fang, F. C., Steen, R. G., & Casadevall, A. (2012). Misconduct accounts for the majority of retracted scientific publications. *Proceedings of the National Academy of Sciences USA, 109*(42), 17028–17033. https://doi.org/10.1073/pnas.1212247109

Faye, C. (2012). American social psychology: Examining the contours of the 1970s crisis. *Studies in History and Philosophy of Science Part C: Studies in History and Philosophy of Biological and Biomedical Sciences, 43*(2), 514–521. https://doi.org/10.1016/j.shpsc.2011.11.010

Felaefel, M., Salem, M., Jaafar, R., Jassim, G., Edwards, H., Rashid-Doubell, F., . . . Silverman, H. (2017). A cross-sectional survey study to assess prevalence and attitudes regarding research misconduct among investigators in the Middle East. *Journal of Academic Ethics*. https://doi.org/10.1007/s10805-017-9295-9

Fiedler, K., & Schwarz, N. (2016). Questionable research practices revisited. *Social Psychological and Personality Science, 7*(1), 45–52. https://doi.org/10.1177/1948550615612150

Franco, A., Malhotra, N., & Simonovits, G. (2014). Publication bias in the social sciences: Unlocking the file drawer. *Science, 345*(6203), 1502–1505. https://doi.org/10.1126/science.1255484

Garfield, E. (1996). What is the primordial reference for the phrase "publish or perish"? *Scientist, 10*(12), 11.

Gelman, A. (2015). The connection between varying treatment effects and the crisis of unreplicable research: A Bayesian perspective. *Journal of Management, 41*(2), 632–643. https://doi.org/10.1177/0149206314525208

Gelman, A., & O'Rourke, K. (2014). Discussion: Difficulties in making inferences about scientific truth from distributions of published p-values. *Biostatistics*. https://doi.org/10.1093/biostatistics/kxt034

Giner-Sorolla, R. (2012). Science or art? How aesthetic standards grease the way through the publication bottleneck but undermine science. *Perspectives on Psychological Science, 7*(6), 562–571. https://doi.org/10.1177/1745691612457576

Ginsel, B., Aggarwal, A., Xuan, W., & Harris, I. (2015). The distribution of probability values in medical abstracts: An observational study. Medical Research Methodology. *BMC Research Notes, 8*(1). https://doi.org/10.1186/s13104-015-1691-x

Goodman, S., & Greenland, S. (2007). Why most published research findings are false: Problems in the analysis. *PLoS Medicine, 4*(4), 773. https://doi.org/10.1371/journal.pmed.0040168

Goodman, S. N., Fanelli, D., & Ioannidis, J. P. A. (2016). What does research reproducibility mean? *Science Translational Medicine, 8*(341), 341–353. https://doi.org/10.1126/scitranslmed.aaf5027

Gorroochurn, P., Hodge, S. E., Heiman, G. A., Durner, M., & Greenberg, D. A. (2007). Non-replication of association studies: "Pseudo-failures" to replicate? *Genetics in Medicine, 9*(6), 325–331. https://doi.org/10.1097/GIM.0b013e3180676d79

Hartgerink, C. H. J. (2017). Reanalyzing Head et al. (2015): Investigating the robustness of widespread p-hacking. *PeerJ, 5*, e3068. https://doi.org/10.7717/peerj.3068

Hartgerink, C. H. J., van Aert, R. C. M., Nuijten, M. B., Wicherts, J. M., & van Assen, M. A. L. M. (2016). Distributions of p-values smaller than .05 in psychology: What is going on? *PeerJ*, *4*, e1935. https://doi.org/10.7717/peerj.1935

Head, M. L., Holman, L., Lanfear, R., Kahn, A. T., & Jennions, M. D. (2015). The extent and consequences of p-hacking in science. *PLoS Biology*, *13*(3), 15. https://doi.org/10.1371/journal.pbio.1002106

Hicks, D., Wouters, P., Waltman, L., Rijcke, S. de, & Rafols, I. (2015). Bibliometrics: The Leiden Manifesto for research metrics. *Nature*, *520*, 429–431. https://doi.org/10.1038/520429a

Hirschhorn, J. N., Lohmueller, K., Byrne, E., & Hirschhorn, K. (2002). A comprehensive review of genetic association studies. *Genetics in Medicine*, *4*(2), 45–61. https://doi.org/10.109700125817-200203000-00002

Hofmann, B., Helgesson, G., Juth, N., & Holm, S. (2015). Scientific dishonesty: A survey of doctoral students at the major medical faculties in Sweden and Norway. *Journal of Empirical Research on Human Research Ethics*, *10*(4), 380–388. https://doi.org/10.1177/1556264615599686

Hofmann, B., Myhr, A. I., & Holm, S. (2013). Scientific dishonesty—a nationwide survey of doctoral students in Norway. *BMC Medical Ethics*, *14*(1), 3. https://doi.org/10.1186/1472-6939-14-3

Hopp, C., & Hoover, G. A. (2017). How prevalent is academic misconduct in management research? *Journal of Business Research*, *80*, 73–81. https://doi.org/10.1016/j.jbusres.2017.07.003

Hüllemann, S., Schüpfer, G., & Mauch, J. (2017). Application of Benford's law: A valuable tool for detecting scientific papers with fabricated data? *Der Anaesthesist*. https://doi.org/10.1007/s00101-017-0333-1

Ioannidis, J. P. A. (2005). Why most published research findings are false. *PLoS Medicine*, *2*(8), e124.

Ioannidis, J. P. A., Ntzani, E. E., Trikalinos, T. A., & Contopoulos-Ioannidis, D. G. (2001). Replication validity of genetic association studies. *Nature Genetics*, *29*(3), 306–309. https://doi.org/10.1038/ng749

Ioannidis, J. P. A., Stanley, T. D., & Doucouliagos, H. (2017). The power of bias in economics research. *Economic Journal*, *127*(605), F236–F265. https://doi.org/10.1111/ecoj.12461

Ioannidis, J. P. A., & Trikalinos, T. A. (2005). Early extreme contradictory estimates may appear in published research: The Proteus phenomenon in molecular genetics research and randomized trials. *Journal of Clinical Epidemiology*, *58*(6), 543–549.

Iqbal, S. A., Wallach, J. D., Khoury, M. J., Schully, S. D., & Ioannidis, J. P. A. (2016). Reproducible research practices and transparency across the biomedical literature. *PLoS Biology*, *14*(1). https://doi.org/10.1371/journal.pbio.1002333

Jager, L. R., & Leek, J. T. (2014). An estimate of the science-wise false discovery rate and application to the top medical literature. *Biostatistics*, *15*(1), 39–45. https://doi.org/10.1093/biostatistics/kxt007

John, L. K., Loewenstein, G., & Prelec, D. (2012). Measuring the prevalence of questionable research practices with incentives for truth telling. *Psychological Science*, *23*(5), 524–532. https://doi.org/10.1177/0956797611430953

Jordan, S. R., & Gray, P. W. (2013). Research integrity in greater China: Surveying regulations, perceptions and knowledge of research integrity from a Hong Kong perspective. *Developing World Bioethics*, *13*(3), 125–137. https://doi.org/10.1111/j.1471-8847.2012.00337.x

Khadem-Rezaiyan, M., & Dadgarmoghaddam, M. (2017). Research misconduct: A report from a developing country. *Iranian Journal of Public Health*, *46*(10), 1374–1378.

Kidwell, M. C., Lazarevic, L. B., Baranski, E., Hardwicke, T. E., Piechowski, S., Falkenberg, L. S., . . . Nosek, B. A. (2016). Badges to acknowledge open practices: A simple, low-cost, effective method for increasing transparency. *PLoS Biology*, *14*(5), 15. https://doi.org/10.1371/journal.pbio.1002456

Klein, R. A., Ratliff, K. A., Vianello, M., Adams, R. B., Bahnik, S., Bernstein, M. J., . . . Nosek, B. A. (2014). Investigating variation in replicability: A "Many Labs" replication project. *Social Psychology*, *45*(3), 142–152. https://doi.org/10.1027/1864-9335/a000178

Krawczyk, M. (2015). The search for significance: A few peculiarities in the distribution of p values in experimental psychology literature. *PLoS One*, *10*(6). https://doi.org/10.1371/journal.pone.0127872

Lakens, D. (2015a). On the challenges of drawing conclusions from p-values just below 0.05. *PeerJ*, *3*, e1142. https://doi.org/10.7717/peerj.1142

Lakens, D. (2015b). What p-hacking really looks like: A comment on Masicampo and LaLande (2012). *Quarterly Journal of Experimental Psychology*. https://doi.org/10.1080/17470218.2014.982664

LeBel, E. P., & Peters, K. R. (2011). Fearing the future of empirical psychology: Bem's (2011) evidence of psi as a case study of deficiencies in modal research practice. *Review of General Psychology*, *15*(4), 371–379. https://doi.org/10.1037/a0025172

Leggett, N. C., Thomas, N. A., Loetscher, T., & Nicholls, M. E. R. (2013). The life of p: "Just significant" results are on the rise. *Quarterly Journal of Experimental Psychology*, *66*(12), 2303–2309. https://doi.org/10.1080/17470218.2013.863371

Levelt, C., Noort, C., & Drenth, C. (2012). Flawed science: The fraudulent research practices of social psychologist Diederik Stapel. http://www.tilburguniversity.edu/nl/nieuws-en-agenda/finalreportLevelt.pdf

Low-Décarie, E., Chivers, C., & Granados, M. (2014). Rising complexity and falling explanatory power in ecology. *Frontiers in Ecology and the Environment*, *12*(7), 412–418. https://doi.org/10.1890/130230

Marinus, A., Boyle, A., & Pearl, J. (2014). 6 shocking studies that prove science is totally broken. http://www.cracked.com/article_20789_6-shocking-studies-that-prove-science-totally-/

Masicampo, E. J., & Lalande, D. R. (2012). A peculiar prevalence of p values just below .05. *Quarterly Journal of Experimental Psychology*, *65*(11), 2271–2279. https://doi.org/10.1080/17470218.2012.711335

Moonesinghe, R., Khoury, M. J., & Janssens, A. (2007). Most published research findings are false—but a little replication goes a long way. *PLoS Medicine*, *4*(2), 218–221. https://doi.org/10.1371/journal.pmed.0040028

Naudet, F., Sakarovitch, C., Janiaud, P., Cristea, I., Fanelli, D., Moher, D., & Ioannidis, J. P. A. (2018). Data sharing and re-analysis for randomised controlled trials in leading biomedical journals with a full data-sharing policy: A survey of studies published in *The BMJ* and *PLoS Medicine*. *British Medical Journal*, in press.

Necker, S. (2014). Scientific misbehavior in economics. *Research Policy*, *43*(10), 1747–1759. https://doi.org/10.1016/j.respol.2014.05.002

Nord, C. L., Valton, V., Wood, J., & Roiser, J. P. (2017). Power-up: A reanalysis of "power failure" in neuroscience using mixture modelling. *Journal of Neuroscience*, *37*(34), 8051–8061. https://doi.org/10.1523/JNEUROSCI.3592-16.2017

Nuijten, M. B., Hartgerink, C. H. J. J., van Assen, M. A. L. M., Epskamp, S., & Wicherts, J. M. (2016). The prevalence of statistical reporting errors in psychology (1985–2013). *Behavior Research Methods*, *48*(4), 1205–1226. https://doi.org/10.3758/s13428-015-0664-2

Okonta, P., & Rossouw, T. (2013). Prevalence of scientific misconduct among a group of researchers in Nigeria. *Developing World Bioethics*, *13*(3), 149–157. https://doi.org/10.1111/j.1471-8847.2012.00339.x

Oxford University Press. (2017). Oxford Living Dictionaries. https://doi.org/https://en.oxforddictionaries.com/definition/jargon

Patil, P., Peng, R. D., & Leek, J. T. (2016). What should researchers expect when they replicate studies? A statistical view of replicability in psychological science. *Perspectives on Psychological Science*, *11*(4), 539–544. https://doi.org/10.1177/1745691616646366

Pautasso, M. (2010). Worsening file-drawer problem in the abstracts of natural, medical and social science databases. *Scientometrics*, *85*(1), 193–202. https://doi.org/10.1007/s11192-010-0233-5

Pupovac, V., & Fanelli, D. (2015). Scientists admitting to plagiarism: A meta-analysis of surveys. *Science and Engineering Ethics*, *21*(5), 1331–1352. https://doi.org/10.1007/s11948-014-9600-6

Pupovac, V., Prijić-Samaržija, S., & Petrovečki, M. (2017). Research misconduct in the Croatian scientific community: A survey assessing the forms and characteristics of research misconduct. *Science and Engineering Ethics*, *23*(1), 165–181. https://doi.org/10.1007/s11948-016-9767-0

Resnik, D. B., Rasmussen, L. M., & Kissling, G. E. (2015a). An international study of research misconduct policies. *Accountability in Research-Policies and Quality Assurance*, *22*(5), 249–266. https://doi.org/10.1080/08989621.2014.958218

Resnik, D. B., Wager, E., & Kissling, G. E. (2015b). Retraction policies of top scientific journals ranked by impact factor. *Journal of the Medical Library Association*, *103*(3), 136–139. https://doi.org/10.3163/1536-5050.103.3.006

Rhodes, E. (2016). What crisis? The reproducibility crisis. *Psychologist*, *29*, 508–509. http://thepsychologist.bps.org.uk/what-crisis-reproducibility-crisis

Rodriguez-Esteban, R., & Loging, W. T. (2013). Quantifying the complexity of medical research. *Bioinformatics*, *29*(22), 2918–2924. https://doi.org/10.1093/bioinformatics/btt505

Rosenthal, R. (1979). The file drawer problem and tolerance for null results. *Psychological Bulletin*, *86*(3), 638–641.

Rubin, M. (2017a). Do p values lose their meaning in exploratory analyses? It depends how you define the familywise error rate. *Review of General Psychology*, *21*(3), 269–275. https://doi.org/10.1037/gpr0000123

Rubin, M. (2017b). When does HARKing hurt? Identifying when different types of undisclosed post hoc hypothesizing harm scientific progress. *Review of General Psychology*, *21*(4), 308–320. https://doi.org/10.1037/gpr0000128

Schooler, J. (2011). Unpublished results hide the decline effect. *Nature*, *470*(7335), 437. https://doi.org/10.1038/470437a

Schweinsberg, M., Madan, N., Vianello, M., Sommer, S. A., Jordan, J., Tierney, W., . . . Uhlmann, E. L. (2016). The pipeline project: Pre-publication independent replications of a single laboratory's research pipeline. *Journal of Experimental Social Psychology*, *66*, 55–67. https://doi.org/10.1016/j.jesp.2015.10.001

Senn, S. (2012). Misunderstanding publication bias: editors are not blameless after all. *F1000Research*, *1*. https://doi.org/10.12688/f1000research.1-59.v1

Sherman, R. C., Buddie, A. M., Dragan, K. L., End, C. M., & Finney, L. J. (1999). Twenty years of PSPB: Trends in content, design, and analysis. *Personality and Social Psychology Bulletin*, *25*(2), 177–187. https://doi.org/10.1177/0146167299025002004

Siegel, D., & Baveye, P. (2010). Battling the paper glut. *Science*, *329*(5998), 1466. https://doi.org/10.1126/science.329.5998.1466-a

Song, F., Parekh, S., Hooper, L., Loke, Y. K., Ryder, J., Sutton, A. J., . . . Harvey, I. (2010). Dissemination and publication of research findings: An updated review of related biases. *Health Technology Assessment*, *14*(8). https://doi.org/10.3310/hta14080

Stanley, D. J., & Spence, J. R. (2014). Expectations for replications: Are yours realistic? *Perspectives on Psychological Science*, *9*(3), 305–318. https://doi.org/10.1177/1745691614528518

Stroebe, W. (2016). Are most published social psychological findings false? *Journal of Experimental Social Psychology*, *66*, 134–144. https://doi.org/10.1016/j.jesp.2015.09.017

Szucs, D., & Ioannidis, J. P. A. (2016). Empirical assessment of published effect sizes and power in the recent cognitive neuroscience and psychology literature. *bioRxiv*.

Szucs, D., & Ioannidis, J. P. A. (2017). Empirical assessment of published effect sizes and power in the recent cognitive neuroscience and psychology literature. *PLoS Biology*, *15*(3), e3001151. https://doi.org/10.1371/journal.pbio.2000797

Tijdink, J. K., Verbeke, R., & Smulders, Y. M. (2014). Publication pressure and scientific misconduct in medical scientists. *Journal of Empirical Research on Human Research Ethics*, *9*(5), 64–71. https://doi.org/10.1177/1556264614552421

Vale, R. D. (2015). Accelerating scientific publication in biology. *Proceedings of the National Academy of Sciences USA*, *112*(44), 13439–13446. https://doi.org/10.1073/pnas.1511912112

Van Aert, R. C. M., Wicherts, J. M., & Van Assen, M. A. L. M. (2019). Publication bias examined in meta-analyses from psychology and medicine: A meta-meta-analysis. *PLoS One*, *14*(4). https://doi.org/10.1371/journal.pone.0215052

Vermeulen, I., Beukeboom, C. J., Batenburg, A., Avramiea, A., Stoyanov, D., van de Velde, B., & Oegema, D. (2015). Blinded by the light: How a focus on statistical "significance" may cause p-value misreporting and an excess of p-values just below .05 in communication science. *Communication Methods and Measures*, *9*(4), 253–279. https://doi.org/10.1080/19312458.2015.1096333

Voelkl, B., & Wurbel, H. (2016). Reproducibility crisis: Are we ignoring reaction norms? *Trends in Pharmacological Sciences*, *37*(7), 509–510. https://doi.org/10.1016/j.tips.2016.05.003

5
Accuracy and Completeness in the Dissemination of Classic Findings in Social Psychology

David A. Wilder and Thomas E. Cuthbert

Over the past decade increasing concerns have been raised about the quality of research generated in the sciences, in general, and social psychology, in particular (e.g., Simmons et al., 2011). Other chapters in this book address a variety of such issues including the transparency of research as well as the appropriateness of statistical analyses and the accuracy of subsequent reports. This chapter initiates an inquiry into a different aspect of the scientific process—the dissemination of research findings to the public. Specifically, our focus is on the accuracy with which core empirical findings are delivered to our most immediate audience (undergraduates enrolled in social psychology courses) and whether that information is retained by them beyond the final exam. The bulk of the chapter focuses on the first point, which is the more important from a best-practices perspective. Are major textbooks used in social psychology courses accurate and relatively complete in their presentation of the findings and implications from core experiments? We also present some data on retention of information from those courses.

Science has historically been divided into two conceptually independent but functionally overlapping concerns. One is basic research that seeks to discover the regularities of nature (natural sciences) and human behavior (social sciences). The other is the application of that research, largely in pursuit of technologies that can aid human life. The strength of science has rested on two pillars: (1) careful observation and experimentation and (2) integrity in the reports and conclusions drawn from those observations. In addition, for science to address human needs outside the lab it must be disseminated, since the practitioners and users are often not the scientists themselves. In the case of social psychology, much of the basic research has direct relevance to how persons interact outside the lab. The most immediate (and captive) audiences for the work of social psychologists are the thousands of students who take social psychology courses in colleges and universities. Many of us who teach these students hope that what we stress is retained and has an impact on their behavior beyond the classroom. We think it is fair to say that most of us are not trying to indoctrinate them in any particular political or social ideology but rather are trying to encourage them to consider how the research findings they learn about may be relevant to their daily lives. This raises two questions. First, are we accurately reporting findings of the field to them? Second, do they retain what we say beyond what is necessary to pass exams?

This chapter focuses on how some classic studies in social psychology are presented in frequently adopted textbooks for basic social psychology courses. We have chosen to focus on textbooks because those outlets are (1) assumed to contain objective and accurate presentations of research findings, (2) designed to cover the field in both breadth and depth, and (3) have a captive audience of students who are exposed to their content. As such, these texts (along with the professor's lectures) are the most direct and potent connection between professional social psychologists and laypeople. Attention to how research is reported in these secondary sources and whether it is retained accurately serves as one gauge of the potential impact that the discipline has on society. The chapter is divided into three sections: (1) identification of a set of core experiments found in the most-used texts; (2) analysis of how accurately and thoroughly their findings have been reported in those books; and (3) assessment of their impact on students' knowledge after leaving the course.

Identification of Core Experiments

We first set out to identify what we term "core experiments" in social psychology. It should be noted at the outset that we are focusing on experiments, not theories or correlational demonstrations or anecdotes. The reasons for this focus are as follows. First, as an empirically based discipline, social psychology experiments provide the bedrock on which theories rest. Second, experiments yield observable, mostly quantitative data, whereas theories are less concrete and more subject to ambiguity. Third, correlational studies and anecdotal observations lack the explanatory power of experiments. Finally, most of the core experiments that we selected have been subject to peer review, whereas other content found in texts, including field observations, news stories, and anecdotes, has often not been vetted beyond the judgment of the text authors.

The core experiments we selected were identified in a series of steps. Initially, we surveyed a number of universities to determine what texts were being used in their introductory social psychology courses. From that list we selected four texts that were most frequently adopted. Then we combed through each to identify experiments that were cited in all and were given sufficient emphasis to indicate that they were considered by the text authors (and by implication course instructors) to be significant and likely to appear on exams.

Selection of Social Psychology Texts

Syllabi for introductory social psychology courses were obtained from psychology department websites. We chose to sample large universities because they teach the most students and should, therefore, impact the largest numbers of undergraduates. We obtained a total of 90 syllabi from 17 universities. These included representatives from major public and private universities in the United States: the Big 10, the Ivy League, the State University of New York system, and the University of California system (Table 5.1). That we obtained the most syllabi from our institution (Rutgers) was not just a matter of convenience or egocentrism but rather due to our department having a policy of making all syllabi publicly available online.

From the syllabi we tabulated the number of times a textbook was adopted. Table 5.2 lists the frequency of adoptions. These data do not tell us the number of students exposed to each text nor the number of different faculty who assigned the text. Our interest here is in identifying a number of frequently used social psychology texts. From that list we selected the top four texts to examine in detail:

Aronson, E., Wilson, T. D., & Akert, R. M. (2012). *Social Psychology* (8th ed.).
Kassin S., Fein, S., & Markus, H. R. (2013). *Social Psychology* (9th ed.).
Kenrick, D. T., Neuberg, S. L., & Cialdini, R. B. (2009). *Social Psychology: Goals in Interaction* (5th ed.).
Myers, D. G. (2012). *Social Psychology* (11th ed.).

Table 5.1 Schools from Which Syllabi Were Acquired

School	Frequency	Percent
Rutgers University	26	28.90
University of Minnesota	17	18.90
Michigan State University	15	16.70
University of Iowa	6	6.70
University of Wisconsin-Madison	4	4.40
Brown University	3	3.30
Purdue University	3	3.30
Columbia University	2	2.20
University of Nebraska-Lincoln	2	2.20
Oregon State University	2	2.20
University of California, Los Angeles	2	2.20
University of Colorado	2	2.20
University of Utah	2	2.20
Arizona State University	1	1.10
Cornell University	1	1.10
Harvard University	1	1.10
University of Albany	1	1.10

Note that more recent editions of these texts have been released since we began this project. Based on examining several editions of the same text, we have found that descriptions of our core experiments tend not to change; later editions are more likely to add new research than to change already written descriptions of the older experiments that formed our core.

Selection of Core Experiments

We defined a core experiment as one that fit the following two criteria: (1) It had to be an experiment (multiple conditions and random subject assignment) and (2) It had to be discussed in some detail in the textbook. We did not require that all texts discuss a core experiment to the same extent. Some of the texts gave more attention to some of these experiments than did the others. But all described the experiments in enough detail for a reader to understand what was done, what was found, and what are the implications

Table 5.2 Textbook Frequency Table

Textbook	Frequency	Percent	Author percent
Aronson, E., Wilson, T. D., & Akert, R. M. (2002). *Social Psychology* (4th ed.)	1	1.11	28.89
Aronson, E., Wilson, T. D., & Akert, R. M. (2006). *Social Psychology* (6th ed.)	2	2.22	
Aronson, E., Wilson, T. D., & Akert, R. M. (2009). *Social Psychology* (7th ed.)	7	7.78	
Aronson, E., Wilson, T. D., & Akert, R. M. (2012). *Social Psychology* (8th ed.)	16	17.78	
Myers, D. G. (2011). *Exploring Social Psychology* (6th ed.)	1	1.11	17.78
Myers, D. G. (2005). *Social Psychology* (8th ed.)	1	1.11	
Myers, D. G. (2007). *Social Psychology* (9th ed.)	3	3.33	
Myers, D. G. (2010). *Social Psychology* (10th ed.)	3	3.33	
Myers, D. G. (2012). *Social Psychology* (11th ed.)	8	8.89	
Kenrick, D. T., Neuberg, S. L., & Cialdini, R. B. (2004). *Social Psychology: Unraveling the Mystery* (3rd ed.)	1	1.11	15.56
Kenrick, D. T., Neuberg, S. L., & Cialdini, R. B. (2007). *Social Psychology: Goals in Interaction* (4th ed.)	1	1.11	
Kenrick, D. T., Neuberg, S. L., & Cialdini, R. B. (2009). *Social Psychology: Goals in Interaction* (5th ed.)	12	13.33	
Kassin, S., Fein, S., & Markus, H. R. (2010). *Social Psychology* (8th ed.)	3	3.33	7.78
Kassin, S., Fein, S., & Markus, H. R. (2014). *Social Psychology* (9th ed.)	4	4.44	
Gilovich, T., Keltner, D., & Nisbett, R. E. (2010). *Social Psychology* (2nd ed.)	1	1.11	5.55
Gilovich, T., Keltner, D., Chen, S., & Nisbett, R. E. (2012). *Social Psychology* (3rd ed.)	4	4.44	
DeLamater, J. D., & Myers, D. J. (2007). *Social Psychology* (7th ed.)	1	1.11	2.22
DeLamater, J. D., Myers, D. J., & Collett, J. L. (2015). *Social Psychology* (8th ed.)	1	1.11	
Baron, R. A., & Branscombe, N. R. (2011). *Social Psychology* (13th ed.)	3	3.33	3.33
Lesko, W. A. (2008). *Readings in Social Psychology: General, Classic, and Contemporary Selections* (7th ed.)	3	3.33	3.33
Smith, E. R. & Mackie, D. M. (2007). *Social Psychology* (3rd ed.)	2	2.22	2.22
Baumeister, R. F., & Bushman, B. J. (2007). *Social Psychology and Human Nature* (1st ed.)	1	1.11	1.11
Breckler, S. J., Olson, J., & Wiggins, E. (2005). *Social Psychology Alive* (1st ed.)	1	1.11	1.11

Table 5.2 *Continued*

Textbook	Frequency	Percent	Author percent
Cahill, S. E., & Sandstrom, K. (2011). *Inside Social Life: Readings in Sociological Psychology and Microsociology* (6th ed.)	1	1.11	1.11
O'Brien, J. (2010). *The Production of Reality: Essays and Readings on Social Interaction* (5th ed.)	1	1.11	1.11
Sanderson, C. A. (2009). *Social Psychology* (1st ed.).	1	1.11	1.11
No textbook	7	7.78	7.78

of those findings. In most cases there were photographs, figures, or tables accompanying the descriptions of the experiments.

Based on these criteria, the following eight studies were culled from the four textbooks (listed in alphabetical order):

Asch (1951, 1952a, 1952b, 1956): Conformity in small groups
Berkowitz and LePage (1967): Weapons effect on aggression
Darley and Latané (1968): Bystander intervention
Festinger and Carlsmith (1959): Cognitive dissonance
Jones and Harris (1967): Correspondent inferences
Milgram (1963, 1965, 1974): Obedience to authority
Rosenthal and Jacobson (1968): Self-fulfilling prophecies
Sherif et al. (1961): Intergroup conflict

Again, it should be noted that this list is empirically derived from attention given to these across four often-used texts. Certainly, some instructors may emphasize some of them more than others in their lectures or on their exams. Moreover, there may be other studies that any given instructor spends more time on in class than these (e.g., research conducted by that particular professor).

What is striking and satisfying about this list is that it spans major topic areas and chapters found in the typical undergraduate text. These include social perception (Jones and Harris), attitude change (Festinger and Carlsmith), social influence (Asch, Milgram, Rosenthal and Jacobson), aggression (Berkowitz and LePage), helping (Darley and Latané), and intergroup relations (Sherif et al.). These studies also span the gamut from small-scale, tightly controlled laboratory experiments of about an hour to broader field experiments lasting multiple weeks.

Another commonality among these studies is that they may be considered "well seasoned." They date from the 1950s (Asch, Sherif et al.), 1960s (Milgram, Rosenthal and Jacobson, Jones and Harris, Berkowitz and LePage), and 1970s (Darley and Latané). Because of their age, they have the advantage of having been on the ground floor as the field grew significantly after World War II as an academic discipline. Once introduced into texts, these experiments have remained in subsequent revisions and have assumed the status, at least in the texts, as being settled knowledge.

In addition, all of these experiments created a rich phenomenal experience for their subjects. High levels of experimental realism were incorporated into the procedures of these core studies, which produced a psychologically involving and powerful experience for the subjects. The procedures often had a touch of theater about them, one that the secondhand reader can vicariously experience in some of the more vivid descriptions of the procedures. None of the culled studies relied heavily on hypothetical situations or imaginary scenarios.

Yet another characteristic that many of these studies share is their sometimes unexpected or surprising findings. For example, both Asch and Milgram did not initially expect the amount of social influence that they observed in their experiments. The surprising, and sometimes counterintuitive, nature of the findings attracts attention in the manner of the journalism cliché that "dog bites man" is not news but "man bites dog" is news. Perhaps the field gives extra attention to unexpected or counterintuitive findings because we social psychologists are sensitive to the complaint that much of our work seems to produce obvious findings that anyone's grandmother could have told us.

Finally, these studies were mostly conducted before the field became concerned about best research practices. As a consequence, they can be challenged, at minimum, on the issue of openness or transparency and, perhaps more seriously, on the grounds of questionable research practices (e.g., no consideration of appropriate sample size, inappropriate or incomplete statistical analyses). Nevertheless, they form an established core that undergraduates are exposed to in lectures and accompanying textbooks. It is also worth pointing out that some of these studies have been successfully replicated (e.g., Smith & Haslam, 2012).

CLASSIC FINDINGS IN SOCIAL PSYCHOLOGY 129

In the following sections we briefly review the most significant findings from the selected experiments. Then we examine the accuracy of their presentations in the four texts. Experiments are discussed in chronological order.

Accuracy of Presentation in the Texts

Asch Conformity (1951)

Asch's conformity experiments form the foundation for the discussion of conformity in social psychology texts. In the Asch paradigm, college students made judgments about lengths of lines (and sometimes about the shade of colors) in the presence of seven to nine other college students. All students, but one, were accomplices of the experimenter and on most trials (the number varied across experiments) gave incorrect responses. The primary dependent measure was whether participants conformed to the incorrect judgments of the others or remained independent. On critical trials subjects could either answer correctly (disagree with the majority), conform to the majority position, or, on some trials, adopt a compromise position (an alternative that was incorrect but not as incorrect as the majority choice). Asch conducted a number of variations of this paradigm. The most comprehensive account of his program of research can be found in *his Psychological Monographs* paper (Asch, 1956).

All four texts devote at least a full page to the Asch studies and accompany their discussions with either photographs or figures. The texts note that, overall, conformity in the face of group pressure occurred in one-third to 37% of the trials (which is accurate given that Asch conducted several replications with slightly varying outcomes in that range). A couple of minor inaccuracies can be found in the Kassin and Kenrick texts. Kassin reports that "50% went along on at least half of the critical presentations" (Chapter 7, p. 219). Actually, 37.6% of subjects went along on half or more of the critical trials (Asch, 1956, Table 3). Kenrick states that no one conformed on all 12 critical trials (Chapter 6, p. 197). However, 4.9% of Asch's subjects conformed on all 12 trials (Asch, 1956, Table 3). To its credit the Aronson text also includes a bar graph (Chapter 8, p. 207) that presents the percentage of subjects who conformed on either 0, 1 to 3, 4 to 6, 7 to 9, and 10 to

12 trials. Although exact percentages are not given, extrapolating from the bars, we arrived at the following: 0 (24%), 1 to 3 (33%), 4 to 6 (14%), 7 to 9 (18%), and 10 to 12 (11%). These are pretty close to the actual percentages from Asch (1956, Table 3): 0 (23.6%), 1 to 3 (28.4%), 4 to 6 (16.3%), 7 to 9 (18.8%), and 10 to 12 (13.1%).

All in all, what was presented in the four texts was mostly accurate. In particular, the Aronson text should be commended for focusing on the distribution of errors among the subjects. The summary statement of conformity occurring in between one-third and 37% of the trials, while accurate, does not give as rich a description of the phenomenon as when conformity is looked at by the number of conforming trials. Those data clearly show that a majority of subjects (52%) either did not conform or conformed less than one-third of the time (0 to 3 conformity responses). Those who conformed one-third or more of the time were distributed nearly evenly (with a noticeable blip at 10 errors) from 4 through 12: 4 (4.9%), 5 (5.7%), 6 (5.7%), 7 (3.3%), 8 (10.6%), 9 (4.9%), 10 (4.9%), 11(3.3%), and 12 (4.9%). Presentation of the number of subjects who conformed at different levels strikes us as a more accurate way to introduce students to the complexity of social influence. The fact that conformity varied substantially among subjects suggests that social pressure in the Asch situation interacted with the personality or self-concerns of the subjects. That may strike seasoned social psychologists as a given unnecessary of commentary, but for novice undergraduates this opens the door to questions about why some subjects conformed often and others less so, and thereby provides an opportunity to talk about the broader person-by-situation interaction that accounts for the variability they see in their lives outside the classroom.

The Asch experiments also offer some interesting findings that do not appear in introductory texts. These outcomes can serve as bridges to other topics. To cite one example, Asch reported that when talking with subjects after the experiment, those who conformed tended to underestimate the number of times they yielded to the majority (self-serving bias?). To cite another example, those who conformed usually conformed early; it was not a process of wearing down a subject's resistance. Moreover, Asch noted that when interviewing subjects afterwards, they seemed more concerned about the negative consequences of nonconformity (e.g., the loneliness of the dissenter) than about the positive feelings one might have when asserting independence. The stick of social disapproval was more powerful than the carrot of independence.

Sherif Intergroup Competition (1954)

Although Sherif and his colleagues conducted several field experiments on the effects of intergroup competition, the one most cited in texts took place in the summer of 1954. It appears in greatest detail in their 1961 book (Sherif et al., 1961). This is an extremely rich mine of data and observations, and, of course, an introductory social psychology text cannot be expected to cover it in great detail. In short, they recruited 24 boys (11 or 12 years of age) from public schools in Oklahoma City for a summer camp at Robbers Cave State Park in Oklahoma. They took great care in recruiting the children to ensure that they came from middle-class backgrounds, were doing well in school, and were generally of average to above-average intelligence. Most importantly, the children were not known to one another before meeting at the camp. On arriving at the camp, they were arbitrarily assigned to two groups with an attempt to match the groups as closely as possible (e.g., height, weight, sports ability, popularity at their home schools). The experiment then consisted of three stages. During the first stage (7 to 8 days) they participated in activities within their own groups to develop a sense of identity (e.g., group name [Eagles, Rattlers], flag, leader). In stage 2 (5 days) they were brought together to interact in a tournament with 15 different competitions (e.g., baseball games, treasure hunt, tent-pitching contest). The group with the highest cumulative score from the competitions would earn a trophy and individual medals and knives for its members. The series of competitions created animosity between the groups, including derogatory name calling and physical altercations. By the end of stage 2, when asked to identify their friends, 94% of Rattler and 93% of Eagle choices were for ingroup members. Consistent with friendship choices, ratings of the outgroup were predominantly negative on a set of traits that appear in the 12-year-old lexicon of that time (brave, tough, friendly, sneaky, stinkers, and smart alecks).

After creating intergroup bias in stage 2, Sherif and his colleagues turned their attention to reducing that hostility in stage 3. For example, they organized a set of contact experiences between the groups (meal together, shooting off fireworks together), but these attempts failed as the groups used those occasions to insult one another. What worked was contact in pursuit of a shared goal (superordinate goal). The experimenters organized a series of eight encounters in which the groups needed to cooperate in order to accomplish a shared goal (e.g., repairing a broken water supply, towing a truck). As the number of shared successful outcomes increased, tension between the groups diminished. On the bus trip home boys sat with members of the once-hated outgroup. As an example of the change of heart, the group that had won $5 in a bean-toss contest voted to use their winnings to buy malts (milk drink, not Scotch) at a refreshment stop for all campers.

Moving from anecdotes to harder data, outgroup members were more frequently chosen as friends following stage 3. For the Rattlers, at the end of stage 2, only 6% of their friendship choices were outgroup members; after stage 3 it had increased to 36%. For Eagles the percentage of outgroup members chosen as friends increased from 7% (stage 2) to 23% (stage 3). Finally, ratings of the ingroup and outgroup on the six traits (see two paragraphs above) did not differ by the end of stage 3.

There are two points that we think are particularly important to take away from the outcomes of this research. First, the effects of the stage 2 competitions were not eradicated even though there was a substantial lessening of hostilities and increase in friendship choices between groups. Friendship choices at the end were still heavily skewed toward the ingroup. Of course, that may have been due as much to the positive feelings developed toward individual ingroup members in stages 1 and 2 as to negative feelings about the outgroup. Note that the traits ratings for the ingroup and outgroup did not differ by the end of stage 3, which suggests that bias had been eliminated for trait ratings if not for friendship choices. Second, the reduction in hostility between the groups did not occur overnight as a result of a single cooperative contact experience. Sherif introduced more than a half-dozen situations in which cooperative interaction was in the interests of both groups. It would be misleading to suggest that a single successful cooperative interaction works as a magic bullet to undo intergroup bias.

The Kenrick and Kassin texts provide a concise and accurate summary of the procedure and major conclusions. The Aronson and Myers texts devote more space to Sherif's research. The authors lay out the procedure in enough detail to give the reader a good sense of what happened. Their conclusions are accurate. Aronson includes a figure that shows the change in friendship choices between stages 2 and 3 (detailed in the last paragraph above). Although Aronson does not present the precise percentages of friendship choices, extrapolation from the figure indicates that it is accurate. Myers, later in the same chapter, presents a graph showing ratings of the groups after stage 2 competition and then again after the cooperative experiences of stage 3. Although exact means are not presented, the graph accurately reflects the change in bias for both groups.

Overall, the four texts do a reasonable job of presenting the major findings from the Sherif study in a clear manner. To its credit, the Myers text explicitly notes that the friction was created between groups of children who did not have economic, cultural, or physical differences—the point being that these were children who ought to get along with one another. This underscores the power of the competitive situation to induce bias. However, none of the summaries addresses the two points that we feel are critical ones to take away from Sherif's studies—the importance of having multiple cooperative encounters and the fact that, even after the successful encounters, there was still preference for one's own group over the other.

Festinger and Carlsmith Forced Compliance Dissonance (1959)

The Festinger and Carlsmith (1959) dissonance study is the prototype for the "forced compliance" dissonance paradigm in which persons are gently coerced into behaving in a manner contrary to their beliefs. To the extent they believe they were free to choose their actions, they should experience dissonance for behaving contrary to their beliefs. Dissonance can be resolved in this situation by bringing their attitudes more in line with their actions. In Festinger and Carlsmith's experiment, the fountainhead of this line of research, all subjects work on repetitive, boring tasks for an hour. Tasks were designed so that subjects would walk away from the experience with the belief that the experiment was not enjoyable or worthwhile. The experimenter then ended the study and told subjects that they were in a control group for an experiment about how expectations affect performance. The next subject would be assigned to a different condition and would be told by an accomplice that the experiment was quite interesting. At this point the experimental manipulation occurred, with subjects being assigned to one of three conditions.

In the control condition subjects were interviewed by a person ostensibly unconnected to the experiment who was evaluating the department's research participation requirement. This person administered the dependent measures. Subjects in the $1 and $20 conditions were told that the accomplice was unable to make it to the next session. Appearing desperate (in the best theatrical vein of dissonance researchers), the experimenter requested that the subject substitute for the absent accomplice and falsely tell the next subject that the experiment was enjoyable and interesting. The experimenter conveniently had written prompts that the subject could use. In addition, he asked subjects if they would be willing to be on call to fill in for the accomplice in the future. They were then told that they would be paid either $1 or $20 for their assistance (and presumably the same for each subsequent session, although that is not entirely clear from their procedure—p. 205). Subjects were then paid and were joined in a waiting room by a female accomplice of the experimenter (posing as a subject). The subject and accomplice were left alone for 2 minutes. During that time the accomplice inquired about the experiment, and the real subject indicated it was enjoyable and interesting. The experimenter then returned and escorted the accomplice to the experimental room. The subject was then interviewed by the person allegedly conducting a survey about the department's experiments.

Dependent measures were four questions asking subjects to rate on 11-point scales "how enjoyable the tasks were," "how much they learned," the "scientific importance" of the research, and their desire to "participate in a similar experiment." Results from three of the four measures (all except "how much they learned") were in the direction of the dissonance prediction. However, only the "how enjoyable the tasks were" item showed significant differences across the conditions such that subjects rated the tasks as more enjoyable when they chose to lie to receive the small payment of $1.

All four texts, of course, describe the experiment relatively briefly and note that subjects in the $1 condition rated the experiment as more enjoyable than those in the $20 and control conditions. Myers presents a bar graph of the "enjoyable" ratings; while the actual means are not presented, the heights of the bars in the graph do closely match the means from the original. Kassin also includes a graph of "task enjoyment." The ordinate for this bar graph is a 25-point scale with bar lengths of 6 (control condition), 9.7 ($20 condition), and 22.4 ($1 condition). It's not clear why a 25-point scale was used given that the original measure was an 11-point scale (−5 to + 5). If we transform Festinger and Carlsmith's data to a 25-point scale, the means would be 11.38 (control condition), 12.38 ($20 condition), and 15.88 ($1 condition). Therefore, although the order of means is correct in Kassin's bar graph, differences among conditions have been exaggerated. In particular, the effect of the $1 high-dissonance condition appears much stronger than the actual data. Given the cliché that a picture is worth a thousand words, their graph incorrectly indicates a much stronger effect than Festinger and Carlsmith reported.

Two things strike us about the Festinger and Carlsmith experiment and its presentation in the texts. First, the method is underreported considering the significance of the study. A critical piece of information missing from reports in the texts is that by agreeing to serve as the backup accomplice, the subject was making a commitment beyond that one instance of lying. How much that may have impacted subjects' dissonance is speculative, of course, but the possibility of further service to the experimenters (in exchange for low or high pay) might have increased behavioral commitment and, therefore, the impact of the manipulation. Second, despite its designation as a classic, the results are not particularly strong. The dissonance effect reached conventional statistical significance on only one measure out of four (granted, that was the primary measure of interest to the researchers). In the spirit of caution, texts might note that the Festinger and Carlsmith findings, while trendsetting, were relatively weak. Attention could then be devoted to later dissonance experiments that appear to have stronger results (e.g., Ashmore & Collins, 1968; Helmreich & Collins, 1968).

Milgram Obedience (1963)

Without fail in our discussions with undergraduates, it is the Milgram obedience research that is most mentioned when we ask students what they recall from their social psychology courses. Not surprisingly, the obedience research commands the most attention and space in the texts: Kassin, Myers, and Aronson devote approximately five pages of text, figures, and photographs to Milgram; Kenrick's discussion is briefer (about two pages).

Milgram's obedience experiments are reported in a number of outlets, beginning with a paper in the *Journal of Abnormal Psychology* (Milgram, 1963). Findings from that initial paper along with subsequent publications are collected in a book titled *Obedience to Authority* (Milgram, 1974). It's that compendium of his research program that we use as a reference point here. Some of the major conclusions from the series of experiments Milgram conducted were as follows:

1. In his initial studies 65% of the subjects fully obeyed the experimenter's commands to administer shocks to the maximum level (allegedly 450 volts). He reported no gender differences in obedience.

2. Obedience significantly declined when the experimenter was physically absent (remote conditions) and when the experiment was moved from Yale to a commercial building in Bridgeport, Connecticut (although the latter decline in obedience from 65% to 48% was not statistically significant).
3. Obedience significantly declined as the victim's distress became more audible (voice feedback— 62.5%) or as the victim became physically closer to the subject—proximity (in the same room—40%) and touch proximity (subject had to touch the victim—30%).
4. Full obedience was lowest (10%) when the subject had social support for defiance (from two confederates posing as subjects). Obedience was greatest (92.5%) when the subject, although part of the experiment, did not administer the shocks. In that scenario a confederate was the one who threw the switches.

In all texts, descriptions of the procedure and results are accompanied by photographs and tables or figures. Because of the richness of Milgram's research program, the texts are not able to discuss all of his findings, nor do they devote equal attention to those they do mention. Nevertheless, all touch upon at least portions of the four points we listed as critical findings. They also note (either in the discussion of the obedience studies or in another chapter on research methods) the ethical concerns generated by the stress placed on subjects in his experiments.

Although there were no errors in the reporting of the findings, we believe that all four texts missed an opportunity to emphasize the critical role of social support in the obedience studies. All report that having confederates who disobeyed led to significantly greater disobedience (full obedience fell to 10% of participants). However, there was no discussion of how this finding relates to the role of social support in social influence more generally (e.g., Asch conformity experiments). This strikes us as a missed opportunity to tie together areas of research that are often presented as separate entities. Furthermore, the texts do not make much of Milgram's finding that the greatest obedience occurred when subjects did not have to flip the shock switches themselves. As Milgram notes in his book (p. 121), this finding fits with obedience observed in organizations where people who are part of the chain of command that ultimately inflicts harm are unlikely to resist because they are not the ones at the end of the chain who inflict the harm. The lack of discussion of the implications of this finding strikes us as a missed opportunity to relate the obedience research to issues such as dissonance, rationalization, and self-serving attributions.

Jones and Harris Correspondent Inferences (1967)

The Jones and Harris (1967) experiments are used in social texts to introduce the related topics of correspondent inferences and the fundamental attribution error. These experiments demonstrated that we attribute persons' actions more to their disposition than evidence warrants. In a set of three experiments subjects either read (experiments 1 and 2) or listened to (experiment 3) a speech in which the writer or speaker was either given a choice of taking a pro or con position or was assigned a pro or con position. In experiment 1 the topic was a pro- or anti-Fidel Castro essay written by a college student for a political science exam. In experiment 2, the topic was the same but this time it was a statement made by a debater. Experiment 2 contained several additional conditions (e.g., having the subject also take a pro- or anti-Castro position) that did not significantly affect the pattern of findings, so the authors collapsed across them for some of the analyses. Finally, in experiment 3 subjects listened to a recording of a pro- or anti-segregation speech. The speaker was either from Georgia or New Jersey (given the year of the study, it was reasonable to suppose that a speaker from a Southern state would be more likely to favor racial segregation than a speaker from a Northern state). In all experiments subjects were asked to infer the true or real beliefs of the writer or speaker.

Results were similar in all experiments, with the strongest pro attitude attributed to the pro writer/speaker in the choice conditions and, likewise, the strongest anti attitude to the anti-writer/speaker in the choice conditions. More importantly, there were similar significant differences, albeit smaller, in the no-choice conditions. Thus, even when subjects were aware that the writer/speaker was assigned a position, they still saw that position as indicative of the person's true attitudes.

All of the texts get the basic finding correct that in the no-choice conditions subjects made correspondent inferences (i.e., attributed the behavior to the writer's beliefs even when choice was absent). However, the Kenrick text (p. 80) does not make it completely clear that the dispositional inferences in the no-choice conditions were less strong than in the choice conditions. None of the texts mentions that the Jones and Harris findings were based on a series of studies conducted on multiple topics with multiple modalities. When details of Jones and Harris are presented (Kassin, Myers, Aronson), references are to either experiment 1 (college essay exam) or experiment 2 (debate positions). Kassin, Myers, and Aronson all provide bar graphs of the attribution findings rather than actual means from the experiments. When we extrapolated numerical means from the bar heights in the graphs, we found that all the relationships among bars in all three graphs closely reflected the numerical outcomes from the Jones and Harris paper.

Berkowitz and LePage Weapons Effect (1967)

This single experiment is a relatively small study that has achieved a great deal of impact due, we suspect, to its relevance to the contentious debate over the role of firearms in violence in the United States. Berkowitz and LePage examined how the mere presence of weapons (in this case a 12-gauge shotgun and a .38-caliber pistol) can function as an excitatory cue to enhance interpersonal aggression. The experiment was a 2×3 factorial with one additional condition. Factors were anger (subject either angered or not by a confederate) and presence of a weapon (no weapon, weapons present that belonged to a confederate, weapons present not associated with the confederate). A seventh condition was run with angered subjects and a non-weapon cue (two badminton racquets and a shuttlecock). Briefly, subjects interacted with a confederate who either angered them by giving them seven electric shocks or only one. Then they spent some time in a room with props that included either guns owned by the confederate, guns unrelated to the confederate, no guns, or badminton racquets. Finally, they had an opportunity to retaliate against the confederate. Dependent measures of interest were the number of shocks subjects administered to the confederate and the duration of those shocks.

As expected, there were no differences across conditions when subjects were not angered. However, subjects delivered significantly more shocks to the confederate when they were in the presence of weapons belonging to the confederate ($M = 6.07$) compared to the no-cue condition ($M = 4.67$) or the nonaggressive cue (badminton) condition ($M = 4.60$). Although trending in the predicted direction, the presence of weapons unrelated to the confederate did not produce a significant increase in the number of shocks relative to the control ($M = 5.67$). The shock duration measure showed the same pattern of means, but differences were not significant.

All four texts reported that the presence of a weapon increased aggression among angry subjects. However, none pointed out that this effect was found only when the weapons belonged to the source of the subject's anger. That does not seem to be a trivial oversight to us. The actual findings suggest that the mere presence of weapons is not sufficient to produce more aggression unless those weapons were associated with the source of the anger. Perhaps it was the cumulative effect of the weapon plus the association that pushed subjects to inflict more pain on the confederate. That's not to say that the weapon's effect as reported in the texts is not correct. (There have been successful replications and failed ones as well; e.g., Ellis et al., 1971; Frodi, 1975). But clearly such a broad conclusion is not warranted from this initial study on the "weapons effect." As a final observation, in the Aronson text, the authors present a figure (Chapter 11, p. 339) that shows data from the duration measure. Considering that this measure did not produce significant differences, it's a bit misleading to present a graph that shows differences without noting that those differences were not statistically significant.

Darley and Latané Bystander Intervention (1968)

Research on helping behavior experienced a boom in the 1970s fueled in large part by the clever experiments on bystander intervention initiated by the team of Latané and Darley. Their work is cited in all the texts and, of the numerous studies, the one that is mentioned in most detail is Darley and Latané (1968). That experiment was inspired by the notorious murder of Kitty Genovese outside her apartment building in New York City on March 13, 1964. Her screams were heard by dozens of building dwellers yet (as initially reported) none immediately came to her aid or called police to report the crime. Subsequent examination of the incident revealed that the bystanders were not as inactive as initially reported (Lemann, 2014). Regardless, the incident was the impetus for Darley and Latané's clever creation of a comparable situation in the lab.

In their experiment subjects were placed in cubicles and thought they were interacting with either one, three, or five others via an intercom system. Actually, subjects were alone and the alleged others were tape recordings created by the experimenter. (Comparable to the situation faced by bystanders in the Kitty Genovese incident, subjects in the experiment could not see the reactions of the alleged others in the experiment. Consequently, Darley and Latané's findings cannot be viewed as indicative of what may occur when bystanders have knowledge of the responses of one another.) Participants took turns talking about adjustment to college life. At a designated point in the conversation one of the others appeared to have an epileptic seizure. The primary dependent measure was "the time elapsed from the start of the victim's fit until the subject left her experimental cubicle" (Darley & Latané, 1968, p. 379). The experiment was terminated if the subject did not respond within 6 minutes. Results as a function of time are presented in Table 5.3.

Darley and Latané noted that all subjects in the group size 2 condition responded by the 3-minute mark, whereas helping in the other conditions plateaued by 3 minutes at 62% (group size 3 condition) and 31% (group size 6 condition). The appropriate conclusion to draw from these data is that the probability of a particular bystander helping (when the behavior of other bystanders is unknown) decreases as the number of bystanders increases from one to two to five.

All four of the texts correctly note that the likelihood of a subject seeking help for the victim decreased with the number of bystanders present. The texts differ in whether they report the data from the first minute or from the asymptote (from 3 minutes to 6 minutes helping did not increase). Kassin presents the 6-minute outcomes while Myers and Kenrick note the 1-minute helping results. Aronson had the most complete presentation of the findings, including a graph showing the cumulative helping over the 6 minutes for each condition (after Figure 1 from Darley & Latané, 1968).

What's more interesting from an accuracy perspective are conclusions drawn from the research. According to Kassin, Darley and Latané concluded, "The more bystanders there are, the less likely the victim will be

Table 5.3 Helping in the Darley and Latané (1968) Study

Group size	% responding in 1 minute after fit begins	Time (sec)
2 (subject + victim)	85	52
3 (subject, victim, 1 other)	62	93
6 (subject, victim, 4 others)	31	166

Adapted from Table 1 in Darley & Latané (1968), p. 380.

helped" (Chapter 10, p. 407). Aronson et al. note that the experiment "found that in terms of receiving help, there is no safety in numbers" (Chapter 11, p. 314). The former statement is incorrect and the latter is somewhat misleading. As Darley and Latané (1968) acknowledge in their paper (p. 380), with an increasing numbers of bystanders, the probability of anyone helping decreases. But that is not equivalent to saying that the likelihood of the victim receiving help decreases, because with more bystanders, there are more combinations of possible helpers. In their detailed report of the study in *The Unresponsive Bystander: Why Doesn't He Help?* (Latané & Darley, 1970), they noted that "by 45 seconds after the start of the fit, the victim's chances of having been helped by the single bystanders were about 50% compared to none in the five-observer condition." (p. 99). In the next sentence, however, they acknowledge that after "the first minute, the likelihood of getting help from at least one person is high in all three conditions" (p. 99). In short, any difference in helping among the conditions vanished by the 1-minute mark. These data suggest that immediate help is more likely when a bystander is alone versus being with four other bystanders, but that effect vanishes by the 1-minute mark.

Our point is made more clearly in the following tables generated from their data. The victim will receive help unless all potential helpers fail to intervene. As the number of bystanders increases, the probability of a victim receiving help (since the bystanders are independent) = (1 − probability of a person not helping) n where n is the number of bystanders (Table 5.4). Note that for both helping after 1 minute and helping after 6 minutes following the onset of the victim's fit, the probability of the victim receiving assistance is virtually the same in all conditions (nearly 90% for all conditions after 1 minute and

Table 5.4 Helping and the Probability of Being Helped After 1 and 6 Minutes

Condition	% who helped	Probability of receiving help	% who helped	Probability of receiving help
	1 min.		6 min.	
Lone bystander	85	0.85	100	1.00
Two bystanders	62	0.86	82	0.97
Five bystanders	31	0.84	62	0.98

From Darley & Latané, 1968.

nearly 100% for all conditions after 6 minutes). Hence, a conclusion or even a suggestion that people are less likely to receive aid with more bystanders is patently wrong based on the data from this classic study.

We may seem a bit shrewish about this point because we have found in our social psychology classes that students often miss the distinction between the probability of a particular person helping and the probability of anyone helping. Over the years we have asked social psychology students about this on multiple-choice exams and even after lecturing on it, we find that a sizeable minority fail to appreciate the distinction (much less appreciate the implications of it).

Rosenthal and Jacobson Teacher Expectations (1968)

The most complete presentation of this ambitious field experiment can be found in the book appropriately titled *Pygmalion in the Classroom* (Rosenthal & Jacobson, 1968). The experiment was conducted in a public elementary school (grades one through six). Teachers in 18 classes (three per grade) were given the expectation that some of their students would show intellectual blooming during the academic year based on testing conducted the previous May. Actually, these "bloomers" were a random subset of the class. Students then completed the intelligence test on three later occasions: midway through the academic year, at the end of the academic year in May, and at the end of the next academic year. Overall, "bloomers" showed a significantly greater increase in intelligence scores (13.33 points) at the end of the first academic year than did controls (9.17). However, as Table 5.5 shows, the effect of teacher expectations was confined to grades 1 and 2.

Turning to the four texts, all of them describe the basic procedure and overall findings accurately. But none of them notes that the effect was limited to the first two grades. This strikes us as a serious omission, not only because it is incomplete reporting of the data, but also because it represents a failed opportunity to consider why the effect was only seen among the younger children. The most obvious possibilities to explore would be differences between what teachers know about younger and older children in their schools and differences between the attitudes of younger and older children toward school. Regarding the former, from the perspective of the teachers, they have less information about the younger than the older children; there are fewer records of past performance and there is no teacher grapevine about how

Table 5.5 Test-Score Gains of Bloomers and Nonbloomers by Grade

Grade	Nonbloomers	Bloomers
1	12	27
2	7	16
3	5	5
4	2.5	5
5	17.5	17
6	11	10
Overall	9.17	13.33

good, dedicated, interested, rebellious, and so forth the student is. Lacking that information, the expectations given by the experimenters may have assumed greater influence. As for children's attitudes toward school, they may not have developed a "good" or "bad student" identity and may be more open to whatever subtle influences the teachers emitted. This is speculation, of course, but it suggests how a more complete and accurate account of the Pygmalion findings might be used to stimulate conversation about other factors at work in the classroom and, perhaps, more accurately place the self-fulfilling prophecy phenomenon as one of several factors that can be at work in that setting.

Unless students are aware of the actual pattern of findings from this study, they are likely to come away with the false impression that teacher expectations have a significant impact on students throughout their time in school. Such a conclusion is clearly not warranted by the data but is implied by the texts. A more accurate presentation of this research would also be helpful to integrate it with later work that has shown relatively modest and nuanced self-fulfilling prophecy effects (e.g., Jussim & Harber, 2005).

Summary

Taken as a whole, these eight core experiments have fared well in the textbooks—as well they should, considering that they frequently serve as introductions to topic areas or as core points in the authors' literature reviews. Presentations of these eight experiments in the texts can be roughly categorized into two groupings. First, some of the experiments have been summarized accurately but significant points are omitted that would enhance the discussion of the findings (Asch, Festinger and Carlsmith, Jones and Harris, Milgram, and Sherif). Second, other experiments are reported with, in our opinion, significant factual or interpretative errors (Berkowitz and LePage, Darley and Latané, and Rosenthal and Jacobson).

Retention of Information

The last question we consider is whether students retain knowledge of the core experiments and their implications once they have completed an introductory course in social psychology. As a first step, we obtained two samples of convenience: students who had just completed social psychology and students who were enrolled in an upper-level history of psychology course at Rutgers. Most students in the latter sample had taken social psychology at least one semester before enrolling in the history course. Data from these samples address the following questions. First, what information do students retain soon after being exposed to the core experiments (social psychology sample)? Second, what information is retained a semester or more later (history of psychology sample)? Third, is there any difference in retention between the samples? Both sets of students completed a set of 19 multiple-choice questions. Eight of the questions asked about the results of the eight core experiments discussed in this chapter (one question per study). Seven questions focused on general conclusions and implications relevant to the core studies. The remaining four items were fillers. For an example of a pair of questions, refer to Box 5.1.

Overall, students in the social psychology course answered more of the questions correctly (M = 10.13, SD = 2.95, n = 93) than those in the history of psychology class (M = 9.39, SD = 2.47, n = 85). The social psychology students were accurate on 68% of the 15 questions; the history of psychology students answered 63% of the items correctly. This difference was marginally significant, $t(176) = 1.81, p = 0.07, d = 0.27$.

We then decided to analyze this further by doing separate analyses for the "findings" questions and the "implications" questions. The social psychology students (M = 5.32, SD = 1.76) answered significantly more findings questions correctly than did the history of psychology students (M = 4.25, SD = 1.30), $t(176) = 4.60, p < 0.001, d = 0.69$. This could have been because the social psychology students had learned the material more recently than

Box 5.1 Example of a "Findings" Question and an "Implications" Question

Findings question: In a study of helping by Darley & Latané, subjects heard a person in an adjacent room apparently have an epileptic seizure. They reported that
A. subjects were more likely to help when they thought there were other subjects in the experiment than when they thought they were alone
B. subjects were more likely to help when they thought they were alone than when they thought there were other subjects in the experiment **(Correct)**
C. the presence or absence of other subjects in the experiment had no effect on a subject's likelihood of helping
D. subjects took longer to help the other person when they thought they were alone than when they thought other subjects were in the experiment

Implications question: Which of the following statements is correct based on social psychological research about helping?
A. A person is more likely to help another the fewer other possible helpers there are in the situation. **(Correct)**
B. A person is more likely to help another the more other possible helpers there are in the situation.
C. Strangers are more likely to receive help from a person than are friends.
D. Helping is unaffected by experience; people are either born helpful or not.

---

the history students and, as such, it was easier for them to remember the finer details of the experiments. The social psychology students (M = 4.81, SD = 1.72) did not differ significantly from the history of psychology students (M = 5.14, SD = 1.58) in terms of the number of implications questions that were answered correctly, t(176) = 1.35, p = 0.18.

Certainly, we don't want to make much of this outcome, as this was a sample of convenience and the mean difference was only about one question. It is a bit discouraging that the performance of students who had just taken social psychology was rather mediocre. The questions were pretty straightforward and were not designed to be deceptive or nitpicky. What is somewhat encouraging is that retention for the history students did not fall off all that much considering that many of them had taken social psychology from 1 to 2 years earlier.

Results of the survey broken down by individual experiments are presented in Table 5.6. Suffice it to say that students from both classes appeared to remember the intergroup conflict, aggression, helping, and obedience studies better than the self-fulfilling prophecy, attribution, dissonance, and conformity experiments if we arbitrarily use two-thirds correct as the criterion

Table 5.6 Percentage of Correct Answers by Course and Experiment

	Experiment results		Implications	
Experiment	Social psychology	History of psychology	Social psychology	History of psychology
Sherif	81.70	78.80	75.30	83.50
Berkowitz and LePage	79.60	60.00	79.60	78.80
Darley and Latané	82.80	75.30	69.60	75.30
Milgram	75.30	77.60	57.00	57.60
Rosenthal and Jacobson	64.50	61.20	54.80	65.90
Jones and Harris	54.80	34.10	52.70	60.00
Festinger and Carlsmith*	51.60	24.70	–	–
Asch	41.90	12.90	91.40	92.90

* Due to a procedural error, data were not collected for implications of the dissonance experiment.

for competence. A similar pattern occurred for the implications questions, with the exception of the Asch experiments. Recalling specific outcomes from the conformity experiments proved most difficult for students in both classes, yet the question about the implications of those experiments for social conformity was answered correctly by nearly all subjects.

Final Remarks

Attention to how research is reported in secondary sources is an important adjunct to concerns about how the research is conducted in the first place. Even excellent research that adheres to best practices is ill served if it is misrepresented when reported to audiences via secondary sources. Errors in the transmission of research findings can be due to both inaccuracies of reporting and inappropriate implications drawn from the research. As an initial stab at investigating this topic, we identified a set of core experiments that have been reported in some detail in four frequently used social psychology textbooks for undergraduates. These experiments were chosen not only because they appear in all of these texts, but also because they date from the post–World War II salad days of experimental social psychology. As such, they have served as touchstones or foundations for later research.

We are not holding all of these experiments up as exemplars of excellent research, although as we noted earlier, they are models of how to do research that involves subjects in settings of strong experimental realism. But from the perspective of best practices, most of them have shortcomings, whether it be transparency of procedures, full disclosure of methods, or appropriateness of analyses. For example, several of the experiments appear to have been underpowered in terms of sample size (Berkowitz and LePage, Festinger and Carlsmith, Jones and Harris). However, the purpose of this chapter is not to critique their procedures; rather, it is to evaluate whether these core experiments have been appropriately presented in textbooks. The succinct answer to that question is "yes." Overall, the major findings and implications of the experiments have been reported accurately, even though there were some minor errors in reporting for most of them. As we noted in our review, including more findings from some of the original experiments would enrich their impact and provide greater connections to other topic areas. However, discussion of two of the core studies (Darley and Latané, Rosenthal and Jacobson) suffered significantly from inferences that were in error.

The second question we addressed is what students retain about these core experiments. (A cynic might wonder if a fuss should be made about accuracy if little is retained by the reader.) As a first step in exploring this issue, we constructed a set of questions that asked about the findings and implications of the core experiments. The performance of students who had just completed social psychology was compared to that of students who had taken social psychology a semester to a year earlier. The good news was that students performed about the same in both groups, suggesting there was little memory loss over the intervening semester to a year. The bad news was that overall performance was in the range of 60% to 70% correct, suggesting that much of the information is lost early or never acquired in the first place.

We will end with a third question not addressed in the chapter. If students are able to retain a moderate amount of accurate information about the core experiments, does this have an impact on their behavior? This is a more difficult issue to assess than the ones of textbook accuracy and information retention. Ultimately, if social psychology shares the goal of many disciplines to have an impact on students and society beyond the classroom, then attention should be given to measuring whether or not there has been movement in that direction. Best practices for research focuses on the design, conduct, and analyses of research. Best practices for a discipline that seeks to be relevant to the outside world must also consider how well that good research is disseminated and what impact it has on those it reaches.

References

Aronson, E., Wilson, T. D., & Akert, R. M. (2012). *Social psychology* (8th ed.). Pearson Education Inc.

Asch, S. E. (1951). Effects of group pressure upon the modification and distortion of judgment. In H. Guetzkow (Ed.), *Groups, Leadership and Men; research in human relations* (pp. 177–190). Carnegie.

Asch, S. E. (1952a). Effects of group pressure upon the modification and distortion of judgment. In G. E. Swanson, T. M. Newcomb, & E. L. Hartley (Eds.), *Readings in Social Psychology* (2nd ed., pp. 2–11). Holt.

Asch, S. E. (1952b). *Social Psychology*. Prentice-Hall.

Asch, S. E. (1956). Studies of independence and conformity: I. A minority of one against a unanimous majority. *Psychological Monographs: General and Applied*, 70(9), 1–70.

Ashmore, R. D., & Collins, B. E. (1968). Studies in forced compliance: X. Attitude change and commitment to maintain publicly a counterattitudinal position. *Psychological Reports*, 22(3), 1229–1234.

Berkowitz, L., & LePage, A. (1967). Weapons as aggression-eliciting stimuli. *Journal of Personality and Social Psychology*, 7(2), 202–207.

Darley, J. M., & Latané, B. (1968). Bystander intervention in emergencies: Diffusion of responsibility. *Journal of Personality and Social Psychology*, 8(4), 377–383

Ellis, D. P., Weinir, P., & Miller, L. (1971). Does the trigger pull the finger? Test of weapons as experimental stimuli aggression-eliciting. *Sociometry*, 34(4), 453–465.

Festinger, L., & Carlsmith, J. M. (1959). Cognitive consequences of forced compliance. *Journal of Abnormal and Social Psychology*, 58(2), 203–210.

Frodi, A. (1975). The effect of exposure to weapons on aggressive behavior from a cross-cultural perspective. *International Journal of Psychology*, 10(4), 283–292.

Helmreich, R., & Collins, B. E. (1968). Studies in forced compliance: Commitment and magnitude of inducement to comply as determinants of opinion change. *Journal of Personality and Social Psychology*, 10(1), 75–81.

Jones, E. E., & Harris, V. A. (1967). The attribution of attitudes. *Journal of Experimental Social Psychology*, 3(1), 1–24.

Jussim, L., & Harber, K. D. (2005). Teacher expectations and self-fulfilling prophecies: Knowns and unknowns, resolved and unresolved controversies. *Personality and Social Psychology Review*, 9(2), 131–155.

Kassin, S., Fein, S., & Markus, H. R. (2013). *Social Psychology* (9th ed.). Wadsworth.

Kenrick, D. T., Neuberg, S. L., & Cialdini, R. B. (2009). *Social Psychology: Goals in Interaction* (5th ed.). Allyn & Bacon.

Latané, B., & Darley, J. M. (1970). *The Unresponsive Bystander: Why Doesn't He Help?* Prentice Hall.

Lemann, N. (2014, March 10). A call for help: What the Kitty Genovese story really means. *New Yorker*. https://www.newyorker.com/magazine/2014/03/10/a-call-for-help

Milgram, S. (1963). Behavioral study of obedience. *Journal of Abnormal and Social Psychology*, 67(4), 371–378.

Milgram, S. (1965). Some conditions of obedience and disobedience to authority. *Human Relations, 18*(1), 57–76.

Milgram, S. (1974). *Obedience to Authority: An Experimental View.* Harper and Row, Inc.

Myers, D. G. (2012). *Social Psychology* (11th ed.). McGraw-Hill.

Rosenthal, R., & Jacobson, L. (1968). *Pygmalion in the Classroom: Teacher Expectation and Pupils' Intellectual Development.* Holt, Rinehart & Winston.

Sherif, M., Harvey, O. J., White, B. J., Hood, W. R., & Sherif, C. W. (1961). *Intergroup Conflict and Cooperation: The Robbers Cave Experiment.* University of Oklahoma Press.

Simmons, J. P., Nelson, L. D., & Simonsohn, U. (2011). False-positive psychology undisclosed flexibility in data collection and analysis allows presenting anything as significant. *Psychological Science, 22*(11), 1359–1366.

Smith, J. R, & Haslam, S. A. (2012). *Social Psychology: Revisiting the Classic Studies.* Sage.

6
Strengths and Weaknesses of Meta-Analyses

Katherine S. Corker

How can researchers and policymakers best come to conclusions about the state of evidence in a research literature? The traditional narrative literature review has largely been supplanted in the social sciences by a quantitative technique known as *meta-analysis*. Meta-analysis summarizes evidence in a research area by taking an average of effect sizes. Effect sizes are weighted prior to averaging, usually using some indicator of precision of an effect size estimate. Researchers can also assess the degree of variability in effects across studies and assess possible explanations for that variability.

Armed with support from meta-analyses, social scientists can refine theoretical models, suggest future research studies, and craft evidence-based policies (Chan & Arvey, 2012). Furthermore, meta-analysis promises a certain degree of objectivity that traditional reviews do not. If a literature search is comprehensive, the meta-analyst is simply left to compute the relevant statistics and average them. Simple, right?

Yet, the quality of the summary that results from a meta-analysis depends crucially on the quality of the included studies. In light of recent concerns about questionable research practices (John et al., 2012), publication bias (Malhotra & Simonovits, 2014), and problems replicating research (Open Science Collaboration, 2015), scholars may wonder how informative meta-analyses actually are and whether they are worth the effort to conduct.

This chapter briefly reviews the history of meta-analysis before turning to an assessment of its strengths and weaknesses, as well as considerations of alternatives to and modifications of traditional meta-analysis. It closes with recommendations to make meta-analyses more informative.

Katherine S. Corker, *Strengths and Weaknesses of Meta-Analyses* In: *Research Integrity*. Edited by: Lee J. Jussim, Jon A. Krosnick, and Sean T. Stevens, Oxford University Press. © Oxford University Press 2022. DOI: 10.1093/oso/9780190938550.003.0006

History of Meta-Analysis in the Social and Behavioral Sciences

It may come as a surprise that modern meta-analysis techniques were just developed in the mid-1970s—only a little over 40 years ago. Although earlier techniques had been derived to combine p-values (Fisher, 1932, as cited in Chalmers et al., 2002), correlation coefficients (Pearson, 1904), and values from contingency tables (Mantel & Haenszel, 1959) from multiple studies, these techniques were not often used. Modern techniques involving synthesis of standardized effect sizes were developed only recently (Borenstein et al., 2009).

At its core, meta-analysis is not a complicated technique: it is simply an average of study effect sizes, weighted by a measure of study precision. Using the principal of aggregation, the meta-analyst assumes that idiosyncrasies and unreliability associated with each small individual study are averaged out, and a more precise—presumably more accurate—estimate is rendered in the aggregate. Beyond an average effect size, meta-analysis also offers the chance to measure variability (termed *heterogeneity* in meta-analysis lingo) in effect sizes and test for moderators that explain this variability (Borenstein et al., 2009).

Although Gene Glass coined the term "meta-analysis" to refer to the quantitative synthesis of effect sizes, several scholars independently derived meta-analytic techniques around the same time (Glass, 2015; Schmidt, 2015; Rosenthal, 2015). Glass and his contemporaries derived meta-analysis out of necessity: Ever-increasing numbers of original studies in the post–World War II era meant that bodies of literature could no longer be adequately summarized using traditional narrative reviews. Subsequently, meta-analysis spread from psychology and education and permeated the biomedical and social sciences.

Promise and Strengths of Meta-Analytic Approaches

Early on, meta-analysis promised that it could serve as an objective arbiter of evidence, helping a researcher or policymaker to see the big picture in a body of literature. Individually fallible studies could be combined to give a summary conclusion that was closer to the Truth (Hunt, 1997).

The objective nature of the technique was important. A key promise was that a comprehensive, quantitative synthesis would be less sensitive to cherry-picking and other biases than traditional narrative reviews (but see Ferguson, 2014). Furthermore, because techniques emphasized effect size estimation (with a focus on magnitude of effects), meta-analysis promised to reduce the emphasis on the problematic yes/no thinking that reliance on null hypothesis significance testing seemingly encouraged (Rosenthal, 2015).

Belief in the ability of meta-analysis to fulfill this early promise has waxed and waned in the 40 years since its modern debut. Almost immediately, challengers and skeptics arose who criticized meta-analysis and its premise (e.g., Eysenck, 1978), but in recent years, meta-analysis has enjoyed an enviable position at the peak of a hierarchy of evidence (Borgerson, 2009), representing the highest possible quality of evidence (perhaps the "platinum" standard of evidence, but see Stegenga, 2011).

In the last few years, however, some of the old doubts have begun to surface again. There is a growing realization that the early recognized problem of publication bias threatens to completely undermine meta-analytic synthesis. Additionally, new challenges have arisen with the recognition that researchers may not be fully reporting the extent of exploration that has created a published finding (Kerr, 1998; Simmons et al., 2011). I explain these challenges to the validity of meta-analysis in detail before examining alternative methods of evidence synthesis, as well as recommendations for valid, informative, and reproducible use of meta-analysis.

Pitfalls of Meta-Analysis in the Context of Reproducibility Issues and Questionable Research Practices

Publication Bias

A fundamental assumption behind meta-analysis is that the selection of studies for inclusion in the analysis is comprehensive or, at least, unbiased. That is, each study is imagined to be a member of a broader population of studies, and in order for the sample average of that population to be an unbiased estimate, the selection rule for inclusion must itself be unbiased. In principle, this means that meta-analysts must attempt to identify and include all studies that have been conducted on a topic (or at least to sample randomly within all studies).

A major threat to the unbiased inclusion of studies in meta-analyses is publication bias (Rosenthal, 1979; Sterling, 1959). Because the publication process serves as a filter through which some studies are generally admitted into the scientific record and other studies are left to languish in "file drawers," studies in the published literature are an unrepresentative sample of studies that have been conducted on a topic. There are many reasons for the nonpublication of studies, but lack of statistical significance is one of the major contributors (Fanelli, 2010; O'Boyle et al., 2017; Scherer et al., 2007).

Selection on statistical significance creates a situation in which published effect sizes are overestimates of true population effect sizes.[1] Overestimation increases as the size of studies in the meta-analysis shrinks and as the true effect size under investigation goes to zero (Bakker et al., 2012; van Assen et al., 2015). Effects on heterogeneity are more complex (Augusteijn et al., 2019). When combined with low statistical power, there may even be a situation in which statistically significant published results are more likely to be false positives than true positives (Ioannidis, 2005), which implies that meta-analytic summaries may not just be overestimates, but instead they may sometimes indicate that an effect "exists" when it actually does not.

A poignant example of this situation comes from a highly influential phenomenon from social psychology known as ego depletion. The idea behind ego depletion is that willpower or self-control is a limited resource and drawing on this resource depletes it. Thus, initial acts of self-control should predict weaker self-control on later tasks. An initial meta-analysis (Hagger et al., 2010) amassed 198 studies on this phenomenon (total sample size = 10,782) and showed a medium to large average effect size with narrow confidence interval (Cohen's d = 0.62, 95% CI: [0.57, 0.67]). Almost no matter how the independent variable was manipulated or the dependent variable was measured, a medium to large effect size was observed, attesting to its generalizability. But a 2014 re-analysis (Carter & McCullough, 2014) of the meta-analytic data with various bias-correction techniques suggested the true effect size could be zero, and this possibility was later shown to be consistent with results from a large-scale preregistered replication attempt (Hagger et al., 2016), which found null results (Cohen's d = 0.04, 95% CI: [−0.07, 0.15]).[2]

---

[1] Publication bias can also affect heterogeneity estimates in somewhat unpredictable ways (see Augusteijn et al., 2019). These authors summarize results stating "the Q-test of homogeneity and heterogeneity measures H^2 and I^2 are generally not valid when publication bias is present" (p. 1).

[2] Work continues on the topic of ego depletion, both methodological and theory related (e.g., Friese et al., 2019; Vohs et al., 2021).

How could the initial meta-analysis have drawn such different conclusions from the preregistered replication? A strong possibility is that the published literature was biased, because it was an incomplete record of the studies that had been done—null or negative results went unpublished. It is notable that the initial meta-analysis (Hagger et al., 2010) did not attempt to locate unpublished studies for inclusion in the analysis, but perhaps even if it had, it is unlikely that all studies would have been located and that their partial inclusion would have been enough to fully eliminate the pernicious effects of publication bias.

The issue of study selection was an early point of contention between meta-analysts and critics. Smith and Glass (1977) amassed over 400 studies investigating the effectiveness of psychotherapy, taking great care to conduct a comprehensive search of existing studies. Eysenck (1978) saw this comprehensiveness as a weakness and accused Smith and Glass of ignoring study quality in study selection: "A mass of reports—good, bad, and indifferent—are fed into the computer in the hope that people will cease caring about the quality of the material on which the conclusions are based" (p. 517). Glass and Smith (1978) retorted that "connoisseurs' distinctions about which studies are 'best' and which ought to be discarded would lead, in this instance, to a profligate dismissal of hundreds of findings" (p. 518).

Issues related to the selection of studies for inclusion in meta-analyses have not abated in the years since these early debates. Some sources advise meta-analysts to be as inclusive as possible in their literature searches, scouring conference abstracts and dissertation databases and personally contacting authors likely to have file-drawered studies (Sterne et al., 2017). Others recommend evaluating study quality (see Sanderson et al., 2007, for a variety of such systems) to exclude studies that do not meet certain quality or design standards (e.g., L'Abbé et al., 1987), to include quality as a meta-analytic moderator (Borenstein et al., 2009), or to weight studies by quality (Doi & Thalib, 2008). Sensitivity analyses (in which a variety of different corrections are performed to allow meta-analysis to determine whether results are sensitive to correction method) have also been recommended (Appelbaum et al., 2018). In the absence of mandatory prospective study registration, it seems unlikely that any literature search will ever be truly comprehensive, but as I discuss later (see "Systematic Review"), there are best practices that meta-analysts can follow to attempt to mitigate selection bias.

Questionable Research Practices

Researchers do not only select which effects to include or exclude from a publication. They may also tweak, edit, and craft the specific analyses that are ultimately included in their published papers in the service of obtaining statistical significance. Many (often ambiguous) study-design decisions must also be made along the way (e.g., how to best measure a variable, which outliers to exclude). Because it is not always clear cut which design or analysis variant is correct or best, researchers have a large amount of leeway to make choices that favor obtaining statistical significance, but ultimately inflate the number of false-positive results. These behaviors have been variously termed questionable research practices (QRPs), p-hacking, exploiting researcher degrees of freedom, and the garden of forking paths (see Gelman & Loken, 2013; Simmons et al., 2011).

For the meta-analyst, the presence of QRPs in the research literature means that meta-analytic data are likely to be biased. Exactly how much effect sizes are biased under various conditions is an active and ongoing area of research (Carter et al., 2019; Simonsohn et al., 2014a; Simonsohn et al., 2014b; van Aert et al., 2016). Results so far can best be summarized by stating that the effects of QRPs can be unpredictable and complex. Van Aert et al. (2016) even went so far as to say: "In case of strong evidence or strong indications of p-hacking, [meta-analysts should] be reluctant in interpreting estimates of traditional meta-analytic techniques and p-uniform and p-curve because their effect-size estimates may be biased in any direction depending on the type of p-hacking used" (p. 714). It is also currently unknown how QRPs affect heterogeneity estimates (Augusteijn et al., 2019).

Carter et al.'s (2019) simulations suggest that the effects of publication bias may be somewhat larger than the effects of QRPs under commonly observed conditions in the social sciences, although the generalizability of this conclusion might depend on how closely the conditions of their simulations do match the real world, as well as which type and combination of QRPs are used. Regardless, Carter et al.'s results need not suggest that QRPs can safely be ignored, because their simulations do show instances where QRPs are quite influential. More broadly, in real research, the effects of publication bias and QRPs will combine to bias meta-analyses in ways that make it extremely challenging to accurately account for their influences.

Selection Bias and Other Coding Issues

Meta-analysts themselves are also likely to encounter ambiguous choices and forking paths, with opportunities for flexibility in meta-analytic coding and analysis. Coding decisions for individual studies carry much ambiguity: Which of two dependent variables should be included in the meta-analysis? Should multiple dependent variables be averaged together or analyzed multivariately? Does this particular operationalization of the independent variable fit inclusion criteria? Should this study be included or excluded? Which key terms should be used, and which databases should be searched? How are unpublished studies to be located, and how is study quality to be assessed? These are only a few of the many possible decisions a meta-analyst must make.

Perhaps the largest opportunity for meta-analyst choice involves the selection and coding of meta-analytic moderators. These moderator variables are selected in order to try to explain variation (i.e., heterogeneity) in study effect sizes. They represent an opportunity to test hypotheses besides the ones that the original authors conceived. For instance, a theory might predict a stronger effect among men than women. A meta-analyst could code the participant gender ratio in existing studies to see whether samples with larger numbers of men show larger effects on average.

These choice points can morph into opportunities for QRPs when decisions are made in a data-contingent way and/or based on their effects on meta-analytic conclusions. Dueling meta-analyses are common (see Ferguson, 2014), suggesting that it is often possible to analyze or interpret meta-analytic data in such a way as to easily support one's preconceptions or theory. Although there are methodological strategies (especially preregistration of meta-analytic protocols) that meta-analysts can use to help protect against such biases, current practices leave ample opportunities for bias (Schmidt, 2017).

Noncumulative Methods and Measurement

A meta-analyst's task is synthesizing findings on a common research question or hypothesis. Sometimes, however, the methods and measures used to investigate a question are so diverse that the resulting synthesis may lack meaning. For instance, Eysenck (1978) argued that Smith and Glass's (1977) decision to combine many very different types of psychotherapy in one analysis was problematic. Although it is possible to compute such an average, Eysenck questioned what meaning could be derived from it.

Critics like Eysenck have termed this problem "mixing apples and oranges," with the idea being that averages of such diverse "fruit" are not meaningful (Feinstein, 1995). Proponents of meta-analysis note that researchers can code methodological features of studies and include those features in the analysis, as Smith and Glass did (1977; see Chan & Arvey, 2012). For example, studies can be classified as experimental or observational, using long-form or short-form measures, adhering to Theory A or competing Theory B, and so on. These codes then become potential moderators that might explain heterogeneity in effect sizes.

One problem is that the methodological features of various studies may end up being mostly confounded. For instance, if proponents of Theory A also tend to use long-form measures and do experiments, whereas proponents of Theory B use short-form measures and do observational studies, it becomes impossible to determine which (if any) of these ingredients is the critical feature that is causing a difference in observed effect size. And as noted earlier, meta-analytic moderators can be selected post hoc in a way that helps a meta-analyst to draw preferred conclusions. Just as in primary research, when meta-analytic moderator variables are not randomized and experimentally controlled, it becomes challenging to draw strong conclusions about the reason for an effect.

Another problem is that in some areas of research, it is possible that coding of methods or measures might reveal that many studies are "loners" or "onlys" (i.e., they are the sole studies that use those methods or measurement). Author-developed or other one-off measures are very common in some research literatures. Flake et al. (2017) found that nearly half of papers published in 2014 in the *Journal of Personality and Social Psychology* (a top journal in its subfield) were either explicitly declared to have been developed on the fly or failed to include references to established scales (suggesting the measures were developed ad hoc). Thus it seems that researchers are not strongly incentivized to work cumulatively using shared paradigms.

As an example of why nonstandard measurement can be problematic for research synthesis, consider Elson (2016), who has catalogued the literature on the CRTT (Competitive Reaction Time Task), a laboratory measure of aggressive behavior (see also Elson et al., 2014). Elson found that there were more ways to score the CRTT (156 scoring strategies) in the published literature than there were papers that used the task ($k = 130$). Interestingly, the modal scoring strategy was unique (no other study used that strategy), with 106 of the 156 strategies being used only once, ever. This is not good news for the research synthesist. A lack of cumulative research design and scoring strategies makes meta-analysis challenging at best, and in some cases, it may render meaningful summaries very difficult.

Alternatives to and Supplements for Meta-Analysis

Given the potential severity of the problems just outlined for meta-analytic conclusions, one might speculate as to whether there are better alternatives to traditional meta-analysis when seeking to synthesize research conclusions. This section considers possible alternatives to, and supplements for, meta-analysis as currently practiced in the social sciences.

Narrative Review

Meta-analytic (or quantitative) reviews can be contrasted with traditional narrative reviews, often simply called literature reviews. Generally, in a narrative review, an author gives an overview of relevant previous work that provides context and justification for a subsequent study or future line of research. These reviews are usually not meant to be comprehensive; rather, they summarize particular features of a research literature (Grant & Booth, 2009). Narrative reviews also do not contain a quantitative synthesis of research evidence.

It is possible that a research community could consider abandoning meta-analyses altogether and return to doing narrative reviews only. But the observant reader might recall that meta-analyses were invented because narrative reviews were found wanting (Borenstein et al., 2009; see also Meehl, 1990). Indeed, narrative reviews are not well suited to summarizing large bodies of evidence, and unlike meta-analysis, there is no explicit weighting of different studies.

Narrative reviews might even encourage a "vote-counting" method in which researchers simply tally up the studies "for" or "against" a hypothesis. Such methods are flawed (Gurevitch et al., 2018) because, among other reasons, they fail to take the precision of estimates into account, implicitly treating all studies as equal.

Another issue is cherry-picking. In a narrative review, there is nothing preventing authors from simply presenting only those studies that support their positions and viewpoints (even unintentionally). For all of these reasons, it seems unlikely that researchers will view narrative review as a viable alternative to meta-analysis.

Systematic Review

Systematic review is a method for transparently conducting rigorous and comprehensive literature reviews (Grant & Booth, 2009). Importantly, systematic reviews are *not* just high-quality qualitative reviews. The term "systematic review" includes a *method* for reviewing research literature that should produce reproducible and unbiased findings. Systematic reviews are likewise not solely quantitative reviews; they can include meta-analyses but are not required to do so (Haddaway & Bilotta, 2016).

Several key ingredients distinguish systematic reviews from traditional narrative reviews (Haddaway et al., 2017). First, systematic reviews must use transparent and reproducible methods to locate relevant studies, and these methods must be described in sufficient detail to allow reproducibility. Best practices include searching multiple databases and naming those databases in the paper, clearly describing strategies used to locate unpublished works, and providing the exact search strings used (in the paper or a supplement).

Second, systematic reviews must have systematic procedures for evaluating studies—both published and unpublished (i.e., gray literature)—for inclusion or exclusion in the review. Researchers first screen titles and abstracts, eliminating studies that obviously don't fit inclusion criteria. The remaining studies are evaluated to ensure they meet inclusion criteria. As a best practice, researchers should have independent coders assess each study for inclusion (and measure interrater reliability), and they must systematically track decisions to include or exclude studies.

Finally, systematic reviews must include critical appraisal, also known as risk of bias assessment or quality assessment, of the constituent studies in the review. Critical appraisal means that studies are evaluated to ensure that they possess certain quality or design features. Many different critical appraisal systems exist; there is not one gold-standard method (Sanderson et al., 2007).

The GRADE system (Guyatt et al., 2008) provides a further scheme for evaluating the quality of evidence and strength of recommendations in whole literatures rather than individual studies.

Additionally, some bodies (Cochrane Collaboration, Campbell Collaboration, Center for Environmental Evidence [CEE]) require publication of a peer-reviewed protocol before starting a systematic review. A protocol serves as a preregistration for the review, which can help to constrain reviewers' researcher degrees of freedom and prevent bias in the review. The Campbell Collaboration accepts reviews that are relevant to social science disciplines, but the reviews need to focus on policy applications. There is no currently existing home for peer-reviewed registered protocols of systematic reviews for basic social science research.

Another related type of review is called a systematic map (James et al., 2015), also known as an evidence map or gap map. Systematic maps use systematic procedures to locate studies on a topic, but they do not synthesize the evidence from these studies (e.g., using meta-analysis), nor do they employ formal critical appraisal. What the maps can do is reveal areas or topics that have been understudied and are therefore missing information. In principle, it would be possible for researchers to evaluate the studies gathered in a systematic map and use this evaluation to support new, preregistered data collection. For instance, if studies showed either a limited evidence base or substantial evidence of QRPs or other biases, researchers could opt not to convert a systematic map to a systematic review (with meta-analysis). Instead, they could simply collect new (less biased) data.

Systematic reviews have become somewhat popular in biomedicine (Bastian et al., 2010), but uptake in the social sciences has been slower. Since 1980 (and as of late 2019), *Psychological Bulletin*, a premier outlet for review papers in psychology, has published 246 (13.4%) original research papers (i.e., not commentaries, retractions, corrections, or editorials) with "meta-analysis" in their titles[3] but just 12 (0.6%) papers with "systematic review" (out of 1,833 original research papers). Of course, a lack of consistency in terminology means that some meta-analyses in psychology might actually be adhering to many or most of the methodological protections that are present in systematic reviews, but they are not being labeled as such. It could also be that some papers with the label "systematic review" are not truly systematic

---

[3] Including the phrase "meta-analysis" or "systematic review" in the title is a best practice, but not one that is always followed. Hand searching of volumes of *Psychological Bulletin* would likely reveal both more meta-analyses and more systematic reviews.

reviews. Haddaway et al. (2017) find that misunderstandings of the term "systematic review" are common in their field (environmental ecology and conservation), a finding that likely extends to the social sciences (see also Petticrew, 2001).

Even if many meta-analyses were already taking great care with search reproducibility and tracking study exclusion (and there is evidence they do not; see Moher et al., 2007), most psychology meta-analyses are missing a formal critical appraisal step (Aytug et al., 2012; Bastian, 2016), rendering them ineligible to be considered true systematic reviews. Again, critical appraisal involves the systematic evaluation of study quality using a tool such as the Cochrane Collaboration's checklist (Higgins et al., 2011). Furthermore, only a handful (e.g., Jones et al., 2018; Woll & Schönbrodt, 2020) have ever been preregistered,[4] and there is no central collaboration akin to Cochrane, Campbell, or CEE in psychology. Taken together, the evidence suggests that although psychology and related social sciences make frequent use of meta-analyses, these meta-analyses are not often of the high methodological rigor required for the use of the label "systematic review."

In sum, systematic reviews hold some promise in terms of their ability to increase quality and decrease bias in research syntheses. Moher et al. (2007) report that Cochrane reviews, which have very rigorous standards for peer review, preregistration, execution, and reporting, are of demonstrably higher quality than non-Cochrane reviews. Moher et al.'s findings provide proof that it is possible for a field to make its meta-analyses more rigorous.

Systematic reviews are unlikely to be a panacea for several reasons. First, low quality and high risk of bias in existing studies may mean that even the most rigorously conducted reviews are ultimately uninformative (at least in terms of yielding an interpretable summary effect size). Second, full systematic reviews are laborious and take even more time than nonsystematic reviews to complete. Critics might correctly wonder whether the tradeoff of quality versus time to completion is worth it. Finally, even Moher et al.'s (2007) evidence shows that systematic review methodology (as employed in Cochrane reviews) still shows a lot of room for improvement. Thus, although preregistration of meta-analyses and coordination by a collaborative body stands to improve methods and reporting substantially, systematic review

---

[4] Reviews with health-related outcomes are eligible for registration in PROSPERO, and some studies have been registered there.

cannot fully solve the problems of publication bias and poor quality of evidence in the literature.

Bias-Corrected Meta-Analysis

The preceding sections have described how biases in individual study estimates (QRPs) and in whole literatures (publication bias) can affect meta-analytic conclusions. Perhaps one way to address these biases is simply to take account of them and apply corrections. This logic undergirds the many bias-correction tools that are available to meta-analysts. I consider the rationale, as well as strengths and weaknesses of the most often used bias correction tools.

Popular But Poorly Performing Methods of Bias Correction: Fail-Safe N and Trim and Fill

Fail-safe N should more realistically be thought of as a bias detector rather than a bias corrector, but I consider it here because of its widespread use. Importantly, even as a bias detector, fail-safe N underperforms relative to alternatives, and it should realistically not be used at all.

Rosenthal (1979) proposed fail-safe N as a way to assess how many results with effect size equal to zero would be needed to nullify a statistically significant meta-analysis. Although computationally simple, Becker (2005) reviews the many problems with this statistic, noting (among other things) the lack of a formal statistical model supporting its use and the lack of a clear criterion for identifying large test values. Furthermore, Becker (2005) notes that the statistic assumes that missing studies are exclusively null, as opposed to negative (Begg & Berlin, 1988; Ferguson & Heene, 2012).

In practice, fail-safe Ns are often large, implying that huge numbers of studies would be needed to change a meta-analytic conclusion. Cases like ego depletion (discussed previously) suggest that fail-safe N offers an overly optimistic take on the problem of publication bias (Hilgard, 2016). Given this lack of validity together with the aforementioned statistical critiques, researchers are well served to avoid using fail-safe N.

Trim and fill (Duval & Tweedie, 2000) is a test that relies on funnel plot asymmetry to detect and correct publication bias. A funnel plot is a graphic that plots study effect sizes (on the x-axis) against the inverse of their precisions (on the y-axis). In unbiased literatures, this results in a symmetrical plot, with more precisely estimated studies closer to the average overall effect size and less precisely estimated studies tending to show more variable effect sizes, symmetrically in the positive and negative direction. In biased literatures, funnel plots show asymmetry; there is a negative correlation between study precision and effect size. (It should be noted that selection bias is not the only cause of funnel plot asymmetry, but it is one major cause.)

In a trim-and-fill analysis, outlying studies are iteratively removed ("trimmed") from one side of the funnel plot until the plot is symmetrical, and the new axis of symmetry is taken as an adjusted estimate of the effect size. The resulting estimate has a variance that is too small, so the studies that were removed are added back and additional studies are then imputed ("filled") to again achieve symmetry (Borenstein et al., 2009).

Moreno et al. (2009) compared trim and fill to various forms of meta-regression (discussed subsequently). They found that trim and fill consistently underperformed relative to these alternative models, especially when there was heterogeneity in effect sizes. Carter et al.'s (2019) simulation agreed, finding that trim and fill gave positively biased effect sizes under publication bias, in addition to having very high type I error rates.

These authors and others (e.g., McShane et al., 2016; Simonsohn et al., 2014a; van Assen et al., 2015) converge in their recommendation to avoid the use of trim and fill as a bias-correction technique. As a bias detector, there are other tools that will do a better job, but researchers can consider trim and fill as one of several tools in a sensitivity analysis (Carter et al., 2019).

Selection Models: P-Curve, P-Uniform, and Three-Parameter Selection Model (3PSM)

Selection models are another class of bias-correction tools. Overall, these models assume that the published literature represents a subset of studies that have been performed, and the analysis attempts to fit parameters that model this selective publication process. Different selection models make differing assumptions about patterns of publication bias. They then use these assumptions to fit a model that corrects for missing studies.

The simplest of these models assumes that the cutoff for statistical significance (i.e., $p < 0.05$) fully determines which results will be published/observed. That is, results that are not statistically significant are not included in the meta-analysis. These models also assume that all of the studies in an analysis measure the same population effect size (i.e., there is no heterogeneity beyond sampling error). The model then estimates one parameter, μ, which is the average effect size adjusting for studies missing due to publication bias. Hence, these models are known as one-parameter selection models (McShane et al., 2016).

After an early introduction (Hedges, 1984), these models have had renewed interest under slightly different specifications under the names p-curve (Simonsohn et al., 2014b) and p-uniform (van Assen et al., 2015). The basic logic behind these models is that p-values are uniformly distributed under the null hypothesis, whereas under non-null models, the distribution of p-values varies based on statistical power. As power increases, the proportion of small p-values (p < 0.01) observed also increases. Therefore, for literatures investigating true effects, small p-values should frequently be observed, whereas p-values near the 0.05 cutoff should be relatively rare.

In terms of strengths, p-curve and p-uniform do a good job of recovering the true effect size when model assumptions are met (i.e., when there is no heterogeneity,[5] when p < 0.05 is a firm selection criterion, and all results with p < 0.05 are equally publishable). They are relatively simple to implement, though researchers frequently make mistakes regarding which p-values to select (Nelson et al., 2017). However, both p-curve and p-uniform perform quite poorly when there is heterogeneity in effect sizes (Carter et al., 2019; van Aert et al., 2016). Additionally, p-hacking can lead to either underestimation (Simonsohn et al., 2014a; Simonsohn, 2014b) or overestimation (Bruns & Ioannidis, 2016; Ulrich & Miller, 2015; van Aert et al., 2016) of corrected effect sizes by p-curve and p-uniform. Van Aert et al. (2016) note that "p-hacking may bias p-uniform and p-curve estimates in any direction depending on the type of p-hacking and (b) p-uniform and p-curve estimates are not necessarily better than those of fixed effect meta-analysis when p-hacking occurs" (p. 721).

These issues have led van Aert et al. (2016) to recommend avoiding meta-analytic synthesis when there is strong evidence of p-hacking. They also recommend using subgroups to try to achieve a homogeneous subset of studies for analysis, addressing the heterogeneity issue. In reality, identifying the appropriate subgroups for analysis is a nontrivial task as the variable(s) needed to mark subgroups may be unknown or unmeasured. Another

---

[5] Simmons et al. (2018; http://datacolada.org/67) disagree that p-curve performs poorly when there is effect-size heterogeneity. They claim, instead, that p-curve accurately recovers the average true effect size "of the studies included in p-curve." This effect size is in contrast to the population effect size that meta-analysis typically attempts to recover.

issue with these models involves selecting the appropriate hypothesis tests for inclusion in the analysis (Simonsohn et al., 2014b). The method does not handle dependent p-values (e.g., tests from related dependent variables taken from the same sample), so meta-analysts must specify a plan ahead of time to help them choose which of the many p-values in a paper to include in the analysis. Neither p-curve nor p-uniform can test moderator variables at present.

More complex selection models exist, such as Iyengar and Greenhouse's (1988) three-parameter selection model (3PSM; see also Hedges & Vevea, 2005). This model has a mean parameter (like p-curve and p-uniform) in addition to a heterogeneity parameter and a selection parameter (thus yielding the eponymous three parameters). The selection parameter applies weights that account for publication bias. In contrast to p-curve and p-uniform, which ignore studies with $p > 0.05$ completely, the 3PSM takes nonsignificant studies into account using a weight function.

On the plus side, the 3PSM has more realistic assumptions behind it than one-parameter models (given that publication bias is unlikely to be acting precisely at the 0.05 cutoff, and heterogeneity is likely to be present in most literatures). Furthermore, the model can be flexibly extended to incorporate formal tests of moderation without the need to rely on subgroup analysis. On the minus side, these techniques are complex enough that they may be difficult to implement for nonspecialists. (A recently developed R package, *weightr* [Coburn & Vevea, 2018], makes the model more accessible, though it makes assumptions to yield higher convergence rates.) Additionally, model convergence may be an issue, particularly when the number of studies in a meta-analysis is small. Further, the weight function, even if estimated, may not be well recovered by the model (Hedges & Vevea, 2005). Crucially, the performance of the model depends on the accuracy of the selection function, which is to some extent unknowable (Augusteijn et al., 2019).

Carter et al. (2019) report that the 3PSM showed reasonable type I error rates but was underpowered under many simulated conditions that match those often observed in the social sciences. In short, p-curve and p-uniform rely on some important assumptions and method limitations that may render them less useful for meta-analysis than one might hope. The 3PSM also suffers from some important limitations, most crucially relying on a large number of studies to reliably converge (unless strict assumptions are allowed). Investigations into these models under various conditions remain ongoing, rendering firm conclusions unwarranted.

Meta-Regression: Egger's Test and PET-PEESE

A final set of bias-correction models again rely on the logic of a funnel plot to examine publication bias. These tools, broadly known as meta-regression techniques, involve using regression to model the association between effect sizes and study precision. Egger et al. (1997) proposed regressing logged odds ratios on study precisions, with statistically significant slope coefficients indicating funnel plot asymmetry and therefore publication bias.

Stanley and Doucouliagos (2014) extended Egger et al.'s (1997) logic to examining not only the slope of this regression, but also using the model intercept as an estimate of meta-analytic effect size after correcting for publication bias. They called this test PET (Precision Effect Test). Another variant of this model uses study variances (i.e., standard error squared) rather than standard errors to predict study effect sizes, yielding a quadratic model called PEESE (Precision Effect Estimate with Standard Error). Stanley and Doucouliagos (2014) recommend using PET-PEESE as a conditional test in which the analyst proceeds to run a PEESE model only after rejecting the null hypothesis of no effect in a PET model. This conditional test was chosen due to the fact that PET is biased downward when the null hypothesis is false, but PEESE is biased upward when the null hypothesis is true. However, PET may be underpowered in many common research scenarios, leading some to recommend that analysts avoid using the conditional test (Hilgard, 2017).

Like the 3PSM, meta-regression models have the possibility to include and test moderating variables, making them more flexible than p-curve or p-uniform. PET-PEESE also showed fairly good type I error rates, but it had low power under many conditions (Carter et al., 2019). Stanley (2017) reviews additional potential problems with PET-PEESE as applied under common scenarios in social science research literatures. Specifically, when all individual studies are underpowered, PET and PEESE do not accurately recover effect sizes. Furthermore, because they are regression models, a large number of studies are needed for the models to perform as intended (though convergence was not as much of an issue as it was for the 3PSM). Thus, Stanley's (2017)[6] results suggest that small-scale meta-analyses may be inappropriate for meta-regression techniques. Finally, PET and PEESE may be underpowered relative to naive (i.e., uncorrected) fixed effects and

---

[6] Readers should note that another technique, known as Top10 (Stanley et al., 2010), proposes to reduce the influence of likely biased small studies by meta-analyzing only the top 10% most precisely estimated studies. Given that many social science meta-analyses involve small numbers of studies, this technique may not be viable under common circumstances; it remains to be seen whether Top10 proves to be useful for bias correction.

random effects meta-analysis, especially when there is little to no publication bias in reality.

Summary

Meta-analysts are faced with many choices when it comes to selecting a technique to correct for the biasing effects of publication bias and QRPs. Several factors are important to consider when choosing a test, including (1) the size of a typical study (2) the number of studies, k, (3) variance in sample sizes, (4) likely severity of publication bias, (5) severity and type of p-hacking, and (6) effect-size heterogeneity. Carter et al. (2019) offer a web application, *metaExplorer*, that researchers can use to assess when a particular technique may or may not be appropriate for their review. Augusteijn et al. (2019) also offer *Qsense*, a web application that can help researchers understand how heterogeneity estimates may be biased under varying conditions.

Note, however, that many of these factors that researchers must take into account to choose a bias-correction tool are precisely the factors that they would like for meta-analyses to estimate (e.g., degree of heterogeneity)! Thus, researchers are left in an unsettling place. Although it would be ideal if applying bias-correction tools led to straightforward recovery of the unbiased meta-analytic effect size, the various simulation studies reviewed here suggest that they are unlikely to do so. Yet, uncorrected (naive) meta-analysis often performs far worse than these bias-corrected tools. When investigating a null effect under conditions of heavy publication bias (perhaps an all-too-frequent occurrence in social science research), random effects meta-analysis nearly always yields a wrong answer. In brief, the best researchers can do is to apply a variety of corrections and assess the sensitivity of their conclusions to the models applied (Appelbaum et al., 2018; Carter et al., 2019). Easy solutions are not forthcoming.

Large-Scale Preregistered Trials, Registered Reports, and Registered Multiple-Laboratory Studies

Bias-correction tools implicitly assume that the magnitude of bias in a research literature is (1) discoverable and (2) correctable. To the extent that these assumptions are unsupported, researchers may be better off collecting new data on a question rather than trying to extract meaning from the existing literature. Two possibilities exist to support the collection and analysis of less biased data: unreviewed preregistration and registered reports.

Preregistration implies the full specification of study design and data analysis prior to commencing a study, and it may also (optionally) involve specification of a priori, theory-derived hypotheses. Unreviewed preregistrations are generated by researchers themselves and submitted to a registry before data collection begins. The preregistration is then later linked in the final journal article so that peer reviewers and later readers can compare the preregistration plan to the ultimately published paper.

By contrast, a registered report involves editor-supervised peer review of a preregistered study proposal at a participating journal, again prior to the onset of data collection (Chambers, 2013). Aside from peer review of study proposals (termed *stage 1 protocols*), a unique feature of registered reports is *in principle acceptance* (IPA). IPA means that participating journals agree to publish accepted registered reports regardless of the statistical significance of the key hypothesis test. Instead, publication decisions are made based on a priori defined conditions, such as whether a study passes certain quality thresholds (termed *positive controls*).

Registered replication reports (RRRs) are another recent innovation, pioneered at the journal *Perspectives in Psychological Science* (Simons et al., 2014) and now rehomed in the newly formed journal *Advances in Methods and Practices in Psychological Science* (Simons, 2018). RRRs are a form of registered report that focus on direct replications (i.e., studies that attempt to duplicate as many features of an original study as possible), involve adversarial collaboration (i.e., input from both proponents and skeptics of an effect), and have data collection distributed over many participating laboratories. It should be noted that multiple-laboratory registered reports can also involve novel research, not just replication studies (Schweinsberg et al., 2016).

Well-powered preregistered studies—perhaps especially those run through the registered reports mechanism—may ultimately be more informative than retrospective meta-analyses. In particular, if researchers want to be able to manipulate and control potential moderators, collecting new data may well be the best mechanism to do so (because researchers can avoid the uncontrolled nature of moderators in existing studies, as well as potential confounding of site-level variables). Furthermore, preregistered multisite studies allow researchers to assess the magnitude of heterogeneity under conditions that are known to have limited researcher degrees of freedom and be free of publication bias.

However, well-done large trials are extremely resource intensive, and the decision to pursue one likely needs to be informed by existing evidence.

Thus, researchers might find themselves in the tricky position of needing to complete a systematic map or a full systematic review (and perhaps meta-analysis) before deciding whether or not to run a large-scale registered replication. Ultimately the decision to pursue a review rather than collect new data will depend on idiosyncratic features of the research question at hand, but researchers should recognize that a directive to simply avoid meta-analysis in favor of new-data collection is unrealistic.

Conclusion and Recommendations for Informative and Reproducible Meta-Analyses

In the 40 years since their modern introduction, meta-analyses have gone from being viewed as mega-silliness (Eysenck, 1978) and statistical alchemy (Feinstein, 1995), to being regarded as a precipitator of Kuhnian revolutions (Chan & Arvey, 2012) and "platinum" evidence (Stenenga, 2011), to once again being regarded with suspicion (Engber, 2016). What this review has hopefully shown is that core issues—related to publication bias, meta-analytic coding decisions, and noncumulative methods and measurement—as well as newly recognized issues, like QRPs, are serious challenges to the validity of meta-analysis. Furthermore, no single suggested change or improvement (abandoning synthesis altogether, switching to systematic reviews, employing bias-correction tools, switching to preregistered trials only) is likely to be sufficient to address these problems.

In combination, these tools would have the chance to improve the quality of meta-analytic synthesis. Lakens et al. (2016) offer six further suggestions for making meta-analyses more reproducible, and readers who are considering undertaking a meta-analysis or systematic review are advised to carefully attend to each of their points.

It may well be the case that spending fewer resources on research synthesis and more resources on improving the quality (and reducing the bias) in the published literature may be a more productive use of researchers' limited time. Yet, the question remains as to how we decide which areas of the literature to invest more resources in and which to abandon. Increasing the quality of meta-analytic synthesis using the strategies described in this chapter, as well as working collaboratively and using multisite methodologies to determine how to move forward (Moshontz et al., 2018), seems to be our only option. Easy solutions are not forthcoming.

References

Appelbaum, M., Cooper, H., Kline, R. B., Mayo-Wilson, E., Nezu, A. M., & Rao, S. M. (2018). Journal article reporting standards for quantitative research in psychology: The APA Publications and Communications Board task force report. *American Psychologist, 73*(1), 3.

Augusteijn, H. E. M., van Aert, R. C. M., & van Assen, M. A. L. M. (2019). The effect of publication bias on the assessment of heterogeneity. *Psychological Methods, 24*, 116–134.

Aytug, Z. G., Rothstein, H. R., Zhou, W., & Kern, M. C. (2012). Revealed or concealed? Transparency of procedures, decisions, and judgment calls in meta-analyses. *Organizational Research Methods, 15*, 103–133.

Bakker, M., van Dijk, A., & Wicherts, J. M. (2012). The rules of the game called psychological science. *Perspectives on Psychological Science, 7*, 543–554.

Bastian, H. (2016, July 5). Psychology's meta-analysis problem. http://blogs.plos.org/absolutely-maybe/2016/07/05/psychologys-meta-analysis-problem/

Bastian, H., Glasziou, P., & Chalmers, I. (2010). Seventy-five trials and eleven systematic reviews a day: How will we ever keep up? *PLoS Medicine, 7*(9), e1000326. https://doi.org/10.1371/journal.pmed.1000326

Becker, B. J. (2005). Failsafe N or file-drawer number. In H. R. Rothstein, A. J. Sutton, & M. Borenstein (Eds.), *Publication Bias in Meta-Analysis—Prevention, Assessment, and Adjustments* (pp. 111–125). John Wiley & Sons, Inc.

Begg, C. B., & Berlin, J. A. (1988). Publication bias: A problem in interpreting medical data (with discussion). *Journal of the Royal Statistical Society, Series A, 151*, 419–463.

Borenstein, M., Hedges, L. V., Higgins, J. P., & Rothstein, H. R. (2009). *Introduction to Meta-Analysis*. John Wiley & Sons.

Borgerson, K. (2009). Valuing evidence: Bias and the evidence hierarchy of evidence-based medicine. *Perspectives in Biology and Medicine, 52*(2), 218–233.

Bruns, S. B., & Ioannidis, J. P. (2016). p-curve and p-hacking in observational research. *PLoS One, 11*(2), e0149144.

Carter, E. C., & McCullough, M. E. (2014). Publication bias and the limited strength model of self-control: Has the evidence for ego depletion been overestimated? *Frontiers in Psychology, 5*, 823. doi: 10.3389/fpsyg.2014.00823

Carter, E. C., Schönbrodt, F. D., Gervais, W. M., & Hilgard, J. (2019). Correcting for bias in psychology: A comparison of meta-analytic methods. *Advances in Methods and Practices in Psychological Science, 2*(2), 115–144.

Chalmers, I. Hedges, L. V., & Cooper, H. (2002). A brief history of research synthesis. *Evaluation and the Health Professions, 25*, 12–37.

Chambers, C. D. (2013). Registered Reports: A new publishing initiative at Cortex [Editorial]. *Cortex: A Journal Devoted to the Study of the Nervous System and Behavior, 49*(3), 609–610. https://doi.org/10.1016/j.cortex.2012.12.016

Chan, M. E., & Arvey, R. D. (2012). Meta-analysis and the development of knowledge. *Perspectives on Psychological Science, 7*, 79–92.

Coburn, K. M., & Vevea, J. L. (2018). weightr: Estimating weight-function models for publication bias in r. R package version 1.1.2. https://CRAN.R-project.org/package=weightr

Doi, S. A., & Thalib, L. (2008). A quality-effects model for meta-analysis. *Epidemiology, 19*, 94–100.

Duval, S., & Tweedie, R. (2000). Trim and fill: A simple funnel-plot–based method of testing and adjusting for publication bias in meta-analysis. *Biometrics, 56,* 455–463.

Egger, M., Smith, G. D., Schneider, M., & Minder, C. (1997). Bias in meta-analysis detected by a simple graphical test. *British Medical Journal, 315,* 629–634.

Elson, M. (2016). FlexibleMeasures.com: Competitive Reaction Time Task. http://www.flexiblemeasures.com/crtt/ https://doi.org/10.17605/OSF.IO/4G7FV

Elson, M., Mohseni, M. R., Breuer, J., Scharkow, M., & Quandt, T. (2014). Press CRTT to measure aggressive behavior: The unstandardized use of the Competitive Reaction Time Task in aggression research. *Psychological Assessment, 26,* 419–432. https://doi.org/10.1037/a0035569

Engber, D. (2016, March 6). Everything is crumbling. http://www.slate.com/articles/health_and_science/cover_story/2016/03/ego_depletion_an_influential_theory_in_psychology_may_have_just_been_debunked.html

Eysenck, H. J. (1978). An exercise in mega-silliness. *American Psychologist, 33,* 517.

Fanelli, D. (2010). "Positive" results increase down the hierarchy of the sciences. *PloS One, 5,* e10068.

Feinstein, A. R. (1995). Meta-analysis: Statistical alchemy for the 21st century. *Journal of Clinical Epidemiology, 48,* 71–79.

Ferguson, C. J. (2014). Comment: Why meta-analyses rarely resolve ideological debates. *Emotion Review, 6,* 251–252.

Ferguson, C. J., & Heene, M. (2012). A vast graveyard of undead theories: Publication bias and psychological science's aversion to the null. *Perspectives on Psychological Science, 7,* 555–561.

Fisher, R. A. (1932). *Statistical Methods for Research Workers* (4th ed.). Oliver and Boyd.

Flake, J. K., Pek, J., & Hehman, E. (2017). Construct validation in social and personality research: Current practice and recommendations. *Social Psychological and Personality Science, 8,* 370–378.

Franco, A., Malhotra, N., & Simonovits, G. (2014). Publication bias in the social sciences: Unlocking the file drawer. *Science, 345,* 1502–1505.

Friese, M., Loschelder, D. D., Gieseler, K., Frankenbach, J., & Inzlicht, M. (2019). Is ego depletion real? An analysis of arguments. *Personality and Social Psychology Review, 23,* 107–131. https://doi.org/10.1177/1088868318762183

Gelman, A., & Loken, E. (2013). The garden of forking paths: Why multiple comparisons can be a problem even when there is no "fishing expectation" or "p-hacking" and the research hypothesis was posited ahead of time. http://www.stat.columbia.edu/~gelman/research/ unpublished/p_hacking.pdf

Glass, G. V. (2015). Meta-analysis at middle age: A personal history. *Research Synthesis Methods, 6,* 221–231.

Glass, G. V., & Smith, M. L. (1978). "An exercise in mega-silliness": Reply. *American Psychologist, 33*(5), 517–519. https://doi.org/10.1037/0003-066X.33.5.517.b

Grant, M. J., & Booth, A. (2009). A typology of reviews: An analysis of 14 review types and associated methodologies. *Health Information & Libraries Journal, 26,* 91–108.

Gurevitch, J., Koricheva, J., Nakagawa, S., & Stewart, G. (2018). Meta-analysis and the science of research synthesis. *Nature, 555,* 175–182.

Guyatt, G. H., Oxman, A. D., Vist, G. E., Kunz, R., Falck-Ytter, Y., Alonso-Coello, P., & Schünemann, H. J. (2008). GRADE: An emerging consensus on rating quality of evidence and strength of recommendations. *British Medical Journal, 336,* 924–926.

Haddaway, N. R., & Bilotta, G. S. (2016). Systematic reviews: Separating fact from fiction. *Environment International, 92*, 578–584.

Haddaway, N. R., Land, M., & Macura, B. (2017). "A little learning is a dangerous thing": A call for better understanding of the term "systematic review." *Environment International, 99*, 356–360.

Hagger, M. S., Chatzisarantis, N. L. D., Alberts, H., Anggono, C. O., Batailler, C., Birt, A. R., Brand, R., Brandt, M. J., Brewer, G., Bruyneel, S., Calvillo, D. P., Campbell, W. K., Cannon, P. R., Carlucci, M., Carruth, N. P., Cheung, T., Crowell, A., De Ridder, D. T. D., Dewitte, S., ... Zwienenberg, M. (2016). A Multilab Preregistered Replication of the Ego-Depletion Effect. *Perspectives on Psychological Science, 11*(4), 546–573. https://doi.org/10.1177/1745691616652873

Hagger, M. S., Wood, C., Stiff, C., & Chatzisarantis, N. L. D. (2010). Ego depletion and the strength model of self-control: A meta-analysis. *Psychological Bulletin, 136*, 495–525.

Hedges, L. V. (1984). Estimation of effect size under nonrandom sampling: The effects of censoring studies yielding statistically insignificant mean differences. *Journal of Educational Statistics, 9*, 61–85.

Hedges, L. V., & Vevea, J. (2005). Selection method approaches. In H. R. Rothstein, A. J. Sutton, & M. Borenstein (Eds.), *Publication Bias in Meta-Analysis—Prevention, Assessment, and Adjustments* (pp. 145–174). John Wiley & Sons, Inc.

Higgins, J. P. T., Altman, D. G., Gøtzsche, P. C., Jüni, P., Moher, D., Oxman, A. D., Savovic, J., Schulz, K. F., Weeks, L., & Sterne, J. A. C. (2011). The Cochrane Collaboration's tool for assessing risk of bias in randomised trials. *British Medical Journal, 343*, d5928.

Hilgard, J. (2016, July 19). The failure of fail-safe N. http://crystalprisonzone.blogspot.com/2016/07/the-failure-of-fail-safe-n.html

Hilgard, J. (2017). Response to Colada. http://datacolada.org/wp-content/uploads/2017/04/Response-by-Joe-Hilgard-to-Colada-59.pdf

Hunt, M. (1997). *How Science Takes Stock: The Story of Meta-Analysis*. Russell Sage Foundation.

Ioannidis, J. P. (2005). Why most published research findings are false. *PLoS Medicine, 2*(8), e124.

Iyengar, S., & Greenhouse, J. B. (1988). Selection models and the file drawer problem. *Statistical Science, 3*, 109–117.

James, K. L., Randall, N. P., & Haddaway, N. R. (2015). A methodology for systematic mapping in environmental sciences. *Environmental Evidence, 5*, article 7. https://doi.org/10.1186/s13750-0059-6

John, L. K., Loewenstein, G., & Prelec, D. (2012). Measuring the prevalence of questionable research practices with incentives for truth telling. *Psychological Science, 23*, 524–532.

Jones, A., Remmerswaal, D., Verveer, I., Robinson, E., Franken, I. H., Wen, C. K., & Field, M. (2018, May 29). Compliance with ecological momentary assessment protocols in substance users: A meta-analysis. https://doi.org/10.31234/osf.io/k4agy

Kerr, N. L. (1998). HARKing: Hypothesizing after the results are known. *Personality and Social Psychology Review, 2*, 196–217.

L'Abbé, K. A., Detsky, A. S., & O'Rourke, K. (1987). Meta-analysis in clinical research. *Annals of Internal Medicine, 107*(2), 224–233.

Lakens, D., Hilgard, J., & Staaks, J. (2016). On the reproducibility of meta-analyses: Six practical recommendations. *BMC Psychology, 4*(1), 24.

Mantel, N., & Haenszel, W. (1959). Statistical aspects of the analysis of data from the retrospective analysis of disease. *Journal of the National Cancer Institute, 22*, 719–748.

McShane, B. B., Böckenholt, U., & Hansen, K. T. (2016). Adjusting for publication bias in meta-analysis: An evaluation of selection methods and some cautionary notes. *Perspectives in Psychological Science, 11*, 730–749.

Meehl, P. E. (1990). Why summaries of research on psychological theories are often uninterpretable. *Psychological Reports, 66*, 195–244.

Moher, D., Tetzlaff, J., Tricco, A. C., Sampson, M., & Altman, D. G. (2007). Epidemiology and reporting characteristics of systematic reviews. *PLoS Medicine, 4*, e78. https://doi.org/10.1371/journal.pmed.0040078

Moreno, S. G., Sutton, A. J., Ades, A. E., Stanley, T. D., Abrams, K. R., Peters, J. L., & Cooper, N. J. (2009). Assessment of regression-based methods to adjust for publication bias through a comprehensive simulation study. *BMC Medical Research Methodology, 9*, article 2. https://doi.org/10.1186/1471-2288-9-2

Moshontz, H., Campbell, L., Ebersole, C. R., IJzerman, H., Urry, H. L., Forscher, P. S., . . . Chartier, C. R. (2018). Psychological science accelerator: Advancing psychology through a distributed collaborative network. *Advances in Methods and Practices in Psychological Science, 1*, 501–515. https://doi.org/10.1177/2515245918797607

Nelson, L. D., Simmons, J. P., & Simonsohn, U. (2017, May 8). Forthcoming in *JPSP*: A non-diagnostic audit of psychological research. http://datacolada.org/60

O'Boyle Jr., E. H., Banks, G. C., & Gonzalez-Mulé, E. (2017). The chrysalis effect: How ugly initial results metamorphosize into beautiful articles. *Journal of Management, 43*(2), 376–399.

Open Science Collaboration. (2015). Estimating the reproducibility of psychological science. *Science, 349*(6251), aac4716.

Pearson, K. (1904). Antityphoid inoculation. *British Medical Journal, 2*, 1667–1668.

Petticrew, M. (2001). Systematic reviews from astronomy to zoology: Myths and misconceptions. *British Medical Journal, 322*(7278), 98–101.

Rosenthal, R. (1979). The file drawer problem and tolerance for null results. *Psychological Bulletin, 86*, 638–641.

Rosenthal, R. (2015). Reflections on the origins of meta-analysis. *Research Synthesis Methods, 6*, 240–245.

Sanderson, S., Tatt, I. D., & Higgins, J. P. T. (2007). Tools for assessing quality and susceptibility to bias in observational studies in epidemiology: A systematic review and annotated bibliography. *International Journal of Epidemiology, 36*, 666–676.

Scherer, R. W., Langenberg, P., & von Elm, E. (2007). Full publication of results initially presented in abstracts. *Cochrane Database of Systematic Reviews, 2*, MR000005. https://doi.org/10.1002/14651858.MR000005.pub3

Schmidt, F. L. (2015). History and introduction to the Schmidt-Hunter meta-analysis methods. *Research Synthesis Methods, 6*, 232–239.

Schmidt, F. L. (2017). Statistical and measurement pitfalls in the use of meta-regression in meta-analysis. *Career Development International, 22*, 469–476.

Schweinsberg, M., Madan, N., Vianello, M., Sommer, S. A., Jordan, J., Tierney, W., . . . Uhlmann, E. L. (2016). The pipeline project: Pre-publication independent replications of a single laboratory's research pipeline. *Journal of Experimental Social Psychology, 66*, 55–67.

Simmons, J. P., Nelson, L. D., & Simonsohn, U. (2011). False-positive psychology: Undisclosed flexibility in data collection and analysis allows presenting anything as significant. *Psychological Science, 22*, 1359–1366.

Simmons, J. P., Nelson, L. D., & Simonsohn, U. (2018, January 8). p-curve handles heterogeneity just fine. http://datacolada.org/67

Simons, D. J. (2018). Introducing *Advances in Methods and Practices in Psychological Science. Advances in Methods and Practices in Psychological Science, 1,* 3–6.

Simons, D. J., Holcombe, A. O., & Spellman, B. A. (2014). An introduction to registered replication reports at Perspectives on Psychological Science. *Perspectives on Psychological Science, 9,* 552–555. https://doi.org/10.1177/1745691614543974

Simonsohn, U., Nelson, L. D., & Simmons, J. P. (2014a). p-curve and effect size: Correcting for publication bias using only significant results. *Perspectives on Psychological Science, 9,* 666–681.

Simonsohn, U., Nelson, L. D., & Simmons, J. P. (2014b). p-curve: A key to the file-drawer. *Journal of Experimental Psychology: General, 143,* 534–547.

Smith, M. L., & Glass, G. V. (1977). Meta-analysis of psychotherapy outcome studies. *American Psychologist, 32,* 752.

Stanley, T. D. (2017). Limitations of PET-PEESE and other meta-analysis methods. *Social Psychological and Personality Science, 8,* 581–591.

Stanley, T. D., & Doucouliagos, H. (2014). Meta-regression approximations to reduce publication selection bias. *Research Synthesis Methods, 5,* 60–78.

Stanley, T. D., Jarrell, J. B., & Doucouliagos, H. (2010.) Could it be better to discard 90% of the data? A statistical paradox. *American Statistician, 64,* 70–77.

Stegenga, J. (2011). Is meta-analysis the platinum standard of evidence? *Studies in History and Philosophy of Science Part C: Studies in History and Philosophy of Biological and Biomedical Sciences, 42,* 497–507.

Sterling, T. D. (1959). Publication decisions and their possible effects on inferences drawn from tests of significance—or vice versa. *Journal of the American Statistical Association, 54,* 30–34.

Sterne, J. A. C., Egger, M., Moher, D., & Boutron, I. (2017, June). Chapter 10: Addressing reporting biases. In J. P. T. Higgins, R. Churchill, J. Chandler, & M. S. Cumpston (Eds.), *Cochrane Handbook for Systematic Reviews of Interventions,* version 5.2.0. www.training.cochrane.org/handbook

Ulrich, R., & Miller, J. (2015). p-hacking by post hoc selection with multiple opportunities: Detectability by skewness test? Comment on Simonsohn, Nelson, and Simmons (2014). *Journal of Experimental Psychology: General, 144,* 1137–1145.

van Aert, R. C. M., Wicherts, J. M., & van Assen, M. A. L. M. (2016). Conducting meta-analyses based on p-values: Reservations and recommendations for applying p-uniform and p-curve. *Perspectives on Psychological Science, 11,* 713–729.

van Assen, M. A., van Aert, R., & Wicherts, J. M. (2015). Meta-analysis using effect size distributions of only statistically significant studies. *Psychological Methods, 20,* 293–309.

Vohs, K. D., Schmeichel, B. J., Lohmann, S., Gronau, Q. F., Finley, A. J., Ainsworth, S. E., ... Albarracín, D. (2021). A Multisite Preregistered Paradigmatic Test of the Ego-Depletion Effect. *Psychological Science, 32*(10), 1566–1581. https://doi.org/10.1177/0956797621989733

Woll, C. F. J., & Schönbrodt, F. (2020). A series of meta-analytic tests of the efficacy of long-term psychoanalytic psychotherapy. *European Psychologist, 25*(1), 51–72. https://doi.org/10.1027/1016-9040/a000385

7
Statistical Inference in Behavioral Research

Traditional and Bayesian Approaches

Alexander Etz, Steven N. Goodman, and Joachim Vandekerckhove

The recent crisis of confidence in psychological science (Pashler & Wagenmakers, 2012) has led to repeated calls for better statistical methods, better study designs, and better social incentive structures. The link of these analytical and inferential issues to research integrity is fairly direct, in that research integrity, writ large, is the fidelity of the scientific process and resulting conclusions to the truth. If it can be shown that the manner in which studies are done, data analyzed, or conclusions drawn is likely to systematically deviate from the truth, then by definition we have a challenge to research integrity. There has been an evolution of professional and scientific norms within the behavioral sciences that have exaggerated and reified some of the most unfortunate misconceptions and misuses to which standard methods using hypothesis tests and p-values (known as "frequentist") are subject; in particular that statistical significance is an arbiter of truth, that the credibility of a claim can be assessed without considering the prior probability of the claim being true, and that nonsignificant studies are uninformative. These misconceptions and misuses include but are not limited to:

- The false belief that a typical experiment yielding $p < 0.05$ is all that is needed to prove a theory;
- Resistance to replication of important experiments;
- The difficulty of publishing research replications;
- Strong selection pressure at journals for significant findings (i.e., publication bias);
- Professional advancement dependent on publications in highly cited journals, with acceptance influenced by statistical significance;
- Widespread use of "p-hacking";

- Failure to use sample sizes that correspond to a priori plausible or scientifically important effect sizes;
- Failure to share data;
- Failure to prepare, share, or publish research protocols.

A number of these practices, particularly those related to replication and publication, can be related directly to practices based on extreme versions of frequentist philosophy. But they also mean, because so many of these practices are deeply entrenched (and indeed institutionalized), that adopting alternative methods (e.g., "Bayesian") cannot solve all of the challenges to scientific integrity in the social and behavioral sciences. Nevertheless, we believe that understanding Bayesian approaches represents a critical piece of a multifaceted strategy that the behavioral sciences must adopt if its findings and claims are to be regarded as reliable. To explain why this is so, in this chapter we will review the fundamentals of both frequentist and Bayesian philosophies and methods.

The Foundations of Inference: Types of Probability

Science starts and ends in uncertainty. As such, it should not be surprising that the properties— indeed, the integrity—of any scientific method depend on how it represents uncertainty. The most basic measure we have for representing uncertainty is probability. Many scientists are surprised to learn that probability is an extraordinarily difficult and complex measure, philosophically and scientifically. We will begin this discussion of methods in statistical inference by outlining how different conceptions of probability lead to different approaches to inference. Many controversies about the proper approaches to statistical inference are in fact derived from controversies about the meaning of probability itself, which we will review here.

The original meaning of probability derived from the same root as "approbation," related to the degree to which an opinion or action was supported by evidence, such as when deciding on the guilt or innocence of a suspect. This kind of probability was "epistemic" in nature; it related to one's degree of belief, or a logical relationship between the opinion and the strength of underlying evidence. This notion was completely distinct from the notion of "chance," as exemplified in games of chance, or gambling. This kind of probability came to be designated "aleatoric," related to games, or "stochastic," which today applies to a random physical process.

Today's dominant approaches to probability can be divided into the "frequentist" and "epistemic" schools. The frequentist notion derives from the aleatoric type, and epistemic probability is sometimes called "Bayesian." The *frequentist approach* to probability is actually the more recent of the two, having only been formalized in the early 20th century. The frequentist approach represented an attempt to make probability as objective and measurable a scientific quantity as physical measurements like height, weight, and mass. This was achieved by defining the probability of event A as being equal to its proportion in a prespecified, in principle observable, "collective" of repeatable random events—equivalent to a "long-run frequency." The idea was that if we could observe this proportion, this probability would be objective, uniquely specified, and observable. This probability was deductive in nature, in that once the collective was specified, the probability of outcomes within it would be set, or as von Mises (1957) famously declared, "First the collective, then the probability."

Two consequences of this definition are worth noting, as the problems with any probability definition are inevitably shared by the systems of inference built upon them. First, the frequentist notion of probability does not apply to individual events, but rather to the collective itself (i.e., the "long run"). Thus, if an experiment is generating a single outcome to which we want to assign a probability, this definition says that we cannot apply a probability to that individual experiment, only to the "long run" of repetitions. This is why virtually every traditional statistical measure, from p-values to confidence intervals to type I and type II error rates, have definitions starting with "if this experiment is repeated." The second problem is that the long run is not actually observed but constructed through a thought experiment. One can "imagine" what might happen if the experiment were repeated many times, but this differs from having the multiple repetitions in hand. There may not be a consensus on why the experiment stopped or how it was run, with consequent uncertainty about which "long run" is relevant; a given result can be a legitimate member of several different long runs (Goodman 1999a; Wrinch & Jeffreys, 1919).

To complicate this further, outcomes within a given long run may not be equiprobable; for instance, the border of a "tail area" used to calculate a p-value is almost always the most probable outcome within that tail, and grouping it with less likely outcomes sometimes violates inferential intuition. So the conditions for using frequentist probability as a foundation for inference come at a price; the resulting numbers cannot be used to apply to an individual experiment, observers must agree on the hypothetical "long run," and demonstrably different elements of a long run may be treated similarly. These properties generate the requirement for rigid prespecification of all experimental procedures, including outcome measures and stopping rules, and cautions that 95% confidence intervals don't mean we have 95% confidence in any individual interval.

In contrast, *epistemic probability* can apply to individual events or to propositions that are not repeatable events. It is a plausibility, or a "degree of justified belief," with the justification arising from underlying evidence. The "logical" subtype of epistemic probability requires that the correspondence between belief and the evidence be unique, based on logical relationships that can be difficult to get agreement on. The "subjective" subtype allows for variation among individuals but raises the question of whether intersubjective variability renders it illegitimate as a scientific tool.

What Makes Probability "Scientific"?

The question of what makes methods based on these types of probability "scientific," or correspond with the truth, is a central issue for science. For the frequentist, a "scientific" or objective probability is based on correspondence with an imagined empirical reality. This reality is not usually observable, and is typically based on statistical models, calculations, or simulations. Even if these models are correct, or agreed upon, they apply only to the data, not to hypotheses, so a frequentist has no language or measure of uncertainty about hypotheses giving rise to the data.

The "scientific" property of epistemic probability is not empirical, but logical. It is that probabilities are (a) consistent (i.e., one would never believe simultaneously that $Pr(A) > Pr(B)$ and $Pr(A) < Pr(B)$), and (b) coherent, in that one would never act based on these beliefs in ways that guaranteed one would be worse off. These properties lead us directly to Bayes' theorem: One can only satisfy these conditions if one's epistemic probabilities are modified by empirical data using Bayes' theorem. Bayes' theorem further guarantees that with accumulating data, any intersubjective differences (such as interindividual differences in the strength of one's prior beliefs) will eventually disappear and probability estimates will typically conform to observable reality (Diaconis & Freedman, 1986). So epistemic probability in some sense ends where frequentist probability tries to start—a correspondence with observed reality. As Kendall (1949) stated, "Neither party can avoid using the ideas of the other to set up and justify a comprehensive theory."

Bayes' Theorem

It was the need to answer fundamental questions about the behavior of games and rational betting strategies that led to developments in the calculus of probabilities (Devlin, 2010). It was the theorem of an amateur scientist, the Rev. Thomas Bayes, that has reverberations today. He set out to answer the question of how much one should bet on one player versus another player in an interrupted game of chance. In solving this, he came up with an equation that is an uncontroversial mathematical expression. It was that the probability of two events occurring together, A and B, could be decomposed into different ways: the probability of A given B, times the probability of B, or the probability of B given A, times the probability of A. This can be written:

$$\Pr(A \& B) = \Pr(A|B) \times \Pr(B) = \Pr(B|A) \times \Pr(A)$$

Equating the two expressions on the right, this can be rearranged to yield Bayes' theorem:

$$\Pr(A|B) = \Pr(B|A) \times \Pr(A) / \Pr(B)$$

This is merely the algebra of conditional probability, subject to no more controversy than $1 + 1 = 2$. The difficulty begins when we assign meanings to A or B such that their probabilities cannot be directly observed. If A is a scientific hypothesis and B is data, Bayes' theorem becomes:

$$\Pr(\text{Hypothesis}|\text{Data}) = \Pr(\text{Data}|\text{Hypothesis}) \times \Pr(\text{Hypothesis}) / \Pr(\text{Data})$$

This equation requires us to define a measure that corresponds to the probability of a hypothesis being true (e.g., Pr(Hypothesis)) without data. This kind of probability falls into the "epistemic" category; logically justified, perhaps, but not necessarily empirically confirmable.

So Bayes' theorem, when applied to the process of inference—drawing conclusions about nature based on observed data—requires an epistemic probability of a hypothesis. This was historically known as "inverse" probability because it allows us to "invert" Pr(Data|Hypothesis) to Pr(Hypothesis|Data), but it is now more commonly called "Bayesian" probability (Fienberg, 2006). The acceptance or rejection of this foundational concept is at the core of the controversy about the use of frequentist and Bayesian methods in statistics.

Statistical Inference

Statistical inference is a subset of the broader subject of scientific inference. An inference from the general (hypothesis) to the specific (data) is called "deductive" and is truth preserving, in that the conclusions are true if the premises are true. This is what makes it an attractive foundation for empirical science; it guarantees—as in pure mathematics—that all statements deriving from the premises are valid if the premises are true. But it comes at the price of not expanding our knowledge beyond what is already in the premises. Making a statement about the truth of a hypothesis based on observed data is a form of inductive inference, also called "ampliative" inference, in that the conclusion (about a hypothesis) has more explanatory power than the premises (the data). So inductive logic "amplifies" our knowledge, but at the price of not knowing if our conclusions about the hypotheses are correct.

In statistical inference, the hypotheses are probabilistic statements about nature (i.e., statistical). Examples of statistical hypotheses are "a response rate is 10%" and "the success rates of two interventions are equal." Under such hypotheses, one can predict the distribution of observations one would expect under specified experimental conditions. A prediction based on probabilistic formulae, of how often various outcomes will arise under a specified statistical hypothesis, is deductive, and the attendant probabilities are "frequentist." Any probabilistic statements about the underlying truth are by definition epistemic, or "Bayesian."

Origins of Frequentist Inference

The central challenge of statistical inference is how to make statements not about observable data, but about the hypotheses that give rise to them, the essence of inductive reasoning. Until the early 20th century, a widely accepted methodology for how to use data to ascertain the truth of underlying hypotheses did not exist. Scientists and statisticians were familiar with the mathematics of probability, but how to use those mathematical properties to draw conclusions about nature from data was far more unsettled. The problem lay in the measure of probability itself; there was a well-known formula that could guide inference about probabilities—Bayes' theorem—but its use required the acceptance of epistemic probability that many rejected as a foundation for sound science. The challenge was whether a method could be constructed, based purely on frequentist probability, that could provide a measure of uncertainty about underlying hypotheses without the machinery of Bayes or attendant Bayesian probabilities.

Frequentist inference as we know it today was really born in the 1920s and 1930s, as a reaction to the Bayesian model. The pioneers in this frequentist revolution were Ronald Fisher, Jerzy Neyman, and Egon Pearson. Fisher was a mathematician, geneticist, and active experimentalist, the latter in the field of agriculture. Neyman and Pearson were mathematical statisticians. The driving motivation was to develop a new framework of inference that was "objective," in the sense that it was not based on epistemic uncertainty. Fisher believed that the theory of Bayesian inference "is founded upon an error, and must be wholly rejected" (Fisher, 1925, p. 10). What was this fatal error? He objected to using Bayes' theorem when there was no basis to estimate the prior probability of a hypothesis, nor an acceptable way to assign probabilities if we claimed prior ignorance (Aldrich et al., 2008; Zabell, 1989). In the 1920s Fisher constructed his own view of how inference could be conducted, without needing to specify prior distributions. These included new approaches to both testing and estimation. He took the idea of a tail-area probability, used by Karl Pearson, and made it his central tool for statistical testing, calling it the "p-value," short for "probability" value, or "associated probability." The use of the p-value sidestepped the topic of prior probabilities by only considering which data might be observed if the null hypothesis were true.

The p-value was originally intended to be used as a measure of evidence against the null hypothesis to be combined with other sources of evidence, and not as an "error rate" associated with a decision. Fisher suggested that the 0.05 level might be a useful benchmark, not for determining whether the null hypothesis was likely to be false, but for deciding whether an experiment was worth repeating (some more history about the origins of the 0.05 level is given in Cowles & Davis, 1982). He stated that the 0.05 threshold represented weak evidence in a single experiment, and that one should consider the null hypothesis to be false only if, upon repeated experimentation, "a properly designed experiment rarely fails to give this level of significance" (Fisher, 1926). So the "one and done" modern practice of declaring theoretical confirmation based on a single significant experiment is antithetical to the practice suggested by its originator.

Fisher's influence expanded immeasurably with the publication in 1925 of his landmark statistical textbook, *Statistical Methods for Research Workers* (Fisher, 1925). This textbook was the first of its kind, aimed at practicing scientists, filled with practical examples showing how to analyze common experimental designs, and served to popularize the use of the p-value. This book, revised 14 times, was a scientific bestseller from the time of its publication until after Fisher's death in 1962.

Fisher's approach to inference had both formal and informal components. Two of Fisher's contemporaries, Jerzy Neyman and Egon Pearson, began to try to reframe Fisher's ideas in a more formal mathematical framework. In 1928 they proposed a modification to Fisher's original testing procedure (Neyman & Pearson, 1928). Their idea was to introduce an alternative hypothesis to contrast to the null hypothesis used by Fisher, and to propose formal decision rules for accepting and rejecting these hypotheses. They introduced the now-familiar notions of type I and II errors and power. They proposed that statistical properties of various decision rules should be studied, and in 1933 they derived the properties of optimal statistical tests (Neyman & Pearson, 1933). Neyman would later turn his sights to the topic of estimation, proposing the now-ubiquitous confidence interval procedure (Neyman, 1937).

The innovations by Fisher, Neyman, and Pearson served as the foundation of modern mathematical statistics. In the following sections we outline the differences between them, discuss the ways in which frequentist testing and estimation are done today, and summarize a number of common criticisms levied at them.

The Basics of Frequentist Testing

In a statistical testing context we are concerned with deciding which of a set of competing hypotheses are true. A statistical hypothesis refers to either population parameter values or the forms of statistical models. Tests of these statistical hypotheses are used as a stand-in for tests of scientific hypotheses. For instance, the statement "the average height of men in the population is not equal to that of women" is a hypothesis about the difference between the averages of populations of men and women. If we let the parameter δ represent the difference in height between populations of men and women, then a translation of our hypothesis into statistical language would be that $\delta \neq 0$.

In the Neyman-Pearson theory of hypothesis testing there are two competing hypotheses: the null hypothesis and the alternative hypothesis. The alternative hypothesis is chosen so that it corresponds with our hypothesis of interest; the null hypothesis is (typically) constructed such that it represents the complement of the alternative hypothesis. In our heights example, the hypothesis that $\delta \neq 0$ would be our alternative hypothesis and our null hypothesis would be its complement, $\delta = 0$. In the Neyman and Pearson framework, the outcome of a hypothesis test is a binary decision: Either reject the null hypothesis and accept the alternative, or accept the null hypothesis. This leads to the possibility of making two types of errors: rejecting the null hypothesis when it is actually true (false positive, "α" or type I error), and not rejecting the null hypothesis when it is actually false (false negative, "β" or type II error). The set of observations that would lead to rejection of the null hypothesis is called the *rejection region* of the test. If the observed data are in the rejection region (e.g., $Z > 1.96$), then one is supposed to "reject" the null hypothesis. In this framework, one chooses the rejection region such that there is no more than $(100 \times \alpha)\%$ chance of making a type I error, while at the same time keeping the chance of making a type II error to a minimum. In practice, the use of 0.05 for the type I error and less than 0.20 for the type II error has become standard.

Fisher's significance test shared many features with that of Neyman and Pearson, with a few key differences. In Fisher's approach, there is no alternative hypothesis; one only considers which data might be observed if the null hypothesis were true. With the data in hand one computes the p-value, which is the probability of the observation plus the probability of any other observations further from the null hypothesis. For example, if one observes a Z-value of 2.5, then the p-value is the probability of observing a Z-value greater than or equal to 2.5. Fisher felt that the exact level of the p-value was informative, whereas in a hypothesis test the only information to be used was whether the result fell in the rejection region, and a p-value was not calculated at all. If the p-value is small then one has evidence to suggest the null hypothesis is not true, with smaller p-values providing stronger evidence. On the topic of whether a given p-value should be considered "significant," in this approach it is "open to the experimenter to be more or less exacting in respect of the smallness of the probability he would require before he would be willing to admit that his observations have demonstrated a positive result" (Fisher, 1971, p. 13). This represented the kind of informality that the Neyman–Pearson hypothesis test was designed to eliminate. As noted previously, Fisher also put a particular premium on replication of significance, an idea revived in the 2000s under the rubric of research reproducibility (e.g., Goodman et al., 2016).

Fisher very strongly rejected hypothesis tests as being too algorithmic and thereby anti-scientific, ironically a criticism that is today aimed at his innovation, the use of p-values. But today, the two approaches are typically taught and practiced as a unified set of methods. For instance, researchers might set up a null and alternative hypothesis and choose a type I error rate of 0.05, and then once the data are observed they report (a) whether the data fall into the rejection region and the null hypothesis was rejected, as well as (b) the strength of the evidence against the null hypothesis in the form of a p-value. More historical detail on that controversy and the rise of frequentist inference can be found in Hald (2008), Goodman (1993), and Gigerenzer (1993, 2004).

Criticisms of Frequentist Testing

A number of criticisms have been levied toward the frequentist approaches to hypothesis testing. First, researchers tend to misinterpret p-values and to use them to draw improper inferences from their data (Greenland et al., 2016). A survey by Oakes (1986) (replicated by Haller & Krauss, 2002) illustrates these misconceptions. Oakes quizzed psychology researchers' interpretations of frequentist hypothesis tests by presenting an experiment that results in $t(18) = 2.7$ and $p = 0.01$. In response, 35% of the researchers marked as true the statement "The probability of the null hypothesis has been found;" 85% endorsed the statement "The probability that the decision taken is wrong is known;" and 60% endorsed the statement "A replication has a 0.99 probability of being significant." Since neither a p-value nor a type I error rate applies to the underlying hypotheses, none of those interpretations is correct.

Other critiques have focused on the statistical properties of the null-hypothesis significance testing procedure. The p-value is defined as the probability, if the null hypothesis were true, of results as extreme or more extreme than those observed in the experiment. That is, a p-value takes into account not only the results that were actually observed in the experiment, but also those that could have potentially been observed but were not. This dependence on unobserved data has been seen as an inherent weakness of the procedure (e.g., Jeffreys, 1961), and many take issue with the ambiguity in the definition of which outcomes are "more extreme" than those observed because this depends critically on the sampling plan (Goodman, 1999a; Lindley, 1993)—and the sampling plan is often arbitrarily chosen (in many research labs) or unknown (in the case of naturally occurring data, meta-analyses, etc.).

Another challenge associated with frequentist testing procedures is that they are not always logically consistent. Schervish (1996) and Royall (1997) demonstrate a number of general cases where the process of using p-values as measures of evidence, as well as the process of strict reject/accept hypothesis tests, can lead to paradoxical inferences. Consider two researchers, Pat and Oliver, who want to test whether men and women have different heights. Both specify a point null hypothesis that the average difference is zero (i.e., $\delta = 0$), but Oliver is only interested in whether men are taller, so decides to use a one-sided test. They both agree to use $\alpha = 0.05$ to determine their rejection region, meaning Oliver rejects his null hypothesis if $Z > 1.64$ and Pat rejects her null hypothesis if $|Z| > 1.96$. If the experiment results in $1.64 < Z < 1.96$, then Oliver rejects his one-sided null hypothesis, $p < 0.05$, and asserts that men are taller on average than women. At the same time, Pat cannot reject her null hypothesis, because her calculated p-value is greater than 0.05, and hence cannot assert the weaker logical claim that men are either taller or shorter than women. Thus we are licensed to conclude that men are taller than women, but, paradoxically, have to withhold judgment about whether they are taller or shorter. Examples like these also challenge the notion that frequentist testing is completely objective; we have the same data, the same null hypothesis, yet we cannot know the p-value (and the decision) without knowing what is in the scientists' minds.

A last issue with p-values as measures of evidence is that they incorporate no information about effect magnitude. A large effect in a small study can have the same p-value as a small effect in a large study. This violates basic scientific intuition that if two observed effects have the same "statistical distance" from the null effect (e.g., the same number of standard errors), the one further from the null contradicts it more strongly. The p-value does not have that property because it is calculated only in relation to one hypothesis. Some statisticians and philosophers (e.g., Evans, 2015; Royall, 1997) object on logical grounds to calling the p-value "evidence," saying that "evidence" must explicitly compare hypotheses, as the purpose of evidence is to modify belief; "evidence" is a construct that elevates data from being a neutral observation to something inferentially relevant. This is the framework for the Bayes factor, an alternative measure to the p-value, discussed later in the chapter.

Frequentist Estimation

Recently the field of psychology has seen efforts to replace the apparently problematic practice of hypothesis testing with a focus on estimation (Cumming, 2014), a practice long advocated (Gardner & Altman, 1986) and now standard in biomedical research (Altman et al., 2013). Estimation has a different goal than hypothesis testing. Instead of accepting or rejecting hypotheses, estimation concerns which parameter values of a model are most consistent with the observed data. For example, instead of testing the difference in heights of men versus women, we would just estimate the average difference. Frequentist estimation problems consist of two components: finding a best guess about a parameter and computing an interval of uncertainty around it. The "best guess" is called the point estimate, and the frequentist uncertainty interval is called a "confidence interval" (CI). While this seems straightforward, the formal definition of a CI is rather convoluted, because of its foundation in frequentist probability. Namely, "An X% confidence interval for a parameter θ is an interval (L, U) generated by a procedure that in repeated sampling has an X% probability of containing the true value of θ, for all possible values of θ" (Morey et al., 2016). It is important to appreciate the subtle implications of this definition. The frequentist paradigm allows us to make statements about the *group* of estimates generated by the CI procedure, but this differs from making statements about the estimates themselves.

To illustrate the distinction, take the following example (due to D. Basu; Ghosh, 1988). To determine a 95% CI, let us ignore the data and instead generate a random number between 0 and 1 from a uniform distribution, deciding as follows: CI = ∅ if the number is 0.05 or smaller and CI = $(-\infty, +\infty)$ otherwise. Note that this odd procedure has the same property: With a probability of 1 in 20 (5%), it will generate the empty interval ∅, which does not contain the true parameter, and with a complementary probability 95%, it will generate the infinite interval that does contain the true parameter. Hence, according to the definition, any interval generated by this procedure is a valid 95% CI. We hope it is clear that these intervals are useless for scientific inference.[1]

This example is artificial, but the same principle applies in situations where we believe strongly in the null hypothesis (e.g., the existence of ESP), or any range of hypotheses. We do an experiment that generates a 95% CI on the ESP effect size of, say, {0.3 to 0.6}. We would recognize this as very unusual and would not accord it a 95% probability of including the truth because that would mean that after this one result we would have a 95% or greater belief in the existence of ESP. This shows that we do not accord every observed interval the same 95% chance of including the truth. If we strongly believe in the null, we will accord every observed interval including the null much higher than 95% chance of including the truth, and every CI not including the null a much lower than 95% chance of including the truth. If our prior evidence/belief is justified, this would be confirmed empirically.

From these thought experiments, we recognize that the properties of a CI generating procedure do not necessarily transfer to the CIs themselves, and that we need another inferential approach to know what credibility to apply to any particular observed interval. This is not a new insight. The subtle distinction between *properties of an interval* and *properties of the process that generated an interval* is why Neyman used the neologism "confidence" instead of "probability" to describe the interval, as he was aware that the confidence level did not accord with the frequentist notion of probability.

---

[1] Note that an exactly analogous procedure can be conceived for null hypothesis significance testing: Reject the null hypothesis if and only if a 20-sided die comes up 1. Such a procedure guarantees that, in the long run, we will falsely reject approximately 5% of all true null hypotheses. The procedure is nevertheless entirely useless.

Criticisms of Frequentist Estimation

Most CIs used in practice can be seen as inversions of one hypothesis test or another, in that the parameter values inside a $1 - \alpha$ CI are precisely those that would not be rejected by a level α hypothesis test. Thus, these CIs necessarily inherit the statistical criticisms of hypothesis tests mentioned earlier.

Like hypothesis tests, CIs are often misinterpreted. Hoekstra et al. (2014) provided researchers and students with a survey about CIs, analogous to the survey conducted by Oakes (1986) about hypothesis testing. This survey presented the result of an experiment with a 95% CI for the mean ranging from 0.1 to 0.4. In response, 86% of the researchers from this sample marked as true the statement "The 'null hypothesis' that the true mean equals 0 is likely to be incorrect"; 59% endorsed the statement "There is a 95% probability that the true mean lies between 0.1 and 0.4"; 47% endorsed the statement "The probability that the true mean equals 0 is smaller than 5%"; and 58% endorsed the statement "If we were to repeat the experiment over and over, then 95% of the time the true mean falls between 0.1 and 0.4." Just as with the previous survey, none of these statements follows from the result of a CI.

Recognition that the p-value was both widely misused in a "bright line" fashion and misinterpreted as an inverse probability led the American Statistical Association to issue a remarkable statement about p-values in 2016 (Wasserstein & Lazar, 2016), the first such statement in its 125-year history. The most important two points of the statement were that $p \leq 0.05$ does not mean that the probability of the null hypothesis is less than 0.05, and that the use of $p \leq 0.05$ as an indicator of the truth or falsity of a scientific claim represented poor scientific practice.

Bayesian Methods

Bayesian Updating

The way in which probabilities are expressed in natural language is prone to misunderstanding. The confusion of the inverse is the cognitive illusion that the very different probabilities $Pr(A|B)$ and $Pr(B|A)$ are similar in magnitude, whereas they can be completely divergent. A common illustration is the case where A = "Jane is a U.S. citizen" and B = "Jane is a member of the U.S. Senate." In that case, Pr(Jane is a citizen | Jane is a senator) is 1, whereas Pr(Jane is a senator | Jane is a citizen) is close to 0. Similarly, if we flip a standard coin five times and get five heads, the probability of getting that is Pr(5 heads | Fair coin) = 1/32, but the probability that the coin is fair given the 5 heads, Pr(Fair Coin|Data), would still be 1 because—outside of statistics textbooks—people do not carry around biased coins (Gelman & Nolan, 2002).

Bayes' theorem provides us a way to properly go from Pr(Data | Hypothesis), a "direct probability" that we can calculate under any model, to Pr (Hypothesis | Data), the inverse probability. The inverse probability is called a "posterior" probability since it is the probability of the hypothesis after considering the data, contrasted with the "prior" probability of the hypothesis before seeing the data. Going from the prior probability to the posterior probability is called Bayesian "updating." To show this, we will write Bayes' theorem slightly differently than before:

Pr(Hypothesis|Data) = Pr(Hypothesis) × Pr(Data|Hypothesis) / Pr(Data)
(Posterior probability) (Prior probability)   (Updating factor)

In this equation, Pr(Hypothesis) is the prior probability of the hypothesis, and Pr(Data|Hypothesis)/Pr(Data) is an updating factor that captures how much more likely the hypothesis becomes once the data are factored in (Carnap, 1950; Keynes, 1921; Rouder & Morey, 2019). This updating factor is a measure of the strength of evidence supporting the hypothesis (Berger & Wolpert, 1988; Edwards et al., 1963; Royall, 1997; Wagenmakers et al., 2018a).

Bayesian methods have a number of attractive properties for use in science. Because they derive directly from epistemic probability theory, they are guaranteed to be internally consistent, and because they are built on a formal system, they do not rely on shortcuts, heuristics, or leaps of logic. Most importantly, because Bayesian methods allow us to calculate the probability that a hypothesis is true, their use is particularly attractive for behavioral scientists (Edwards et al., 1963; Etz & Vandekerckhove, 2018; Vandekerckhove et al., 2018).

Bayesian Testing

The power of Bayesian methods comes with certain requirements. Because the system of inference is formal, researchers are required to be similarly precise in the specification of their statistical assumptions—as in any formal system, the conclusions are only as good as the assumptions. It is important for analysts to make only assumptions that are reasonable, defensible, or otherwise tenable (e.g., because it can be demonstrated that the conclusions are invariant under multiple sets of assumptions). This can be challenging to researchers accustomed to statistical analyses that work "out of the box" and do not appear to demand such efforts, but classical methods are equally or more assumptive, just not transparently so.

How to represent the prior probability of the hypothesis, Pr(Hypothesis), is often the most contentious in model comparison exercises. Scientists conduct their research to determine the probability that a hypothesis is true (or false), so quantifying that probability before they start is sometimes difficult, particularly if it is an unfamiliar exercise. Of course, there is nothing illogical about factoring prior information into our ultimate evaluation of a hypothesis, but sometimes that information is difficult to quantify. In such cases, it might be desirable to instead limit the scope of the calculation and *assess first only how much is learned from the data at hand*. This is where a new quantity, the *Bayes factor*, becomes useful.

Consider the case where there are two competing hypotheses, Ha and Ho, and where we have some relevant data D. For this case, there will exist two posterior probabilities: Pr(Ha|D) and Pr(Ho|D). A handy way of expressing which hypothesis is more likely than the other is the posterior odds Pr(Ha|D)/Pr(Ho|D). Using Bayes' theorem, we know that

$$\Pr(Ha \mid D) = \Pr(D \mid Ha) \times \Pr(Ha) / \Pr(D)$$

Substituting Ho into the same equation and dividing the two gives us the "odds form" of Bayes' theorem:

$$\underbrace{\Pr(Ha \mid D) / \Pr(Ho \mid D)}_{\text{(Posterior odds)}} = \underbrace{(\Pr(Ha) / \Pr(Ho))}_{\text{(Prior odds)}} \times \underbrace{\Pr(D \mid Ha) / \Pr(D \mid Ho)}_{\text{(Bayes factor)}}.$$

We can read this expression in an intuitive way: The relative posterior probability of two hypotheses is their relative prior probability multiplied by the relative strength of evidence provided by the data. This relative strength of evidence is the ratio of the predictive success of the two hypotheses and is called the *Bayes factor*. In other words, how much better each hypothesis predicts the observed data determines how much more we believe in one than the other after seeing the data.

Mathematical Likelihood

The Bayes factor is the ratio of two probabilities that are important to understand on a deeper level. They are derived from calculating the direct probability of the data under a given model, Pr(Data|Hypothesis), which is also the basis of the likelihood function (Etz, 2018; Goodman & Royall, 1988; Royall, 1997), sometimes written as L(Hypothesis | Data). The reason we rewrite it in that way is that the likelihood function treats the data we observe as fixed and varies the parameter of interest of the probability model generating the data, whereas a probability density function holds the parameters fixed and calculates the probability of all possible data. We interpret the probability of the observed data under a given model as the support the data give to that model, captured in the simple relationship:

$$L(\text{Hypothesis} \mid \text{Data}) = C * \Pr(\text{Data}|\text{Hypothesis})$$

The likelihood function has two critical properties that differ from p-values. First, it uses to the probability of the data in hand, not the often unknowable "more extreme data" used in frequentist methods. Second, for inferential purposes, it is always used in a comparative fashion, as in the Bayes factor mentioned earlier. The arbitrary constant C cancels when ratios are taken and shows that the likelihood has no unique value. So instead of being a probability under only one hypothesis (e.g., p-values), we compare instead how well two hypotheses predict the observed data; it is the *relative* support given to different hypotheses that is interpreted as evidence, not the degree to which the data are incompatible with just one hypothesis. Finally, likelihood functions provide a formal framework (viz., Bayes' theorem) for interpreting their inferential meaning, whereas frequentist methods do not.

Bayesian Testing with Likelihood Ratios

Consider the case of bistable perception. In this phenomenon, a single perceptual stimulus can be seen or heard two different ways. A figure might look like a vase one moment but look like two faces the next moment; or a drawing might look like a duck one second, a rabbit the next.

Some ambiguous percepts differ between individuals: A dress in a photograph might appear blue and black to some people, gold and white to others; or a sound clip might sound like "YANNY" to some and like "LAUREL" to others.[2] Suppose that a researcher claims that teenagers are more likely to hear YANNY than LAUREL—three times more likely, in fact (i.e., 75% chance of YANNY). Another researcher claims there is no preference (i.e., 50% chance of YANNY). Because both of these claims are quite specific, let us call the latter claim the "point null hypothesis" and the former claim the "competing point hypothesis." Further suppose that the researchers collected data from 30 teenagers and found that Y = 20 heard YANNY while L = 10 heard LAUREL.

We can now calculate how strongly either hypothesis had predicted this outcome. In both cases, the probabilities are obtained with the binomial formula. For the point null hypothesis, the probability is

$$\Pr(Y = 20, L = 10 \mid \text{point null}) = (Y + L, \text{choose } Y) \times 0.50^Y \times 0.50^L$$
$$= (30, \text{choose } 20) \times 0.50^{20} \times 0.50^{10}$$
$$= 0.0280,$$

while for the competing point hypothesis, the probability is

$$\Pr(Y = 20, L = 10 \mid \text{competing point})$$
$$= (30, \text{choose } 20) \times 0.75^{20} \times 0.25^{10}$$
$$= 0.0909.$$

Hence, the competing point hypothesis is supported more strongly by these observations by a factor of .0909/.0280 = 3.247. Figure 7.1 illustrates this comparison graphically.

A Bayes factor of 3.247 is generally considered to be only weak evidence (Goodman, 1999b; Kass & Raftery, 1995; Wagenmakers et al., 2018c).

---

[2] This example is based on a real debate caused by an audio clip that went viral on social media in the spring of 2018. In the audio clip, a male voice is clearly heard saying "LAUREL," but many perceived it as saying "YANNY." The clip, some variations, and background, can be found on CNN (May 16, 2018).

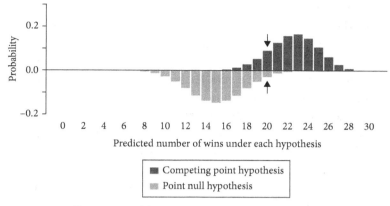

Figure 7.1. An illustration of the computation of the Bayes factor using visualizations from Etz et al. (2018). Shown are the predictive distributions of two competing hypotheses: one "point null hypothesis" under which some event happens with a 50% probability (lighter bars, upside-down) and one "competing point hypothesis" under which it happens with a 75% probability (darker bars, upright). The predictions are for an experiment with 30 trials in which the event can either occur or not. The arrows indicate the case where the event happened 20 times out of 30. This outcome is predicted with a probability of 0.0280 under the point null hypothesis and with a probability of 0.0909 under the competing point hypothesis. The Bayes factor between these two models is simply the ratio of these probabilities, here 3.247.

Combined with a perfectly ambivalent prior (50% on either claim, or a prior ratio of 1), this Bayes factor brings us to a posterior probability of only about 76% in favor of the competing point hypothesis—not a very high probability.

Bayesian Estimation

In the Bayesian framework, the distinction between testing and estimation is less clear-cut than it is in the frequentist framework. It is useful to think of the two practices as the ends of a continuum. The continuum captures how many possible states of the world are being considered. If we are interested in the probability θ that a coin comes up heads, we might limit our possible hypotheses to A: θ = 0.5 and B: θ = 1.0. This has all the bearing of a testing scenario. Alternatively, we might consider A: θ = 0.0, B: θ = 0.5, C: θ = 1.0, which still has the appearance of a testing context. However, if we permit that θ might be any of (0.01, 0.02, ..., 0.99, 1.00), then it is less clear if we are estimating a parameter or selecting between 101 models. If we allow θ to be anywhere from 0.5 to 1.0, or from 0.0 to 1.0, then we are more obviously dealing with an estimation scenario. Hence, the Bayesian estimation task can be seen an extension of Bayesian hypothesis testing, in which truth value is reallocated among many possible parameter values.

Behavioral researchers rarely have strong quantitative theories that permit statements such as "the probability that a teenager will hear YANNY is 75%." Instead, much behavioral research is conducted in a context of discovery: We seek to quantify effect sizes or estimate parameters (Cumming, 2014), rather than to discriminate between a set of competing theoretical accounts. The simplest way to illustrate Bayesian estimation is to use conjugate families of distributions. A prior distribution and likelihood for the data are said to be conjugate when the resulting posterior distribution is in the same class as the prior distribution. For example, updating a normal prior distribution with normally distributed data results in a normal posterior distribution with a new mean and standard deviation. In what follows we will illustrate conjugate updating and estimation using the conjugate family that includes beta prior distributions and binomial likelihood functions.

Continuing with the bistable perception phenomenon, we might consider two researchers interested in estimating the fraction θ of teenagers who hear YANNY versus LAUREL. The two researchers, independently from one another, retrieve the data from the previous example (a sample of 30 teenagers, 20 of whom hear YANNY) and use it to estimate θ. However, the two researchers differ in their prior conceptions of this proportion. Researcher 1 believes that teenagers are relatively homogeneous and will to a large extent either all hear LAUREL or all hear YANNY (i.e., θ will be close to 0% or 100%). Researcher 2 believes that the population is more likely to be split, and θ is most likely close to 50%. This difference in prior beliefs is displayed with the dashed lines in both panels of Figure 7.2. Researcher 1's prior is well captured by a beta(0.5,0.5) distribution while Researcher 2's prior is best described with a beta(2,2) distribution. Finding the set of prior parameters that best captures one's prior beliefs is known as *prior elicitation*. In practice this is often a matter of experience, but intuitions about the effect of parameter changes can be

STATISTICAL INFERENCE   195

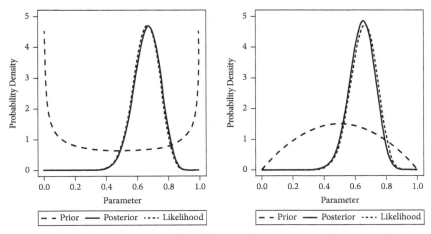

Figure 7.2. Prior and posterior distributions of two independent researchers seeing the same data. Researcher 1 (left) expects the ratio parameter to be extreme, either close to 0 or close to 1. Researcher 2 (right) expects the parameter to be closer to 0.5. Both researchers observe the same data: A sample of 30 yields 20 observations in one category and 10 in the other. When these data are factored in, the differences between the two researchers dissipate—even the dramatic difference in priors is easily overwhelmed by a modest amount of data.

built by visualizing the prior density, by experimenting with its effect on the model's data predictions, and through mathematical analysis—an example of that is given in what follows, and Kadane and Wolfson (1998) provide a comprehensive review.

The beta(a, b) prior is defined as

$$\Pr(\theta | a, b) = \theta^{a-1} (1-\theta)^{b-1} \times C_{prior}$$

where C_{prior} is a scaling parameter independent of θ that ensures the function describes a proper distribution (i.e., one whose mass totals 1). The interpretation of the parameters a and b will be revealed once we compute the posterior distribution.

To obtain the posterior distribution of θ, we multiply the prior with the binomial likelihood of the data, which is:

$$\Pr(Y,L\mid\theta) = \theta^Y \times (1-\theta)^L \times C_{\text{likelihood}}$$

where we again capture all factors that do not contain θ into a single scaling parameter. The posterior is then, by Bayes' theorem,

$$\Pr(\theta\mid Y,L) = \Pr(Y,L\mid\theta) \times \Pr(\theta\mid a,b) \times C_{\text{posterior}}$$
$$= \left[\theta^Y \times (1-\theta)^L\right] \times \left[\theta^{a-1} \times (1-\theta)^{b-1}\right] \times C_{\text{posterior}}$$

Some algebraic rearrangement yields

$$\Pr(\theta\mid Y,L) = \theta^{a-1+Y}(1-\theta)^{b-1+L} \times C_{\text{posterior}} = \theta^{a'-1}(1-\theta)^{b'-1} \times C_{\text{posterior}}$$

where we have first collected all scaling factors into a new factor $C_{\text{posterior}}$ and then introduced the updated parameters a' = a + Y and b' = b + L. This rearrangement illustrates the conjugacy of the beta prior and the binomial likelihood: The posterior distribution of θ again follows a beta distribution. Due to the conjugacy, adding further observations is easy: Simply increment a' with the number of new YANNY observations and increment b' with the number of new LAUREL observations.

The way in which a and b absorb the number of observations of each type also reveals an interesting interpretation of these parameters: The value of a and b *prior to seeing the data* can be interpreted as the (possibly hypothetical) number of times the researcher had already observed YANNY and LAUREL occurrences (respectively). The "effective prior sample size" a + b expresses the strength of the available prior information. Note that this remains true if we were to add a second batch of observations: The effective sample size after the first batch is a' + b', and upon observing new data (Y_2, L_2) the new parameters would be a'' = a' + Y_2 and b'' = b' + L_2. Updating the probability density with new data is a matter of incrementing the parameters of the distribution and (in this case) does not require complex mathematical exercises.

It is also easy to see how the data will quickly overwhelm the prior: Researcher 1 has the equivalent prior information of one observation and Researcher 2 has the equivalent of four observations. These quickly pale when incremented by 30 observations.

With the parameters of the posterior distribution Pr(θ|Y,L) in hand, we can now compute a number of interesting quantities, such as the most "plausible" value of θ (the posterior mode):

$$(a'-1)/(a'+b'-2)$$

which is 0.672 for Researcher 1 and 0.656 for Researcher 2. We could also compute the posterior probability that θ > 0.5, which is 0.970 for Researcher 1 and 0.960 for Researcher 2. Here, again, the dramatic difference in the prior distribution makes little difference in the ultimate quantities of interest. Both researchers conclude that θ is close to two-thirds and is very likely greater than one-half.

Software

Some of the most common Bayesian methods require no more computational effort than standard approaches. To illustrate the use of Bayesian computation we will recreate the estimation analysis given earlier using the software JASP (JASP Team, 2018). JASP is a statistical program with a graphical user interface, meaning no knowledge of scripting or coding is necessary to perform a Bayesian analysis. We have created a data file containing 20 YANNY and 10 LAUREL responses, available for download at https://osf.io/ksvdp/. If we open this file in JASP and select "Bayesian binomial test" from the frequencies drop-down button we are brought to an options menu. In this menu we can specify that the success counts are in the YANNY column of the data, and also specify that we wish to use a beta(2,2) prior distribution for the success parameter (indicating that we expect the population to be split in two groups, as in the previous section). JASP will then generate the results of the Bayesian analysis in the right-most panel, in the form of a plot of the prior and posterior distributions of the probability of success, which we present in Figure 7.3 (right panel). Note that this posterior distribution exactly matches that from the right panel of Figure 7.2. JASP provides a 95% credible interval for the parameter, which in this case ranges from 0.482 to 0.796.

Whereas Bayesian analysis of common designs is possible in software such as JASP, Bayesian calculation for complex modeling is often computationally

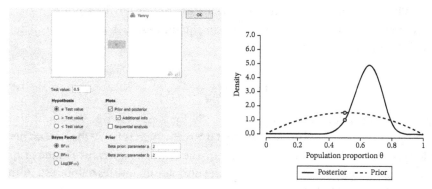

Figure 7.3. A Bayesian binomial test in JASP. Left: The interface for the Bayesian binomial test. Right: Default output from the test applied to the YANNY/LAUREL dataset.

intensive. Fortunately, user-friendly tools for Bayesian analysis have emerged in recent years and have been incorporated into virtually all standard statistical software (e.g., Stata, SPSS, SAS, and R), as well as in new specialized software specifically for Bayesian analyses (e.g., JASP). Introductions to the use of general-purpose Bayesian software can be found in Matzke et al. (2018), van Ravenzwaaij et al. (2018), and Wagenmakers et al. (2018b), but more tutorials appear on a regular basis.

Conclusion

It is not critical for the entire analytical approach of the behavioral sciences to move to Bayesianism to prevent bad inferential practices. It is interesting to look at the methodological evolution within biomedicine, which has not given up frequentist methods but has avoided some of the particularly egregious practices seen in the behavioral sciences. Most importantly, in clinical biomedicine there is a culture of disbelief in small, one-off single studies, particularly small ones, and knowledge is not regarded as established until a sufficiently large body of data collection of studies generates convincing evidence, typically as shown in systematic reviews and meta-analyses. Poorly informative, underpowered studies are strongly disfavored at the major journals, and strong emphasis is put on estimation together with testing, particularly for nonsignificant studies with equivocal findings. Study protocols are now routinely requested by the major journals, and the law requires that randomized trials must be preregistered at clinicaltrials.gov within 21 days from when the first patient is enrolled, and the results of randomized controlled trials must be reported in clinicaltrials.gov regardless of outcome, with government penalties for noncompliance.

This is not to suggest that the field of clinical research has solved or avoided all of the issues of research integrity or proper statistical design and interpretation that are now plaguing the behavioral and social sciences. As a field, it went down similar paths of awareness and reform starting three to four decades ago and has since adopted a number of practices that have blunted some of the worst potential effects of frequentist philosophy and methods. That said, problems remain. Interestingly, many of the innovations currently being suggested for the behavioral sciences are now being adopted within the biomedical sciences as ways to accelerate progress there, particularly the move to open science.

Short of moving completely to a Bayesian paradigm, major progress can be made within the current frequentist paradigm by eliminating claims based only on statistical "bright lines" (i.e., significance), understanding that marginal significance (e.g., $0.01 \leq p \leq 0.05$) represents fairly weak statistical evidence, moving to a cumulative evidence model, and basing conclusions more on CIs than on "testing."

Changes in the practices of an entire discipline require far more than a change in analytical philosophy; these must be accompanied by changes in education, professional norms and expectations, funding, promotion criteria, and publication. But understanding how the dominant analytical philosophy contributes to some of the most harmful practices is critical to make the right changes and thereby improve the trust that those inside or outside the behavioral sciences put in the field and its findings.

Acknowledgments

This work was supported by National Science Foundation grants #1534472 and #1658303 to JV and National Science Foundation Graduate Research Fellowship Program #DGE-1321846 to AE.

References

Aldrich, J. (2008). R. A. Fisher on Bayes and Bayes theorem. *Bayesian Analysis, 3*(1), 161–170.

Altman, D., Machin, D., Bryant, T., & Gardner, M. (2013). *Statistics with Confidence: Confidence Intervals and Statistical Guidelines.* John Wiley & Sons.

Berger, J. O., & Wolpert, R. L. (1988). *The Likelihood Principle* (2nd ed.). Institute of Mathematical Statistics.

Carnap, R. (1950). *Logical Foundations of Probability.* University of Chicago Press.

CNN. (2018, May 16). Laurel or Yanny? What science has to say. https://www.cnn.com/2018/05/15/health/yanny-laurel-audio-social-media-trnd/

Cowles, M., & Davis, C. (1982). On the origins of the .05 level of statistical significance. *American Psychologist, 37*(5), 553.

Cumming, G. (2014). The new statistics: Why and how. *Psychological Science, 25,* 7–29.

Devlin, K. (2010). *The Unfinished Game: Pascal, Fermat, and the Seventeenth-Century Letter That Made the World Modern.* Basic Books.

Diaconis, P., & Freedman, D. (1986). On the consistency of Bayes estimates. *Annals of Statistics, 14*(1), 1–26.

Edwards, W., Lindman, H., & Savage, L. J. (1963). Bayesian statistical inference for psychological research. *Psychological Review, 70,* 193–242.

Etz, A. (2018). Introduction to the concept of likelihood and its applications. *Advances in Methods and Practices in Psychological Science, 1*(1), 60–69.

Etz, A., Haaf, J. M., Rouder, J. N., & Vandekerckhove, J. (2018). Bayesian inference and testing any hypothesis you can specify. *Advances in Methods and Practices in Psychological Science, 1*(2), 281–295.

Etz, A., & Vandekerckhove, J. (2018). Introduction to Bayesian inference for psychology. *Psychonomic Bulletin & Review, 25,* 5–34.

Evans, M. (2015). *Measuring Statistical Evidence Using Relative Belief.* Chapman and Hall/CRC.

Fienberg, S. E. (2006). When did Bayesian inference become "Bayesian"? *Bayesian Analysis, 1*(1), 1–40.

Fisher, R. A. (1925). *Statistical Methods for Research Workers.* Oliver and Boyd.

Fisher, R. A. (1926). The arrangement of field experiments. *Journal of the Ministry of Agriculture, 33,* 503–513.

Fisher, R. A. (1971). *The Design of Experiments* (7th ed.). Hafner.

Gardner, M. J., & Altman, D. G. (1986). Confidence intervals rather than p-values: Estimation rather than hypothesis testing. *British Medical Journal (Clinical Research Edition), 292*(6522), 746–750.

Gelman, A., & Nolan, D. (2002). You can load a die, but you can't bias a coin. *American Statistician, 56*(4), 308–311.

Ghosh, J. K. (Ed.). (1988). *Statistical Information and Likelihood: A Collection of Critical Essays by Dr. D. Basu.* Springer New York. doi: 10.1007/978-1-4612-3894-2

Gigerenzer, G. (1993). The superego, the ego, and the id in statistical reasoning. In G. Keren & C. Lewis (Eds.), *A Handbook for Data Analysis in the Behavioral Sciences: Methodological Issues* (pp. 311–339). Erlbaum.

Gigerenzer, G. (2004). Mindless statistics. *Journal of Socio-Economics, 33,* 587–606.

Goodman, S. N. (1993). P values, hypothesis tests, and likelihood: Implications for epidemiology of a neglected historical debate. *American Journal of Epidemiology, 137,* 485–496.

Goodman, S. N. (1999a). Toward evidence-based medical statistics. 1: The p-value fallacy. *Annals of Internal Medicine, 130*, 995–1004.

Goodman, S. N. (1999b). Toward evidence-based medical statistics. 2: The Bayes factor. *Annals of Internal Medicine, 130*, 1005–1013.

Goodman, S. N., Fanelli, D., & Ioannidis, J. P. (2016). What does research reproducibility mean? *Science Translational Medicine, 8*(341), 341ps12.

Goodman, S. N., & Royall, R. (1988). Evidence and scientific research. *American Journal of Public Health, 78*(12), 1568–1574.

Greenland, S., Senn, S. J., Rothman, K. J., Carlin, J. B., Poole, C., Goodman, S. N., & Altman, D. G. (2016). Statistical tests, p-values, confidence intervals, and power: a guide to misinterpretations. *European Journal of Epidemiology, 31*(4), 337–350.

Hald, A. (2008). *A History of Parametric Statistical Inference from Bernoulli to Fisher, 1713–1935.* Springer Science & Business Media.

Haller, H., & Krauss, S. (2002). Misinterpretations of significance: A problem students share with their teachers? *Methods of Psychological Research, 7*, 1–20.

Hoekstra, R., Morey, R. D., Rouder, J. N., & Wagenmakers, E.-J. (2014). Robust misinterpretation of confidence intervals. *Psychonomic Bulletin & Review, 21*, 1157–1164.

JASP Team. (2018). JASP (Version 0.9). https://jasp-stats.org/

Jeffreys, H. (1961). *Theory of Probability* (3rd ed.). Oxford University Press.

Kadane, J., & Wolfson, L. J. (1998). Experiences in elicitation. *Journal of the Royal Statistical Society: Series D (The Statistician), 47*(1), 3–19.

Kass, R. E., & Raftery, A. E. (1995). Bayes factors. *Journal of the American Statistical Association, 90*, 773–795.

Kendall, M. G. (1949). On the reconciliation of theories of probability. *Biometrika, 36*, 101–115.

Keynes, J. M. (1921). *A Treatise on Probability.* Macmillan & Co.

Lindley, D. V. (1993). The analysis of experimental data: The appreciation of tea and wine. *Teaching Statistics, 15*, 22–25.

Matzke, D., Boehm, U., & Vandekerckhove, J. (2018). Bayesian inference for psychology. Part III: Parameter estimation in nonstandard models. *Psychonomic Bulletin & Review, 25*, 77–101.

Morey, R. D., Hoekstra, R., Rouder, J. N., Lee, M. D., & Wagenmakers, E.-J. (2016). The fallacy of placing confidence in confidence intervals. *Psychonomic Bulletin & Review, 23*, 103–123.

Neyman, J. (1937). Outline of a theory of statistical estimation based on the classical theory of probability. *Philosophical Transactions of the Royal Society of London, Series A, Mathematical and Physical Sciences, 236*, 333–380.

Neyman, J., & Pearson, E. S. (1928). On the use and interpretation of certain test criteria for purposes of statistical inference: Part I. *Biometrika, 20A*(1/2), 175–240.

Neyman, J., & Pearson, E. S. (1933). On the problem of the most efficient tests of statistical hypotheses. *Philosophical Transactions of the Royal Society A, 231*, 289–337.

Oakes, M. W. (1986). *Statistical Inference.* Epidemiology Resources.

Pashler, H., & Wagenmakers, E.-J. (2012). Editors' introduction to the special section on replicability in psychological science: A crisis of confidence? *Perspectives on Psychological Science, 7*, 528–530.

Rouder, J. N., & Morey, R. D. (2019). Teaching Bayes' theorem: Strength of evidence as predictive accuracy. *American Statistician, 73*, 186–190.

Royall, R. M. (1997). *Statistical Evidence: A Likelihood Paradigm.* Chapman & Hall.

Schervish, M. J. (1996). P values: What they are and what they are not. *American Statistician, 50*, 203–206.

van Ravenzwaaij, D., Cassey, P., & Brown, S. D. (2018). A simple introduction to Markov chain Monte-Carlo sampling. *Psychonomic Bulletin & Review, 25*, 143–154.

Vandekerckhove, J., Rouder, J. N., & Kruschke, J. K. (Eds.). (2018). Editorial: Bayesian methods for advancing psychological science. *Psychonomic Bulletin & Review, 25*, 1–4.

von Mises, L. (1957). *Probability Statistics and Truth* (6th ed.). Dover.

Wagenmakers, E. J., Gronau, Q. F., Dablander, F., & Etz, A. (2018a). *The Support Interval.* https://psyarxiv.com/zwnxb/

Wagenmakers, E.-J., Love, J., Marsman, M., Jamil, T., Ly, A., Verhagen, A. J., Selker, R., Gronau, F., Dropmann, D., Boutin, B., Meerhoff, F., Knight, P., Raj, A., van Kesteren, E-J., van Doorn, J., Šmíra, M., Epskamp, S., Etz, A., Matzke, D., . . . Morey, R. D. (2018b). Bayesian inference for psychology. Part II: Example applications with JASP. *Psychonomic Bulletin & Review, 25*, 58–76.

Wagenmakers, E.-J., Marsman, M., Jamil, T., Ly, A., Verhagen, A. J., Love, J., Selker, R., Gronau, Q. F., Šmíra, M., Epskamp, S., Etz, A., Matzke, D., Rouder, J. N., & Morey, R. D. (2018c). Bayesian inference for psychology. Part I: Theoretical advantages and practical ramifications. *Psychonomic Bulletin & Review, 25*, 35–57.

Wasserstein, R. L., & Lazar, N. A. (2016). The ASA's statement on p-values: Context, process, and purpose. *American Statistician, 70*, 129–133.

Wrinch, D., & Jeffreys, H. (1919). On some aspects of the theory of probability. *Philosophical Magazine, 38*, 715–731.

Zabell, S. (1989). R. A. Fisher on the history of inverse probability. *Statistical Science, 4*(3), 247–256.

8
Stimulus Sampling and Research Integrity

James J. Cummings and Byron Reeves

Introduction

Psychological experiments most often have a sample of people respond to a sample of stimuli in two or more conditions. This means that there are two random factors in an experiment, people and stimuli, and that there is interest in generalizing to other possible samples of people *and* other samples of stimuli that might have been used in the research. Among those two samples, design decisions about participants get the most emphasis. Should subject samples be broad or narrow? Should subjects participate in only a single condition or in all conditions? Is there appropriate diversity of people? And how many subjects should be sampled? The last question—how many people?—is the most prominent in discussions of statistical power and scientific integrity. Too often, results or experiments are jeopardized by issues with subject sampling that make it difficult to detect effects, especially when the size of an effect may be interesting but small. Underpowered experiments with ill-chosen subjects hurt science, as discussed elsewhere in this volume.

Problems with *stimulus* samples, discussed far less than issues related to subjects, may be equally consequential for research, and especially consequential for studies that hope to generalize findings to large categories of complex stimuli that are important in the real world. This would be true, for example, for research about how violent video games might influence aggressive behavior, how medical interventions in diet might affect health, or how use of social media might influence political ideology and voting. Each of these areas defines a collection of real-world objects, messages, or practices that may have global similarities (e.g., all video games might share some common features like scoring systems, virtual currencies, and personalized characters). But the individual examples in each category may vary considerably in details that could influence the outcomes of research (e.g., specific video games may be unique with respect to graphics, characters, pictorial realism, type of violence, or devices used for play). When researchers select a single example, or even a sample of two or three different stimuli, the research could easily produce misleading generalizations, no less so than research that used a single subject or a small subject sample based on convenience.

A lack of attention to stimuli makes the sampling of them a hidden, even if critical, integrity issue. Stimuli are often given cursory treatment in scientific literature, especially in meta-analyses, and in public and policy uses of science. In the example of video games, researchers rarely qualify results as applicable only to a particular segment of one game that was used in research. Rather, researchers are likely, as we review in this paper, to inappropriately generalize to the larger category of *all* video games. The external validity of subject samples is often mentioned (e.g., the results apply or not to a diverse, gender-balanced group of adolescents), but there is less expectation that results will be evaluated based on the external validity of stimuli. This is particularly worrisome because investment in a good stimulus sample may often be more essential to addressing a given research question than an investment in subjects. In the video game example this would be true if there is *more* variance between different examples of games (a broad category of commercial products that range across numerous psychological properties) than variance between people who might respond to any particular single example. A similar problem exists broadly regarding the stimulus manipulations found in social and cognitive psychology, as highlighted later in this chapter.

This chapter is about the asymmetry between subject and stimulus sampling, and the potential consequences of underinvesting in stimuli. We first link problems in stimulus sampling to other integrity issues in this volume. Next, we review the sampling decisions researchers make when creating a study with samples of subjects and stimuli. As an example, we present empirical findings on stimulus sampling from the field of media psychology.[1] We close with a review of strategies for addressing problems of stimulus

---

[1] While this chapter emphasizes media stimuli in illustrating stimulus sampling as an integrity issue, the concerns discussed apply to a wider field of behavioral science, including not only media psychology but also literatures in social and cognitive psychology. Direct examples beyond media psychology are referenced below.

sampling investments, ranging from better stimulus definitions to consideration of stimuli as a random factor in statistical analyses to alternative sampling paradigms that may balance sampling investments.

Stimulus Sampling Connections to Research Integrity

Stimulus sampling is a concern that is most often discussed separately from other integrity issues, and when it is discussed it is most often associated with solutions that address primarily statistical issues (Judd et al., 2012; 2017; Westfall et al., 2014; Westfall et al., 2015). Beyond statistical concerns, however, stimulus sampling touches many other integrity issues examined in this volume. We name them here to emphasize the connections, ahead of discussion about their consequences and possible solutions.

Replication

Failures to replicate in social science may be attributable in part to changes in stimuli used in research, even when all other specifications of a study are identical to original efforts (Shrout & Rodgers, 2018; Westfall et al., 2015). The goal in replication should be to reach conclusions that are applicable to *both* random factors—stimuli as well as subjects. When single examples of stimuli are used or when responses to several stimuli are averaged, type I statistical errors are inflated, leading researchers to claim effects that may not generalize to other possible examples of the stimulus category. For example, the results for an experiment that uses 20 minutes of violent video game play to study influences on physiological arousal (e.g., Ivory & Kalyanaraman, 2007) could change substantially if different game examples were substituted in conceptual replications, even if all other measures and procedures remained unchanged. When a conceptual replication fails to reproduce past findings, it may indicate that the previously observed "effect" is not particularly robust or perhaps is even nonexistent. But alternatively, a legitimate effect may fail to replicate due to a misconception within the methods and procedure of a new study (Schmidt, 2009). In the case of relatively simple stimuli, if the "effect" hinges on a very specific manipulation, its generalizability may be particularly limited. However, in the case of complex stimuli, a failure to replicate may relate more to a lack of precision in manipulations. The understanding of what the manipulation actually captured in the original study can be mistaken, with levels of the actual causal element being relatively lesser or even entirely absent in an intended conceptual replication. It would be desirable to represent as much of the stimulus variance as possible in a single study (i.e., use multiple game titles in the research), but also useful to catalog the extent to which unique stimulus samples are responsible for different results as replications are attempted and accumulated.

Researcher Biases

When stimuli are convenience samples from large categories, researcher biases, even though unintended, may influence stimulus selection. One possible bias is that stimulus selection could favor examples that maximize differences by condition, even if the stimuli used are unrepresentative of a larger category (e.g., choosing the single unique video game that causes modeling of aggressive behavior). Sometimes biases are explicit (e.g., "we wanted to find the most violent game currently on the market") but often the selection criteria are unstated. This leaves considerable room for bias, for example, with respect to political ideology (Jussim et al., 2015) or culture (Van de Vijver & Poortinga, 1997). Without a stimulus sampling plan that dealt with these biases, research could be adversely affected (e.g., choosing a video game that represented a political argument, one biased toward male rather than female play, or one that was culturally narrow and played only within a particular subculture or country).

P-hacking

When researchers manipulate analyses in an attempt to achieve statistical significance (p-hacking; see Simonsohn et al., 2014 and elsewhere in this volume), one possible "hack" is to alter analysis in favor of certain stimuli, picking a subset of examples for which results are significant and eliminating others that did not show differences. Conversely, stimuli may be manipulated by averaging across several examples to show an overall effect when a single stimulus in the collection is exclusively responsible for the differences. In that case, the averaging may seem to justify a generalizable conclusion but in fact the repetitions of the results across the examples would show effects isolated to a single or few examples.

Overstatement of Results

A common strategy in designing experiments is to create stimuli that maximize variance on features highlighted in the research. That might be a good strategy to the extent that it allows differences to be uncovered, especially in the first studies of a stimulus category (e.g., "are there any video games that cause aggressive behavior?"). If that strategy begins to characterize a literature, however, the collection of stimuli to which the summaries depend, even when averaged across several studies, will be biased toward stimuli that cause the biggest differences in favor of qualities of the stimuli that exist across examples. Concluding, for example, that most video games are benign but there is one that is troublesome is quite different than concluding that video games as a category are consequential.

Publication Bias

This bias is most often considered with respect to emphasis on significant findings relative to unpublished, and possibly more numerous, studies that find no differences and are consequently ignored by authors and journals because they are not interesting (e.g., Franco et al., 2014). There is also the possibility of publication bias toward research deemed to be newsworthy, irrespective of scientific quality (e.g., Callaham et al., 2002). This is an understudied bias in social science publication but it may be of increasing concern as citation statistics create pressures to favor popular topics that are magnets for citation. Engaging stories about research, and hence the newsworthiness of publications, may be centered on stimuli that are of particular public interest, and their noteworthiness alone may influence publication. Following the video game example, a disproportionate amount of research in that literature favors a handful of popular game titles (*Grand Theft Auto, Mortal Kombat*), known in part because they are extreme examples of violent game content and in part because they are favorites among politicians and public advocates trying to minimize game influences (Reeves et al., 2016).

Research Transparency

Reporting details about subjects is increasingly a requirement for publication. Similar details about stimuli, however, are often more difficult to find, as are journal guidelines about what stimulus information needs to be reported. This includes information about stimulus examples that were *excluded* from the research, either from pre-tests or because they did not produce interesting results, as well as information about how the particular examples that are eventually used were selected. A lack of transparency may hurt the chances for replication, except in cases where the exact same stimuli are coincidentally used. Research that attempts to replicate a study with new samples for both random factors will be jeopardized. There is one new proposal for stimulus transparency that parallels subject information (Simons et al., 2017). Although the authors devote most of their attention to the conditions of generalizability that relate to subject samples, they do specify a need for researchers to define, and register prior to conducting the research, the class of materials or stimuli to which findings are expected to generalize. This means defining the critical features of stimuli that must be maintained for a new study to be about the same constructs. It isn't useful to find a failure to replicate if the conflicting results are simply due to the use of new stimuli, outside the bounds of original definitions.

Why Are Good Stimulus Samples Important?

In part, stimulus selection is a technical issue about external validity, sampling, and statistics. Technical solutions, especially sophisticated analytical strategies to examine the effects of random stimulus variance against the fixed effects of treatments, make up the bulk of writing about stimulus problems. Many early challenges to researchers about stimulus sampling cited these technical issues in warnings about the integrity of research. For example, the most cited warning (Clark, 1973) was about the choices of particular words and sentences—out of all possible combinations in the English language. Less frequent, however, have been warnings about overgeneralization of particular stimuli that had currency in public or policy discussions. We review here three reasons to focus on stimuli *in and of themselves*.

First, stimuli are often the entrée to research. Much of social science is devoted to studying the effects of messages, practices, interventions, and the like on important social criteria. In these cases, integrity of results depends as much on stimulus definitions and generalizations as on any other attribute of the research. Medical researchers care about particular advice given about specific illnesses. Media designers care about the specific public service announcement created to change one health behavior. Political scientists care about the specific news stories that might alter voting behavior during one particular election. Getting the stimuli wrong, even if the subject sample is excellent, will mean errors in an important use of the research—namely, the ability to advocate for or against particular stimuli, sometimes the exact ones employed in the research but even more likely ones that are similar in the real world. Consider, for example, research that seeks to understand the relationship of negative emotional experiences and memory. Psychologists focused on emotion and memory might want show a negative video game segment to subjects but with little or even no interest in the particular game segment used. They might only seek to find *any* stimulus that could produce the emotion of interest so they could examine the relationship of that experience to other concepts. A *media* psychologist, however, with a primary interest in whether specific types of games should be regulated or critiqued would be substantially more invested in the stimulus sample.

Second, researchers who emphasize stimuli in their work may find that enhanced investments in stimuli, as opposed to other sources of variance, may best benefit external validity. The amount of variance in a population to which a sample hopes to generalize helps determine the size and diversity of samples. We choose many people for research because we know they are not all the same. The more variance between people with respect to characteristics of interest in the research, the more people that should be included in research to adequately capture that variance. A good investment question is whether between-person variance exceeds variance that exists between stimuli. Imagine 10 different health messages that are possible examples of persuasive appeals about healthier diets, and imagine that they are each seen by 10 different people (men and women of different ages, politics, geographical regions). Should one expect more variance between people in responses to any one message, or more variance between messages for any given person? We believe the answer is often that there is more stimulus variance. Stimuli, and especially ones like media, health interventions, educational curricula, or political messaging, are infinitely complex (Cappella, 2006; Reeves & Geiger, 1994). They are rarely an example of only one feature and nothing else. That complexity will often dwarf the complexity of the people who view any given example. Putting investments where the variance is, as a matter of research application as well as research integrity, will often mean investing in stimuli, sometimes even at the expense of investments in subjects.

Third, stimulus variance in many areas of social research is growing. One important source of that growth is the ability to use technology to generate different examples of messages and interventions, and to experiment, sometimes in real time, with different stimulus configurations. Digital technology makes it possible to create stimuli quickly and cheaply, enabling large collections of possible stimuli to compete for inclusion in research. In addition to allowing researchers to sample more easily, large stimulus collections allow researchers to define more explicitly the population of stimuli that need to be sampled. The ability to quickly prototype stimuli is useful because researchers can experiment with different definitions of a stimulus category. Sophisticated analytics can be used to test different stimulus configurations; for example, rapidly evaluating stimuli via A/B testing (Kohavi & Longbotham, 2017). This and similar strategies could allow for more powerful stimuli to be part of research with the advantage that results would more likely be significant and interesting as stimuli are fine-tuned. Importantly, however, the easy configurations and changes using technology make research transparency a critical concern. Imagine, by comparison, the integrity interest if researchers pretested subjects to see which ones enabled the largest significant differences to emerge.

Example Literature: Media Psychology

We have presented the case of video games and their effects in reviewing several potential integrity concerns with respect to stimulus sampling. Our attention to that example was inspired by a recent study of stimuli in the wider field of media psychology, an area that includes research about how people think and feel in relation to different content and forms of media. Empirical studies in the field typically include samples of participants (the people viewing, listening to, reading, playing with, or interacting with a piece of media), while some also include stimulus variance (different pieces of media themselves). The populations of people who respond to media and the populations of media are both tremendously diverse, with large and varied groups of users sometimes engaging a large and varied assortment of messages.

The extent of stimulus variance in this research, however, was unknown. While there have been critiques of stimulus issues in communication (e.g., Brashers & Jackson, 1999; Jackson & Jacobs, 1983; Reeves & Geiger, 1994), those arguments are older and there were no summaries of stimuli used in research conducted since the year 2000. To update the characterization of stimuli used in research, we analyzed 306 empirical studies conducted between 2004 and 2016 that looked at how people processed media information in various categories, from video games to international news to persuasive public-service announcements (PSAs) about health (Reeves et al., 2016). The studies represented all of the research published in the journal *Media Psychology* over the last 10 years, as well as the most-cited media experiments published across the social sciences in that same period.

Our analysis revealed that the majority of experiments (65%) used only single examples of media messages per condition, yet study conclusions were typically discussed with respect to large categories of real-world media experiences. The majority of the remaining studies used three or fewer stimuli, but none of those studies analyzed stimulus repetitions as a random effect, a commonly suggested corrective statistical procedure (Jackson & Jacobs, 1983; Judd et al., 2012; Judd et al., 2017). While subject sampling in these studies was generally acceptable, the media selections across the entire literature were limited, increasing the probability that idiosyncratic choices were being used to characterize a complex population of real-world experiences. Our conclusion was that this represented a significant research integrity issue.

The same under-sampling of stimuli may characterize any literature, creating problems for the external validity of stimulus generalizations, but is particularly egregious when single examples are used to represent complex stimulus categories that are the entrée for research—for example, in research about teaching strategies, health interventions, or behavior change initiatives about the environment or civic participation.

The threat to research integrity posed by single-stimulus studies, like those in media psychology, is also an issue of construct validity. That is, the inability to generalize the results of a study with few or even a single stimulus exists because we do not know whether the effects observed are due to an unstated stimulus feature. In some cases, this may lead to type I or type II errors, in which a confounding attribute of the stimulus accentuated or suppressed the effect of the intended attribute of study. Either error could be avoided with larger samples of the stimuli that better represented the population distribution of the hidden construct.

Worse perhaps, single-stimulus experiments raise the potential for a type III error. This occurs when research provides essentially a right answer but for the wrong question by mistakenly rejecting the null hypothesis for reasons other than the predicted difference (Linnan & Steckler, 2002; Shaffer, 2002). Imagine a study examining how stimuli that contain either fear appeals or humor appeals compare to one another in influencing compliance with a desired behavior. For sake of example, let us contend that humor appeals are truly more effective at eliciting the desired behavior than are fear appeals. That is, the populations of possible stimuli representing each appeal type have a distribution of effects on behavior, and in this case the mean level of effect for humor appeals is greater than that of the mean level of effect for fear appeals. It is quite plausible that these distributions overlap, in such a manner that while means are significantly different, a particularly powerful fear appeal may actually be more effective than a particularly weak humor appeal, due to a conceptually unassociated factor (say, level of realism) rather than the variable in question. In the case of single-stimulus samples, in which only one member of each distribution is used for implementing the intended manipulation, it is possible that the stimulus choices of the researcher capture these extremes. In such cases there is a possibility of correctly rejecting the null hypothesis but for the wrong reason (Reeves et al., 2016). That is, it is possible that a single stimulus could lead to a conclusion that is not just wrong in that it suggests a result when there are actually no differences, but a conclusion that is diametrically opposed to a result that could be found with a better, more robust stimulus sample.

Media psychology serves as a particularly worrisome example of how entrenched issues of stimulus sampling, and resulting injury to research integrity, may be within a given field of study. Notably, an alarm about stimulus selection in communication science was sounded decades ago (Jackson & Jacobs, 1983), and many scholars have since advocated for the need for multiple-message samples when designing experiments (O'Keefe, 2014; Reeves & Geiger, 1994; Thorson et al., 2012). The 2016 analysis of hundreds of recent studies, however, suggests that changing standards within an established field may be a long, slow process.

While the media psychology literature may provide a particularly apt example of the issue of single-stimulus experiments and resulting concerns regarding research integrity, it is by no means a special or unique case. Even a cursory examination of the wider psychology literature—including experiments in social and cognitive psychology—reveals common and even highly cited cases of studies employing a single stimulus. Within social psychology studies on stereotype threat often include only a single operational manipulation of threat. Indeed, the most highly cited of such studies (Steele & Aronson, 1995) employed a single-stimulus manipulation: At the outset of the study each participant received a single sheet of paper describing the purpose of the study, with the description for the diagnostic condition containing an altered phrasing that suggested the study's intent was to observe how "personal factors" influence performance. A more recent but similarly highly cited piece examining gender bias in hiring faculty in the sciences also drew upon a single operationalization (Moss-Racusin et al., 2012). In this case, participants were asked to evaluate a purported application for a student lab manager position, in which the applicant's first name was set to either "John" or "Jennifer" and male or female pronouns were inserted respectively. Notably, the landmark work by Festinger and Carlsmith (1959) that launched the development of cognitive dissonance theory itself contained a single instantiation of relative levels of pressure for eliciting overt behaviors that contradict one's private opinion: monetary compensation in the form $0, $1, or $20. Studies like these showcase that the use of single-stimulus samples to generalize claims about the effects of hypothetical constructs are not restricted to the field of media psychology. Rather, the practice and its attendant concerns are to be found in the wider psychology literature, even among some of the most notable and potentially influential works.

Making Stimulus Samples Better

Beyond raising awareness of the potential for underinvestment in stimulus sampling to impair research integrity, we identify here different decisions that researchers can make to help mitigate this impact. Specifically, in this section we examine four points of consideration for researchers conducting experiments on the effects of samples of stimuli on samples of respondents: (1) how stimuli are defined; (2) choosing the right number of stimuli; (3) treating stimulus repetitions as a random factor; and (4) alternative designs that intensively gather robust stimulus experiences for individuals.

Specifying "What Is One"

Fixing the inadequacies of subject samples has one clear advantage over fixing stimulus issues. When individuals are the units of analysis, it is obvious what constitutes one example in a population: It is one person. There can be subsequent considerations of gender, age, life experiences, and a multitude of other differences, but the units of inclusion in a final sample are individuals. Researchers sample multiple individuals in numbers that hopefully capture their diversity in the population and the size of their expected differences by condition.

Stimulus sampling is often more difficult with respect to identification of *what constitutes one example*. While there is a parallel concern about number of stimuli (e.g., do we have enough examples to represent the diversity of stimuli that could possibly be included), it is often harder in the first place to specify the exact boundaries of one stimulus that might be chosen for inclusion in research. We comment below on stimulus definitions with respect to their conceptual boundaries, volume, and context.

Continuing the video game example, there are a number of possible definitions of *one stimulus*. A definition might rely on commercial boundaries (e.g., one product for sale or download), but that definition could include games of radically different complexity, length of play, backstories, characters, graphics, age appropriateness, and many other qualities. Regardless of those differences, should they all be considered examples of the same stimulus category? The answer is more conceptual than methodological. It depends on how concepts are defined in the research (i.e., what *exactly* are the units of experience to which concepts apply?). Violent game play might be defined as an attribute of a game narrative that unfolds over days or weeks, or it might be defined as a collection of specific behaviors that players confront in minutes, or it could be associated with any number of other game elements. Without guidance on the specific features that are required for a stimulus to be included in a sampling plan, the choice of stimuli could lead to a hodgepodge collection of examples that may not really belong together.

Another conceptual issue concerns the *volume* of stimuli. What is the amount or dosage of a particular stimulus that should constitute "one experience" that could be sampled? Volume is often defined in terms of duration, with decisions about samples of particular durations determined by logistics and feasibility. In the video game literature, stimuli are typically experienced for about 11 to 20 minutes in the lab. The issue for stimulus generalization is that those minutes are then used to generalize findings to a much more varied collection of game play that includes much longer sessions as well as sessions accumulated over days and months. Often, the volume of a stimulus is itself a variable in research (e.g., the dosage of a drug, the number of repetitions hearing a health recommendation, as well as short vs. long periods of video game play). This is useful in that data can be used to calibrate stimulus definitions in a literature over time.

In addition to the volume or dosage, an important aspect of defining a single stimulus might be the *context* in which it is experienced. When sampling subjects, attention to the contexts in which individuals live is important; it is understood that subject samples are good to the extent that they include people from diverse neighborhoods, communities, organizations, regions, schools, and any other contextual influence that might change how they respond in research. The same is true for research stimuli. They are often influential (or not) because of the context in which they are presented; for example, the location of the experience (e.g., arrangements of a room or building, neighborhood or city in which responses were collected) or the presentation context (e.g., presentation formats, screens, viewing devices). Most often, stimulus effects are investigated in controlled conditions that are designed to eliminate or at least standardize context effects. It is possible, however, that context may be an important part of how stimuli should be defined, and the contexts should be included in the stimulus samples. For example, the sequencing of information (i.e., what precedes and follows any given piece of information) is a key consideration for studying processing phenomena like priming (Hermans et al., 2001; Tulving & Schacter, 1990; Vorberg et al., 2003), framing (Scheufele & Tewksbury, 2007; Seo et al., 2010; Tversky & Kahneman, 1981), and primacy and recency effects (Murphy et al., 2006). When sequence is preserved as part of a stimulus definition, qualities like pacing and rhythms of presentation can be examined (Cutting et al., 2012; Zacks & Swallow, 2007). These may not be examples of one stimulus influencing another (e.g., what comes before influencing what is presented next) but rather a case where the entire sequence should be considered the stimulus. Sampling that considers contextual variance, and the sampling of it, is difficult. But the integrity of the research may depend on at least some attention to the unitization of experiences—that is, when does one meaningful unit of experience end and another begin?

Problems of stimulus definition and specificity exist in any research area that considers complex phenomenon. To enhance research integrity, exact specification of stimulus categories should be standard in research reports, and even in the preregistration of research interests and hypotheses. This would have a theoretical advantage in that researchers would have to consider the exact features of complex stimuli that are the subjects of their work, allowing better stipulation of the population of messages, interventions, and experiences from which to sample.

Choosing the Right Number of Stimuli

In research that seeks to generalize results to people as well as stimuli, it is the case, not surprisingly, that the more examples of each that are included in the research, the greater the statistical power of the experiment *for both factors*. But just how many examples should be included? A first answer is easy: more than one. Studies that use single stimuli cannot be generalized to larger categories of stimuli from which other examples might have been chosen. Unfortunately, there are many studies that use single stimuli (e.g., the majority of experiments in media psychology over the last 10 years, as we reported on earlier). The integrity of research is seriously at risk when researchers use single stimuli but then subsequently comment on an entire population of experiences from which the single example was chosen.

A more detailed and practical answer to the question of "how many" is to consider how to balance investments *between* the two random factors. Should researchers try to include more subjects or include more stimuli? In the literature, the dominant consideration is number of subjects, with the resulting advice being the more the better. Between the two factors, however, a good answer is that researchers should increase the sample size of whichever factor is contributing more variation to the data (Westfall et al., 2014). And as we have argued, there are frequently stimulus categories (e.g., video games, medical interventions, school curricula) for which the variance may be larger than that found for random samples of the people responding to those categories.

Consider these two examples. One experiment measures reaction times that people have to secondary cues (auditory tones) that are presented every 15 seconds while playing a video game. This is a measure of the amount of attention people give to the primary task of paying attention to the game, with longer reaction times indicating greater primary task attention (Basil, 2014). While there is likely large variance in the quickness with which different people can respond to the tone, there may not be substantial variance overall in how people respond to any given tone. Consequently, the best method to increase power in the experiment would be to add subjects, not adding more places in the game where the tones were placed. In a second example study, people are asked to make a subjective judgment, after they had played a video game for 30 minutes, about how much attention they gave to the game play. In this case, it would be likely that different game selections could elicit considerably different subjective judgments about attention, even though there might not be considerable differences between people in how they judged any given game example. In this experiment, there would be more benefit in adding video game segments than adding subjects.

Adding either subjects or stimuli to research has diminishing returns as the sample sizes of each increase (Westfall et al., 2014), and this has particular relevance to research that typically has one or just a few stimulus examples. A study with 100 subjects and two stimuli cannot be improved much, if at all, by doubling the number of subjects, at least when one considers the power calculations for both random factors. But the power of the overall experiment can be increased substantially by doubling the number of stimuli, because the number of stimuli is so low absolutely as well as relative to the number of subjects. (This advantage is related to the diminishing returns of larger samples that advantage increases in smaller number, and to the multiplicative effect of the two samples sizes on power; see Westfall et al., 2014.) It is also worth noting that increasing the number of stimuli may actually be the most cost-effective way to increase power. If the stimulus in the study was a 10-minute video game experience, it would likely take less effort to have 100 people play two extra video game examples than it would be to invite 100 additional subjects to the lab.

Additionally, it is useful to consider stimulus sampling that may accrue over time and across studies rather than sampling that occurs only within a single research effort. Practical reasons may limit the number of stimuli researchers can reasonably include within the sample of a given study. Testing a new course textbook, for example, may take a full semester. An intervention over months may be too long of a treatment period for participants to serially engage multiple instances. Similarly, cost may be a concern. Limited funds could result in the need to decide on producing and testing the effects of only a single PSA message versus the dozens of different options brainstormed. In each of these cases, the selection of a primary or even single stimulus might be done to complement a literature and not just one study. It is also worth noting that occasional use of prominent single stimuli may be justified, and without consideration of sampling at all. A single prominent political debate, for example, may be such a cultural touchstone that it is itself a topic of study, without message sampling being an issue.

Analysis and Replication of Stimulus Samples

We have noted that when a sample of people respond to a sample of stimuli, there are two random factors, and researchers need to consider the quality of *each* sample because they both affect the integrity of research. To achieve this statistically requires different statistics than are commonly used, and there is a robust literature growing that demonstrates why and how statistical analyses need to be changed to accommodate stimulus samples (Judd et al., 2012; Judd et al., 2017; Westfall et al., 2014; Westfall et al., 2015). For research that considers subject and stimulus samples, analyses needs to shift away from t-test and ANOVA procedures that treat stimuli as a fixed factor (often by averaging across stimuli), and instead use an analytical approach in which both sources of random variation are estimated within the models tested (Judd et al., 2017). Mixed models should be used when both factors are treated as random, whether crossed with one another or with one random factor nested within the other (Judd et al., 2012; Judd et al., 2017). The results of these models are particularly important because they provide evidence about the relative contribution of subject versus stimulus variance in explaining results. Our prediction, based on our own look at stimulus variance in media psychology, is that stimulus variance would often trump subject variance in effects on study criteria. Having better information about stimulus variance, obtainable because research included multiple examples and statistics were available on which ones worked, would help to balance emphasis on people versus on stimuli.

Testing random effects of stimulus variance also has important implications for dealing with a replication crisis in psychology (Westfall et al., 2015). Failures to replicate are often attributed to limited statistical power in replication attempts (Maxwell et al., 2015), and low power is attributed almost exclusively to the fact that replications have too few subjects. In their diagnosis of the replication crisis in psychology and behavioral sciences, Shrout and Rodgers (2018) emphasize that the effect-size values required for power analyses stem from the distribution of effects observed in a given literature. One key source of effect variation between studies may be the relative "intensity and purity" of stimuli—that is, as independent instances of the underlying population, a given intervention or study stimulus may produce a non-representative effect size (Shrout & Rodgers, 2018). Similarly, Westfall et al. (2015) forcefully state that direct replications of research need to resample stimuli to increase confidence in the research. They also note that virtually all of the published guidelines and recommendations about direct replications fail to ensure that stimuli are considered in replication designs.

Designs That Observe Multiple Stimuli in Natural Settings

In the laboratory, time is often a practical constraint in the use of multiple stimuli. People can't be expected to participate in research for more than a couple hours, and usually they participate for a much shorter time period. For stimuli that take even 10 to 20 minutes to experience, it would be difficult to include a large number of examples or to increase the total time allowed to experience any one example. One design solution is to move the experiment into the field, allowing stimulus experiences to occur naturally during the course of everyday life. While it has been difficult to exercise controls in field experiments (e.g., when stimuli are experienced, measurement of immediate and delayed responses that are linked to stimuli), it is now possible to arrange laboratory-type control using increasingly ubiquitous and pervasive digital technology. For example, a smartphone or laptop might be used to present stimuli at algorithm-determined moments, and to assess responses that are both immediate and delayed (e.g., Reeves et al., 2021; Yeykelis et al., 2017).

Research that uses intensive experience-sampling techniques to track individuals over extended time periods and to provide well-timed interventions has several advantages, not the least of which is the ability to present more and different stimuli over longer periods of time (reviewed in Reeves et al., 2021). This offers an unprecedented ability to create multiple stimuli that can be tested as a random factor using the statistical procedures outlined previously. Such an approach inverts the conventional asymmetry in sampling investments placing more focus on within-person dynamics and elaboration of theories about how single individuals change over time. While issues of subject generalization will depend on accumulating data across individuals, the integrity of research is substantially helped by detailed knowledge of how particular individuals respond to multiple stimuli in natural contexts, and from the ability to present, over extended time periods, multiple examples of stimuli that are part of a single category.

Conclusion

We have highlighted problems of stimulus sampling in the behavioral sciences that influence the integrity of research. In part, these issues parallel similar concerns about the sampling of people; namely, whether samples represent well the expected variance in populations and whether there is reason to expect that the sample would be similar to other possible samples not used in the research. In spite of parallel issues, however, there is asymmetry in the investment in stimulus sampling relative to sampling of people, an imbalance, we believe, that comes at the expense of confidence that research may be used to evaluate stimuli that were not chosen for a study.

The problem with stimulus sampling in the behavioral sciences is not only one of cleaning up results so that weak findings become strong or of increasing the confidence we already have in applying results beyond specific studies. Rather, the limited representation of highly variant stimuli may cause results, and discussions about their applications, to be wrong. Our most important conclusion is that researchers should be mindful of stimulus variance. Stimuli, much like people, bring with them a degree of heterogeneity that should be factored into designs and resource investments. Recognizing that random variation occurs when constructing a stimulus sample is a requisite first step. There are good and sophisticated remedies for sampling and statistics that, if used, will improve research. It's also true, however, that those remedies are premature in literatures where stimuli are not sampled at all. So perhaps the most important admonition is to consider more than one stimulus: Invest in as many stimuli as the expected variance in concepts demands and that the logistics of research reasonably permits.

References

Basil, M. D. (2014). Secondary reaction-time measures. In A. Lang (Ed.), Measuring psychological responses to media messages (pp. 97–110). Routledge.

Brashers, D. E., & Jackson, S. (1999). Changing conceptions of "message effects": A 24-year overview. *Human Communication Research, 25*(4), 457–477.

Callaham, M., Wears, R. L., & Weber, E. (2002). Journal prestige, publication bias, and other characteristics associated with citation of published studies in peer-reviewed journals. *Journal of the American Medical Association, 287*(21), 2847–2850.

Cappella, J. N. (2006). Integrating message effects and behavior change theories: Organizing comments and unanswered questions. *Journal of Communication, 56*(suppl_1), S265–S279.

Clark, H. H. (1973). The language-as-fixed-effect fallacy: A critique of language statistics in psychological research. *Journal of Verbal Learning and Verbal Behavior, 12*, 335–359.

Cutting, J. E., Brunick, K. L., & Candan, A. (2012). Perceiving event dynamics and parsing Hollywood films. *Journal of Experimental Psychology: Human Perception and Performance, 38*(6), 1476.

Festinger, L., & Carlsmith, J. M. (1959). Cognitive consequences of forced compliance. *Journal of Abnormal and Social Psychology, 58*(2), 203.

Franco, A., Malhotra, N., & Simonovits, G. (2014). Publication bias in the social sciences: Unlocking the file drawer. *Science, 345*(6203), 1502–1505.

Hermans, D., De Houwer, J., & Eelen, P. (2001). A time course analysis of the affective priming effect. *Cognition & Emotion, 15*(2), 143–165.

Ivory, J. D., & Kalyanaraman, S. (2007). The effects of technological advancement and violent content in video games on players' feelings of presence, involvement, physiological arousal, and aggression. *Journal of Communication, 57*(3), 532–555.

Jackson, S., & Jacobs, S. (1983). Generalizing about messages: Suggestions for design and analysis of experiments. *Human Communication Research, 9*, 169–191.

Judd, C. M., Westfall, J., & Kenny, D. A. (2012). Treating stimuli as a random factor in social psychology: A new and comprehensive solution to a pervasive but largely ignored problem. *Journal of Personality and Social Psychology, 103*(1), 54.

Judd, C. M., Westfall, J., & Kenny, D. A. (2017). Experiments with more than one random factor: Designs, analytic models, and statistical power. *Annual Review of Psychology, 68*, 601–625.

Jussim, L., Crawford, J. T., Anglin, S. M., & Stevens, S. T. (2015). Ideological bias in social psychological research. *Social Psychology and Politics, 17*.

Kohavi, R., & Longbotham, R. (2017). Online controlled experiments and A/B testing. In C. Sammut & G. I. Webb (Eds.), *Encyclopedia of Machine Learning and Data Mining* (pp. 922–929). Springer US.

Linnan, L., & Steckler, A. (2002). *Process Evaluation for Public Health Interventions and Research* (pp. 1–23). Jossey-Bass.

Maxwell, S. E., Lau, M. Y., & Howard, G. S. (2015). Is psychology suffering from a replication crisis? What does "failure to replicate" really mean? *American Psychologist, 70*(6), 487.

Moss-Racusin, C. A., Dovidio, J. F., Brescoll, V. L., Graham, M. J., & Handelsman, J. (2012). Science faculty's subtle gender biases favor male students. *Proceedings of the National Academy of Sciences USA, 109*(41), 16474–16479.

Murphy, J., Hofacker, C., & Mizerski, R. (2006). Primacy and recency effects on clicking behavior. *Journal of Computer-Mediated Communication, 11*(2), 522–535.

O'Keefe, D. J. (2014, April). Evidence-based persuasive message design: Specifying the evidentiary requirements. Paper presented at the annual Kentucky Conference of Health Communication, Lexington, KY.

Reeves, B., & Geiger, S. (1994). Designing experiments that assess psychological responses to media messages. In A. Lang (Ed.), *Measuring Psychological Responses to Media Messages* (pp. 165–180). Routledge.

Reeves, B., Ram, N., Robinson, T., Cummings, J. J., Giles, L., Pan, J., Chiatti, A., Cho, M, Roehrick, K., Yang, X., Gagneja, A., Brinberg., M., Muise, D., Lu, Y., Luo, M., Fitzgerald, A., & Yeykelis, L. (2021). Screenomics: A framework to capture and analyze personal life experiences and the ways that technology shapes them. *Human–Computer Interaction, 36*(2), 150–201.

Reeves, B., Yeykelis, L., & Cummings, J. J. (2016). The use of media in media psychology. *Media Psychology, 19*(1), 49–71.

Scheufele, D. A., & Tewksbury, D. (2007). Framing, agenda setting, and priming: The evolution of three media effects models. *Journal of Communication, 57*(1), 9–20. doi:10.1111/j.0021-9916.2007.00326.x

Schmidt, S. (2009). Shall we really do it again? The powerful concept of replication is neglected in the social sciences. *Review of General Psychology, 13*(2), 90–100.

Seo, M. G., Goldfarb, B., & Barrett, L. F. (2010). Affect and the framing effect within individuals over time: Risk taking in a dynamic investment simulation. *Academy of Management Journal, 53*(2), 411–431.

Shaffer, J. P. (2002). Multiplicity, directional (type III) errors, and the null hypothesis. *Psychological Methods, 7*(3), 356.

Shrout, P. E., & Rodgers, J. L. (2018). Psychology, science, and knowledge construction: Broadening perspectives from the replication crisis. *Annual Review of Psychology, 69*, 487–510.

Simons, D. J., Shoda, Y., & Lindsay, D. S. (2017). Constraints on generality (COG): A proposed addition to all empirical papers. *Perspectives on Psychological Science, 12*(6), 1123–1128.

Simonsohn, U., Nelson, L. D., & Simmons, J. P. (2014). P-curve: A key to the file-drawer. *Journal of Experimental Psychology: General, 143*(2), 534.

Steele, C. M., & Aronson, J. (1995). Stereotype threat and the intellectual test performance of African Americans. *Journal of Personality and Social Psychology, 69*(5), 797.

Thorson, E., Wicks, R., & Leshner, G. (2012). Experimental methodology in journalism and mass communication research. *Journalism & Mass Communication Quarterly, 89*, 112–124.

Tulving, E., & Schacter, D. L. (1990). Priming and human memory systems. *Science, 247*(4940), 301–306.

Tversky, A., & Kahneman, D. (1981). The framing of decisions and the psychology of choice. *Science, 211*(4481), 453–458.

Van de Vijver, F. J., & Poortinga, Y. H. (1997). Towards an integrated analysis of bias in cross-cultural assessment. *European Journal of Psychological Assessment, 13*(1), 29–37.

Vorberg, D., Mattler, U., Heinecke, A., Schmidt, T., & Schwarzbach, J. (2003). Different time courses for visual perception and action priming. *Proceedings of the National Academy of Sciences USA, 100*(10), 6275–6280.

Westfall, J., Judd, C. M., & Kenny, D. A. (2015). Replicating studies in which samples of participants respond to samples of stimuli. *Perspectives on Psychological Science, 10*(3), 390–399.

Westfall, J., Kenny, D. A., & Judd, C. M. (2014). Statistical power and optimal design in experiments in which samples of participants respond to samples of stimuli. *Journal of Experimental Psychology: General, 143*(5), 2020.

Yeykelis, L., Cummings, J. J., & Reeves, B. (2017). The fragmentation of work, entertainment, e-mail, and news on a personal computer: Motivational predictors of switching between media content. *Media Psychology, 21*(3), 377–402.

Zacks, J. M., & Swallow, K. M. (2007). Event segmentation. *Current Directions in Psychological Science, 16*(2), 80–84.

9

Questionable Interpretive Practices

Data (Mis)Interpretation and (Mis)Representation as Threats to Scientific Validity

Lee J. Jussim, Sean T. Stevens, and Stephanie Anglin

Science is about generating knowledge—and for something to constitute "knowledge" it has to actually be true (Funder et al., 2014). The scientific investigation of a phenomenon can tolerate a great deal of error and imperfection, but only if a scientific field has reliable mechanisms for efficient self-correction. Unfortunately, science is not always self-correcting (Ioannidis, 2012) and psychology, in particular, has recently faced increased methodological scrutiny (for reviews see Jussim et al., 2019a; Spellman, 2015). For decades, psychologists and scholars from related fields have been sounding the alarm about the prevalence of suboptimal practices in the field. These criticisms accomplished little until the "replicability crisis" (Gelman, 2016; Spellman, 2015, which triggered a wave of critical re-examination and some reforms (see Jussim et al., 2019a; Spellman, 2015). For example, research from 2009 to 2012 central to triggering the replication crisis included:

- Findings of impossibly high, "voodoo" correlations in fMRI (Vul et al., 2009) and other areas of research (Fiedler, 2009);
- A purported demonstration of ESP in the laboratory (Bem, 2011). Many interpreted this more as an indictment of conventional methods and practices in psychological science than as showing of the reality of ESP (e.g., Gelman, 2016; Nelson et al., 2018; Spellman, 2015);
- A failure to replicate (Doyen et al., 2012) an influential study purporting to show behavioral effects of priming social stereotypes (Bargh et al., 1996);
- A survey showing widespread use of questionable research practices, such as selective reporting of studies and analyses (John et al., 2012);

- A revelation of how common methodological and statistical practices can produce invalid and illusory results (Simmons et al., 2011);
- Research showing that psychological phenomena once thought to be universal did not reliably appear outside of Western college students (Heinrich et al., 2010); and
- A survey showing that many social psychologists endorsed discriminating against other scientists, and scientific findings, based on politics (Inbar & Lammers, 2012).

These are some examples of research that sparked what has been called the replication crisis (Spellman, 2015). However, whether the term is justified is debatable. Failed replications are a part of normal science (Simons, 2014). Furthermore, different scientists disagree not only about whether psychology's replication success rate is inadequately low, but also about what even constitutes successful or failed replications (compare, e.g., Aarts et al., 2015 with Gilbert et al., 2016).

The term "replication crisis" is also too narrow because psychological science can go wrong for many reasons other than failed replications. Even if the methods and practices are pristine, and the statistics correctly computed and reported, scientists can and do sometimes still reach erroneous conclusions. Indeed, elsewhere, we have argued that canonization is the key problem in psychological science, not replication. Canonization refers to the process by which some claim or conclusion is taken to be both true and important (Jussim et al., 2019a). The bottom line for scientific research is the creation of new knowledge. Thus, the most central product of science is not a study or even a replicated study; it is what is taken to be valid new knowledge. What gets canonized (taken to be new knowledge) can go wrong either because valid new discoveries are ignored or because invalid research is widely accepted as true. Obviously, the goal of the scientific enterprise is to canonize new knowledge that is actually true, not to ignore true conclusions or canonize false ones.

This chapter, therefore, reviews questionable interpretive practices (QIPs), which can contribute to and demonstrably have contributed to the canonization of false claims. Prior to canonization, however, is reaching conclusions based on data provided by individual studies. We first review the theoretical bases for expecting systematic errors and biases in scientists' interpretations of data; we then review some specific types of QIPs. Next, we provide several examples from published research demonstrating how QIPs produced erroneous or unjustified conclusions. Last, we provide some recommendations to researchers for how to limit QIPs in their own work. We start by reviewing two cases of the entirely scientific creation of mythic beliefs.

The Creation of Scientific Myths

Is the term "scientific myth" too strong, perhaps too pejorative? We do not think so. "Myth" usually refers to some sort of story that is at least partially false. Myths may hold some grain of truth, surrounded by exaggerations and compelling yet unjustified stories and narratives. For example, although it is pretty clear that the Loch Ness Monster is not some sort of surviving dinosaur, it is distinctly possible that some sort of very real modern sea creatures explain the endless sightings (sharks, eels, etc., e.g., BBC, 2019; Huffington Post, 2013). A myth is plausibly called "scientific" when it is promoted, endorsed, and advocated by people who meet conventional descriptions of scientists—they have advanced degrees in scientific fields, they conduct systematic studies, and they publish in peer-reviewed journals.

Bacteria, Not Stress, Cause Ulcers

The history of science is filled with such myths—beliefs widely held by scientists that seemed to have a "scientific" or "evidentiary" basis, but that were eventually shown to be false (e.g., geocentric universe, young Earth, bleeding to cure disease, stress causes ulcers). The case of ulcers (which are actually caused by bacteria) is perhaps most relevant to the present chapter because it occurred in the modern era during a time in which experimental methods were well understood and major advances in biology had been made (including the germ theory of disease), and after widespread adoption of peer-reviewed journals as gatekeepers supposedly ensured that only the highest-quality evidence made it into the scientific canon.

It took the biomedical community about 25 years from the discovery that bacteria, not stress, are the primary cause of ulcers, to actually accept this fact (Weintraub, 2010). Why did it take so long? First, Barry Marshall, the researcher who discovered this, was about as low in fame and prestige as possible: He was a medical student from the Australian Outback, working in a university in western Australia (Weintraub, 2010). Scientific acceptance of new ideas may hinge to some extent on evidence, but it also hinges to some extent on the fame and prestige of those promoting those ideas (e.g., Merton, 1968; Tomkins et al., 2017). Barry Marshall lacked both. Perhaps unsurprisingly, by some reports he was also something of an "unpolished" scientist with an unconventional style that included what some might have viewed as insufficient deference to his senior colleagues (Levitt & Dubner, 2014). Doctors had been treating ulcers as a psychosomatic problem resulting from stress for so many years that a multimillion-dollar pharmaceutical industry had been built around "stress as cause." Thus history, tradition, status, and prestige all conspired to make it exceedingly difficult for Marshall to even get a serious hearing, let alone succeed at impacting the practice of medicine. Thus, the longstanding claim that stress causes ulcers was a myth—a canonical claim, made by real scientists, taken for granted as being true among most real scientists, that was unjustified.

The Curious Case of Antidepressant "Effectiveness"

How do full-blown scientific myths emerge? Given oft-expressed confidence in the ability of conventional scientific norms and practices to produce valid findings (e.g., Jost, 2011; van Bavel et al., 2020), this is a pressing question. A recent paper provides a very clear and interesting answer. De Vries et al. (2018) followed academic scholarship production from the creation of new knowledge to the reaching of a bogus consensus in a field. Specifically, they first identified 105 trials assessing the effectiveness of various antidepressant interventions. This included many in a U.S. Food and Drug Administration (FDA) database. Because the FDA requires clinical trials before rollout to the general public, this database includes studies regardless of whether they were published or not; that is, it includes many unpublished studies.

De Vries et al. (2018) found that about half the studies showed intervention effectiveness and about half showed the intervention studied was ineffective. However, because of publication biases, nearly all of the "effective" studies but only about half the "ineffective" studies were published. Thus the *published* literature indicated far more effectiveness than did the *conducted* studies.

Bias then became more extreme from there, because of selective reporting of outcomes. As they put it, "Ten negative trials became 'positive' in the published literature, by omitting unfavorable outcomes or switching the status of the primary and secondary outcomes" (De Vries et al., 2018, pp. 2453–2454). On top of reporting bias, there was "spin"—by emphasizing the effectiveness of treatment despite nonsignificant results or by switching a primary result with no significant effect for a secondary result that had a significant effect. After publication biases, reporting biases, and spin, the published literature indicated that about 90% of the literature showed that the antidepressant interventions were effective.

But we are not done yet. De Vries et al.'s (2018) final analysis concerned which papers were cited, and it was almost exclusively the papers showing effective interventions. Therefore, the "scientific" literature based on studies that were half effective and half ineffective almost entirely emphasized that the interventions were effective. This is how mixed results are laundered into a beautiful consensus, and how scientific myths are created.

Questionable Interpretive Practices

One largely overlooked source of unjustified conclusions are what we call QIPs, the ways in which scholars reach unjustified conclusions even when the theoretical, methodological, and statistical characteristics of the research are sound and presented transparently (see Jussim et al., 2016c, for an introduction of this idea; see Jussim et al., 2016b, for a fuller review of ways in which interpretations go awry but one that never uses the term "QIP"). To be clear, results rarely explain themselves and there is usually more than one plausible explanation for a set of results. Yet, there are cases where a scientific interpretation is demonstrably false or unjustified. We use the term "false" to refer to a scientific interpretation that is demonstrably wrong. The term "unjustified," on the other hand, refers to a situation where the scientific observation offered cannot be considered false but is also not justified by the data presented.

For example, an inference that different seasons occur because the Earth moves closer to the sun is false, and not just unjustified. This is because seasons are determined by the tilt of the Earth, not its closeness to the sun. In contrast, an inference that a UFO is an alien visitation is unjustified. The "U" in UFO stands for "unidentified" and, as long as something is unidentified, it means that "we do not actually know what it is, so we cannot conclude that it is an alien visitation" (or anything else, really; if we could identify what it was, it would no longer be unidentified).

In other words, the researcher plays a pivotal role in every decision made in the research process (see Stevens et al., 2018). Empirical data need to be framed, presented, and interpreted by someone. Yet, identical data, evidence, or facts are routinely interpreted differently by different people. As a result, people with different interpretations may make different analytical decisions and draw different conclusions. Thus, even though good arguments have been made for stronger theories (Fiedler, 2017; Smaldino, 2019), better measurement (Flake & Fried, 2019; Reyna, 2017), statistical reform (Nelson et al., 2018), and greater transparency (e.g., Jussim et al., 2019a; Nosek et al., 2012; Spellman, 2015), we are skeptical they will be effective if QIPs are left unaddressed. Therefore, the rest of this section reviews the bases and manifestations of QIPs:

1. Theoretical bases for predicting QIPs among scientists; and
2. Some clear types and examples of QIPs from actual psychological research.

Theoretical Bases for Predicting Errors and Biases in Scientific Interpretations of Data

Motivated reasoning constitutes one basis for explaining why researchers misinterpret and miscommunicate their findings in ways that advance their favored conclusions. As discussed in seminal work on motivated reasoning (Kunda, 1990), two types of goals can influence information processing: accuracy goals and directional goals. Accuracy goals motivate people to reason objectively to arrive at the correct or best conclusion possible, whereas directional goals motivate people to reason selectively in order to reach particular, preferred conclusions. Preferred conclusions may be those that one would like to be true (desirability bias; Tappin et al., 2017) and/or those that one believes are in fact true (confirmation bias; Nickerson, 1998).

Although researchers are motivated to be accurate, the directional goals they possess can influence their reasoning. People evaluate evidence more favorably when it supports their beliefs and preferences, and more strongly critique evidence when it opposes their expected or desired views (Ditto &

Lopez, 1992; Edwards & Smith, 1996; Munro & Ditto, 1997; Taber & Lodge, 2006). In addition, people often use confirmatory hypothesis testing strategies and seek out evidence supporting a favored conclusion while failing to search for evidence opposing that view (Klayman & Ha, 1987; Wason, 1968). People are also more likely to interpret results as supporting (vs. challenging) their beliefs (Kahan et al., 2017). Researchers are not immune to these kinds of reasoning (Lilienfeld, 2010; Redding, 2001). In fact, some evidence suggests that those with stronger knowledge and expertise are more susceptible to directionally motivated reasoning (i.e., applying their skills selectively to reach desired conclusions; Kahan et al., 2017; for a failure to observe this effect see Ballarini & Sloman, 2017).

These processes are assumed to be directionally motivated because researchers consistently make errors and distort their results when claiming to find support for their theories, rather than evidence against them (Jussim et al., 2016b; Lilienfeld, 2010). Although people are prone to these biases, they are often unintentional, and can even be quite logical and justified. Beliefs and expectations are based on experience and prior exposure to evidence; therefore, it can be rational for people to more easily accept belief-consistent evidence and be more skeptical of evidence challenging their views (Jern et al., 2014; Koehler, 1993; Tversky & Kahneman, 1974). Nonetheless, it is one thing to *judge* the same evidence differently, based on past experience, and it is quite another to systematically *skew the process of interpretation* by cherry-picking, selectively criticizing work of which one disapproves, and leaping to unjustified conclusions. These and other sorts of QIPs are discussed next.

Types of Questionable Interpretative Practices

QIPs all have the effect of masking a valid conclusion beneath a plausible-seeming yet actually unjustified one. Masked phenomena may constitute alternative explanations for a pattern of results, reasons to believe the published interpretations are true but exaggerated, or reasons to believe the published interpretation is simply incorrect. Conclusions are typically masked because the original report does not even consider or acknowledge them, and because the data that are presented usually create the superficial appearance of support for the presented conclusions. In this section we focus on a number of QIPs that we will first define and then discuss in greater detail:

- Blind spots/cherry-picking: The overlooking of data (either one's own or from the wider literature) that conflict with one's conclusions. These QIPs are discussed together because they are rarely distinguishable from reading papers alone. Blind spots occur when a researcher truly is simply unaware that some evidence exists; cherry-picking occurs when a researcher is aware the evidence exists but purposely avoids it.
- Selective calls for rigor: This QIP occurs when work that one dislikes, disagrees with, opposes, or finds offensive is objected to on grounds of lack of rigor, whereas research that one likes, agrees with, values, and finds edifying is given a pass even though it suffers the exact same deficiencies in rigor (see Alexander, 2014). Often, the claims of scientific flaws or limitations regarding the criticized work may well be justified; but by not applying the same standards to work one supports, the failings of the latter work remain masked. This creates the unjustified impression that the work one supports has stronger scientific support than the work one opposes.
- Mythmaking/wow effects: Mythmaking refers to promoting findings in a dramatic way as if they are true when they are either false outright or, at best, not justified by the data. We refer to these dramatic findings as "wow" effects because they seem intended to "wow" readers and lead them to believe an amazing, possibly world-changing discovery has been made.
- Phantom facts: This QIP refers to instances when scientists declare something true without sufficient evidence to support that declaration.

Blind Spots and Cherry-Picking

Blind spots and cherry-picking both refer to overlooking data. As we have discussed, blind spots occur when a researcher truly is simply unaware that some evidence exists, whereas cherry-picking occurs when a researcher is aware that the evidence exists but purposely avoids it. Absent a confession by an author, however, distinguishing one from the other requires mindreading and is therefore impossible. Yet, it is often possible to identify the behavioral evidence of systematically failing to include evidence that conflicts with one's conclusion. This is one of the main reasons for recent innovations like preregistration, registered reports, and multiverse analyses, all of which make it far more difficult for researchers to selectively report data without being transparent about it (Jussim et al., 2019a; Steegen et al., 2016).

Example 1: Simpson's Paradox, Admissions at Berkeley

Simpson's paradox occurs when a valid statistical conclusion for an entire sample is invalid for all or some subsamples (Simpson, 1951). It is a classic example of a masked phenomenon and was at the core of a famous sex-discrimination lawsuit. At the University of California, Berkeley, admissions data revealed that about 44% of men but only 35% of women were admitted to graduate programs; Berkeley was then sued for gender bias (see Bickel et al., 1975). This difference is close to meeting legal standards for the possibility of discrimination (Greenwald et al., 2015), and an interpretation consistent with that of some scientists (e.g., Ledgerwood et al., 2015; Shen, 2013).

In the case of Berkeley, however, there was no bias. Women were at least as likely as men to be admitted to the departments to which they applied (Bickel et al., 1975). This was possible because *women disproportionately applied to the departments with lower admissions rates*. Within departments, women were *not* less likely to be admitted. The Wikipedia page on Simpson's paradox provides the information on admissions for the six largest departments; more detail can be found in Bickel et al.'s (1975) report, and Jussim et al. (2016b) walk readers through a simple hypothetical case.

A recent review concluded that "Simpson's paradox is more common than conventionally thought, and typically results in incorrect interpretations—potentially with harmful consequences. We support this claim by reviewing results from cognitive neuroscience, behavior genetics, clinical psychology, personality psychology, educational psychology, intelligence research, and simulation studies" (Kievit et al., 2013, p. 1). The authors argue that people, including scientists, are particularly poor at recognizing Simpson's paradox unless they explicitly engage in diagnostic tests to identify it (which they also recommend and describe). Because the data may *appear* to support some conclusion, but, in fact, do not, and the data themselves actually do provide the basis for identifying the correct conclusion (e.g., there is no data fraud), Simpson's paradox is the quintessential "masking" problem.

Example 2: Simpson's Paradox, Dutch Grant Funding

An investigation into Dutch grant funding found that male scientists received more grants than did female scientists, a result interpreted as "evidence of gender bias" (p. 12349; van der Lee & Ellemers, 2015). However, when Albers

QUESTIONABLE INTERPRETIVE PRACTICES   233

(2015) reanalyzed the data by discipline, he found, much like the Berkeley admissions data, women were more likely to apply to fields where funding was more difficult. In four disciplines, women had higher rates; in five, men had higher rates. However, when controlling for multiple comparisons, none of those differences was statistically significant.

Example 3: Citation Biases

One of the simplest ways researchers can mask the existence of contradictory evidence is by simply not citing it. For example, in 2012 and 2015, two papers reporting studies assessing gender biases in STEM hiring were both published in the same journal, *Proceedings of the National Academy of Sciences USA*, yielding opposite findings. One found evidence of biases favoring men (Moss-Racusin et al., 2012); the other found evidence of biases favoring women (Williams & Ceci, 2015).

This is plausibly viewed as a quasi-experiment: Would both papers be cited at similar rates? Table 9.1 (adapted from Honeycutt & Jussim, 2020) summarizes their key characteristics and citations, and shows that the paper finding biases against women has been cited at a vastly higher rate even though, by most conventional methodological quality metrics, it was of lower quality (fewer participants and studies). Not shown are other relative weaknesses, such as the fact that Moss-Racusin et al. (2012) only used a single method, whereas Williams and Ceci (2015) used several methods (e.g., between- and within-subjects designs), and when multiple methods produce the same result, one can be more confident in its validity.

These results are particularly striking for several reasons. First, the rightmost column reports only citations after the Williams and Ceci (2015) study

Table 9.1 Citations to Two Papers in the Same Journal Finding Opposite Patterns of Gender Bias

	Number of experiments	Total sample size	Main finding	Total citations (Google Scholar, 3-18-21)	Citations since 2015 (Google Scholar, 3-18-21)
Williams & Ceci (2015)	5	873	Bias favoring women	315	305
Moss-Racusin et al. (2012)	1	127	Bias favoring men	2,558	2,204

was published. This means that almost 1,200 papers have been published *after it came out* that did cite Moss-Racusin et al. (2012) but did not cite Williams and Ceci (2015). It also rules out alternative explanations: (1) It rules out prestige or visibility of journal effects (because it is the same journal); (2) It rules out topic differences (it was the same topic); and (3) Absent a selective call for rigor (see next section), it also rules out methodological quality, inasmuch as the Williams and Ceci (2015) study was superior to that of Moss-Racusin et al. (2012) with respect to most well-established metrics of methodological quality (sample size, replications; also Williams and Ceci used multiple methods in their five studies). The dramatically higher number of citation of the Moss-Racusin et al. (2012) study strongly indicates that the "scientific" literature on gender bias will itself be biased in the direction of overstating evidence for gender bias by virtue of the fact that so many papers overlooked or ignored contradictory evidence.

Is this pattern unique to these two papers? Quite the contrary. Table 9.2 reports a similar analysis for every study of gender bias in academic peer review that we could find. It shows two striking patterns: (1) Studies finding bias favoring men are cited at vastly higher rates than those finding either unbiased responding or biases favoring women and (2) The studies finding bias against women have vastly smaller sample sizes.

In an even more egregious case of simply overlooking relevant evidence, a review of gender by Ellemers (2018) appeared in *Annual Review of Psychology*, one of the outlets of record for our field. It concluded that gender stereotypes were mostly inaccurate: "Thus, if there is a kernel of truth underlying gender stereotypes, it is a tiny kernel" (p. 278). She reached this conclusion *without citing a single one of the 11 papers reporting 16 separate studies that actually assessed the accuracy of gender stereotypes* (see Jussim, 2018, for

Table 9.2 Citations to Papers Based on Whether or Not They Found Gender Bias Favoring Men

	Main result: Biases favoring men (4 papers)	Main result: Egalitarian responding or biases favoring women (6 papers)
Median sample size	182.5	2,311.5
Citations per year	51.5	9.0

Based on results reported in Jussim, 2019.

the full list of papers). Those 11 papers consistently found that gender stereotypes ranged from moderately to highly accurate (with some correlations between stereotype and criteria of 0.9 or higher; see reviews by Jussim et al., 2015; Jussim et al., 2009).

Selective Calls for Rigor

Selective calls for rigor constitute a different manifestation of the masking problem. By criticizing some disfavored body of work for failing to meet some standards, but by failing to apply the same standards to favored work, one effectively *masks* the weaknesses of the favored work and strongly implies or explicitly states that those weaknesses *only* apply to the disfavored work. Of course, any particular criticism may or may not be justified, and all such criticisms themselves need to be carefully scrutinized and evaluated on their merits. However, in our experience there are many times when criticisms of work are more flawed than the work being criticized (see, e.g., Jussim, 2005, and Jussim, 2012, for arguments that criticisms of work on social perceptual accuracy were more flawed than the work on social perceptual accuracy being criticized).

For example, an essay published in the *Chronicle of Higher Education* extolled the Moss-Racusin et al. (2012) paper described earlier (hence just "M-R") for finding bias against women in academic STEM hiring as "rigorous," but criticized on ostensibly methodological grounds the Williams and Ceci (2015; hence just "W&C") studies that found bias favoring women (Williams & Smith, 2015, hence just "W&S"). From the *Chronicle*: "The 2015 study, performed by Wendy M. Williams and Stephen J. Ceci, isn't rigorous. It's plagued by five serious methodological flaws." These are all worth considering on *their* merits:

1. W&S wrote: "Bias goes beyond the hiring hurdle." Of course it does. It is, however, logically impossible for this to constitute a reason to view M-R as superior to W&C. That is because biases beyond hiring were not addressed by *either* M-R or W&C. That M-R also fails this "test of rigor" is masked.
2. W&S claimed that W&C were subject to social desirability biases—that is, that their participants knew the study assessed gender bias, so they basically lied or distorted their responses to appear unbiased. M-R

used no special methods to avoid social desirability: Participants rated applicants for a lab manager position based on summary résumé information (GPA, GREs, excerpts from recommendations, and a personal statement); W&C's participants rated applicants for a faculty position based on a search committee chair's narrative summary of the scholarly record, job talk, and interviews in several studies; and based on their CV in one study). This criticism masks the fact that neither sets of procedures took any unusual steps to limit social desirability, beyond use of between-subjects designs.

3. W&S stated: "Williams and Ceci fail to pinpoint the effect of bias triggered by motherhood, which is a particularly strong form of gender bias." They referred to their findings as "mud" (i.e., effectively meaningless). This takes "selective call for rigor" to a whole new level. W&S did, in fact, perform two studies (Experiments 2 and 3) that examined biases due to parenthood. It was the M-R study that did not address these issues.

Thus, W&S's critique of W&C on "rigor" grounds smacks far more of bias on W&S's part than of any lack of rigor on W&C's part.

Mythmaking and "Wow" Effects

Mythmaking refers to promoting dramatic findings as if they are true when they are either false outright or, at best, not justified by the data. We refer to these "dramatic findings" as "wow" effects because they often seem to "wow" readers and to lead scientists to believe an amazing, possibly world-changing discovery has been made. A "wow" effect is some novel result that comes to be seen as having far-reaching implications, both for the conduct of science and for the real world. It is the type of work likely to be emulated, massively cited, and highly funded. But how can our stories be sufficiently compelling and persuasive to draw attention and be considered important when the average effect size in our field corresponds to a correlation of $r = 0.20$ (Richard et al., 2003), an estimate that may be exaggerated due to publication biases and questionable research practices (e.g., Bakker et al., 2012; Ioannidis, 2008)? How can scientists create beautiful narratives from data that are usually messy, only partially support their claims, are difficult to replicate, and are typically subject to alternative explanations? Although researchers may rarely intentionally misrepresent their findings, a witch's brew of suboptimal theories, methods, practices, and motivations other than seeking unvarnished truths (Jussim et al., 2019b), may have led to a slew of mythic "wow" effects entering the canon in social psychology. We briefly review two here.

Example 1: "But for Stereotype Threat, African Americans and Whites Would Have Equal Standardized Test Scores"
This common interpretation of the early classic (Steele & Aronson, 1995) research on stereotype threat can still be regularly found in the peer-reviewed literature (e.g., Pigliucci, 2013) despite having been debunked (e.g., Sackett et al., 2004). In the original paper (Steele & Aronson, 1995), three studies examined the effects of racial stereotype threats on the test performance of African American and White college students (one simply examined priming effects without assessing achievement and is not discussed here).

All three studies did show that, after controlling for prior SAT scores, there was no difference in test scores between African American and White students. This, however, is like showing that, after controlling for prior temperatures, there is no difference in the mean temperatures of Nome, Alaska, and Miami, Florida (something we actually demonstrated; Jussim et al., 2016b). Conceptually, the point is quite simple: "Controlling for prior achievement" means "removing differences due to prior achievement." So, if you remove differences due to prior achievement, and nothing else changes, there will be no apparent differences—not because there are no real differences but because you have already removed them! Equal *adjusted* means are not equivalent to *equal means*.

This unjustified interpretation was once common. In referring to the original study (Steele & Aronson, 1995), Aronson et al. (1999, p. 30) stated that African American students performed "about as well as Whites when the same test was presented as a nonevaluative problem solving task." Wolfe and Spencer (1996, p. 180) declared that, "One simple adjustment to the situation (changing the description of the test) eliminated the performance differences between Whites and African-Americans."

After Sackett et al. (2004) exposed the erroneous nature of this interpretation, Steele and Aronson (2004, p. 48) acknowledged that the gap was not eliminated: "In fact, without this [covariate] adjustment, they [referring to the African American students in their studies in the no-threat conditions] would be shown to perform still worse than Whites." One could view this exchange as science functioning well. When errors are made, normal processes of skeptical criticism identify them, and scientific self-correction occurs.

Unfortunately, subsequent characterizations of Steele and Aronson's (1995) results did not change as much as this exchange suggests they should have. For example, Schmader et al. (2008, p. 336) stated that Steele and Aronson (1995) showed that: "African American college students performed worse than their White peers on standardized test questions when this task was described to them as being diagnostic of their verbal ability but that their performance was equivalent to that of their White peers when the same questions were simply framed as an exercise in problem solving (and after accounting for prior SAT scores)." Similarly, Walton et al. (2013, p. 5) wrote: "In a classic series of studies, Black students performed worse than White students on a GRE test described as evaluative of verbal ability, an arena in which Blacks are negatively stereotyped. But when the same test was described as nonevaluative—rendering the stereotype irrelevant—Blacks performed as well as Whites (controlling for SAT scores; Steele & Aronson, 1995)."

These statements are technically true, and there are plenty of others like them in the peer-reviewed psychological science literature (e.g., Appel & Kronberger, 2012; Walton & Spencer, 2009) and a general statement by one of the major professional psychology societies (American Psychological Association, 2006). The language is, however, highly convoluted. This is necessary because to render the statements technically true, the declaration that African American and White scores are "equivalent" in nonthreatening conditions needs to be qualified by what is plausibly viewed as sleight of hand in plain sight—adding the parenthetical regarding "controlling for prior SAT scores." The actual result that preexisting differences continued even under no-threat conditions is not stated and is not apparent absent a very close reading of the text and a deep understanding of what analysis of covariance does and does not show.

It would not have been difficult to avoid nearly all of these misrepresentations and distortions. All that would have been needed is for the original report to have presented the actual cell means rather than (or in addition to) the adjusted cell means. Sunshine remains one of the best disinfectants.

Example 2: "90% of Americans Are Unconscious Racists!"
That may seem like an absurd, extreme claim, probably because it is, especially considering that it was made shortly after the publication of a single peer-reviewed paper reporting a single study investigating racism that included a grand total of 26 Washington University students (Greenwald et al., 1998). Nonetheless, this was the statement made by Greenwald and Banaji at a press conference in 1998 (Schwartz, 1998).

In fairness, they had begun collecting data from an online source with far larger numbers, so the statement was not based solely on the publication. Also in fairness, however, is the fact that the scientific community had, at that point, literally zero opportunity to critically or skeptically evaluate the validity of such extreme claims. Over the subsequent 20 years, nearly every part of that claim has proven false or unjustified. Implicit Association Test scores are not unconscious, clear measures of prejudice, or even clear measures of associations; they are unstable and have low predictive validities for behavior; they are scored in such a way as to overstate the extent and pervasiveness of prejudice; and their construct validity is low (Blanton et al., 2015a; Blanton et al., 2015b; Jussim et al., in press; Schimmack, 2019). In short, they provide no evidence of anything unconscious, and the evidence they provide about any sort of racism remains unclear even after over 20 years of research. Of course "90% of Americans are unconscious racists!" is far more of a "wow" effect than "We found some interesting results with the Implicit Association Test, and we look forward to doing the hard work necessary to fully understand them."

Phantom Facts

One example of a long-held and widely believed phantom fact is that "stress causes ulcers" (discussed earlier in this chapter). It is probably impossible to develop an exhaustive list of sources for phantom facts, but many of them seem to be derived from:

- Overconfidence in the conclusions reached by uncertain methods
- Leaping to conclusions by underestimating the uncertainty surrounding one's methods, statistics, and their interpretations
- Failure to consider alternative explanations
- Misunderstanding statistics
- Wishful thinking

Additionally, many "wow" effects also constitute phantom facts. The claim that "remove threat and eliminate the gap in African American and White standardized test scores" is a phantom fact because there was never any evidence supporting it. Similarly, the claim that 90% of Americans are unconscious racists was also a phantom fact. Next, we provide additional evidence of two other phantom facts in psychology.

Example 1: Inaccurate Stereotypes
In science, the convention is to support empirical claims with evidence, typically via a citation. This is a very important norm because scientists should not be in the business of presenting speculations as if they are facts. In the case of stereotypes, however, this scientific norm has been repeatedly violated. Claims that stereotypes are "inaccurate" pervade the social sciences (see Jussim, 2012; Jussim et al., 2016a, for reviews). However, such claims *almost never* cite empirical research assessing stereotype accuracy because most of that work shows moderate to high levels of accuracy (Jussim, 2012; Jussim et al., 2016a). Instead, scientific articles have declared stereotypes to be inaccurate either *without a single citation* or by citing an article that declares stereotypes to be inaccurate without itself citing empirical evidence. We have called this "the black hole at the bottom of declarations of stereotype inaccuracy" (Jussim et al., 2016a). For example:

> "[S]tereotypes are maladaptive forms of categories because their content does not correspond to what is going on in the environment" (Bargh & Chartrand, 1999, p. 467): No evidence was cited to support this claim.
>
> "If there is a kernel of truth underlying gender stereotypes, it is a tiny kernel" (Ellemers, 2018, p. 277): This claim was made without citing a single one of the 11 papers reporting 16 studies published in peer-reviewed journals that actually assessed the accuracy of gender stereotypes.

Sometimes, researchers may define stereotypes as inaccurate, rather than concluding that, empirically, they are inaccurate. This, however, would require them to first report empirical evidence showing that any given belief they have labeled as a "stereotype" is inaccurate—something that, as far as we can tell, has almost never been done (Jussim, 2012; Jussim et al., 2009, 2015, 2016a). Thus, although empirical evidence may occasionally uncover specific stereotype beliefs that are highly inaccurate, any claim that stereotypes are *generally* inaccurate is a phantom fact.

Example 2: Curious Cases of Confusing Correlations with Means

Lewandowsky et al. (2013) published a paper titled "NASA Faked the Moon Landing—Therefore (Climate) Science is a Hoax"—a title that strongly implies that people who doubt global warming believe bizarre conspiracy theories. As Lewandowsky et al. (2013, p. 622) put it, "[C]onspiratorial thinking contributes to the rejection of science." Their evidence for this conclusion comprised 1,145 respondents' beliefs in various conspiracies and their acceptance of science conclusions (HIV causes AIDs, burning fossil fuels increases atmospheric temperatures, etc.). Lewandowsky et al. (2013) subjected these measures to latent variable modeling and did indeed find that "conspiracist ideation" negatively predicted (−0.21, standardized regression coefficient) acceptance of climate science. So, where is the problem?

The title explicitly draws a link between belief in the moon landing hoax and belief in a climate science hoax, even stipulating a causal direction or cognitive process. However, they had *no data to support such a claim*. This is a classic *phantom fact, where something is stated as true without evidence*. Ten participants (out of 1,145) endorsed the moon landing hoax. But it gets worse: 134 believed climate science was a hoax, but *only three of them endorsed the moon landing hoax* (there was no midpoint or neutral option in their survey, just a four-point scale of Strongly Disagree, Disagree, Agree, and Strongly Agree—we are treating both "Agree" and "Strongly Agree" responses as "agreeing that climate science is a hoax"). The number of people who believed the titular claim that the moon landing was faked and therefore climate science was a hoax was trivially small.

The authors also performed some sophisticated structural equation modeling. They are still, however, correlational analyses from correlational data. Lewandowsky et al.'s (2013) interpretations of their findings conflated the sign of the correlational results with participants' actual placement on the items. Correlations resulted from covariance in levels of agreement among reasonable positions. Specifically, there were varying levels of *disbelief* in hoaxes—and the correlation occurred entirely because *strength* of *disbelief* in one hoax covaried with *strength of disbelief* in other hoaxes—but *almost no one* actually *believed* in these hoaxes. Their findings do show that the more people disbelieved hoaxes, the more they believed in climate science. However, too few believed in most of the hoaxes to warrant reaching *any general* conclusions about people who believe in conspiracy theories.

Potential Solutions to QIPs

Error is an inherent feature of the research process, but erroneous conclusions are not, in and of themselves, indicative of an unhealthy science. By revising conclusions in the face of new information, mistakes are corrected and knowledge advances. A healthy science attempts to minimize errors and is motivated to quickly self-correct when they are discovered.

As noted earlier in the chapter, accuracy goals and directional goals can influence information processing (Kunda, 1990) and although researchers are motivated to be accurate, directional goals can still influence their reasoning (Ditto & Lopez, 1992; Edwards & Smith, 1996; Munro & Ditto, 1997; Taber & Lodge, 2006). Furthermore, cognitive confirmation biases and social norms can also lead conclusions to go astray (Jussim et al, 2019a). This is what makes limiting QIPs so challenging. We identify two different classes of ways to limit one's vulnerability to QIPs:

1. Strategic approaches, defined as broad and general ways of approaching every aspect of science, from choosing collaborators and topics, to conducting and interpreting studies. Such approaches articulate broad principles that can undergird strong science, and may have direct implications for specific practices, but are not, themselves, specific practices.
2. Specific practices, which represent concrete, specific, actionable steps that researchers can take to limit their vulnerability to QIPs.

Strategic Approaches

In this section we recommend the adoption of two principles that may help limit the influence of QIPs in the social sciences:

1. Embrace skepticism and, acknowledge and recognize uncertainty; and
2. Increase viewpoint diversity.

Embrace Skepticism, and Acknowledge and Recognize Uncertainty

As we previously noted, a key problem in psychological science is canonization. One of the main sources of canonization is excessive reliance on null hypothesis significance testing. Obtaining a statistically significant result (or p < 0.05) remains one of the most important gatekeepers for publication (Simmons et al., 2011), and for much of its existence, psychological scientists have treated results obtained as p < 0.05 as having established a new scientific fact (Jussim et al., 2019b).

However, in recent years, an entire cloud of controversies has emerged around the concept of "statistical significance." Many statisticians and methodologists have argued that the p < 0.05 cutoff for "statistical significance" is too lenient, and that p < 0.005 should be used before considering something "statistically significant" (Benjamin et al., 2017). Others, however, have argued that there is no one-size-fits-all statistical threshold (Lakens et al., 2018). Yet others argue against using *any threshold at all*, nicely captured by a paper titled "The Difference Between 'Significant' and 'Not Significant' Is Not Itself Statistically Significant" (Gelman & Stern, 2006).

In this context, it should not be surprising that the executive director of the American Statistical Association was the first author of a paper (Wasserstein et al., 2019) including the following quotes (all on p. 2):

- "Don't Say 'Statistically Significant'" (section heading)
- "[A] declaration of statistical significance today has become meaningless."
- "[T]he statistical and ordinary language meanings of the word [significance] have become hopelessly confused."
- "A label of statistical significance adds nothing to what is already conveyed by the value p; in fact, this dichotomization of p-values makes matters worse."
- "[N]o p-value can reveal the plausibility, presence, truth, or importance of an effect."
- "[A] label of statistical significance does not mean or imply that an association or effect is highly probable, real, true, or important."

Numerous techniques have been nominated as improvements. Some argue that Bayesian analyses can be used to address some of the issues with p-values by virtue of making researchers' often hidden subjective assumptions explicit and by requiring comparison of alternative models (see Chapter 7 in this volume). Lakens (2017, 2021), however, has argued that null hypothesis tests and p-values can be used to test alternative models and even to accept a hypothesis that an effect is too small to matter (something intended to replace "accepting the null"). Multiverse analyses require researchers to perform and report every possible way of testing some hypothesis or answering some question, thereby eliminating the uncertainty that comes from not knowing whether different analytical approaches produce different results (Steegan et al., 2016).

Methodological approaches to reducing uncertainty are also being developed or are experiencing a renaissance. Chapter 8 in this volume reviews the need for stimulus sampling—testing multiple operations of potential causes (e.g., through experimental manipulations) so that results are not an idiosyncratic function of some unique stimulus (an old concept that goes back to Brunswik's [1952] call for ecological design). Blinded data analysis (i.e., conducting statistical analyses without knowing which variables are which; Chapter 11 in this volume) can dramatically reduce researchers' tendencies toward confirmation biases. Although most of these techniques are themselves controversial or too new to conclude that they are inherently superior, researchers interested in improving statistical inference should familiarize themselves with them for consideration of possible adoption.

Intellectual Diversity

As this entire book suggests, much research in the social sciences is shrouded in various degrees of uncertainty. Our view is that embracing intellectual diversity is one of the best approaches toward resolving that uncertainty. Intellectual diversity refers to the idea that, especially when the truth is uncertain, people are justified in holding alternative views or perspectives regarding what the truth actually is. Until science resolves those differences through strong tests that permit falsifying some of them, lots of views may be "wrong," but there is no way to know which ones. Therefore, the shortest path to truth is often by pitting alternative views against each other (Platt, 1964; Washburn & Skitka, 2018).

Our view is that intellectual diversity can be viewed as having four major components: skepticism, theoretical diversity, demographic diversity, and political diversity (especially for many of the politicized topics in the social sciences). Skepticism is a form of intellectual diversity because it involves treating some scientific claim to truth with doubt that then challenges the claimants to either produce stronger evidence or change the claim. As such, Merton (1973) argued that skepticism was one of four key norms of science. Some of the worst features of psychology's replication crisis might have been averted had the field embraced a norm of skepticism much earlier.

Theoretical diversity is also important because, until the data are so clear and compelling that one theory "wins," competition between alternative views can highlight the strengths and weaknesses of each and thereby motivate researchers to either recognize that the differences between theories are irresolvable, or identify ways to resolve them. Either conclusion advances science. If the differences are irresolvable, then at least scientists can realize they should not be in the business of making strong truth claims; if it is resolvable, then perhaps it will actually be resolved. Loeb (2014), writing in *Nature: Physics*, captured this dynamic beautifully:

- "Discoveries in astronomy—or, in fact, any branch of science—can only happen when people are open-minded and willing to take risks." (p. 616)
- "Uniformity of opinions is sterile; the co-existence of multiple ideas cultivates competition and progress. Of course, it is difficult to know in advance which exploratory path will bear fruit." (p. 617)
- "[F]unding agencies should dedicate a fixed fraction of their resources (say, 10–20%) to risky explorations. This can be regarded as affirmative action to promote a diversity of ideas, which is as important for the progress of science as the promotion of gender and ethnic diversity." (p. 617)

Of course, gender and ethnic diversity are also components of intellectual diversity, especially in the social sciences. People from different backgrounds bring different experiences to bear on understanding the human condition—which obviously involves all people, not just those from selected ethnic, economic, or regional groups. This argument is now commonplace throughout academia, and, although this idea has only recently been subject to empirical tests, those tests have generally supported it (e.g., Hofstra et al., 2020).

Less commonplace and widely accepted is the need for political diversity—although the substantive arguments and analysis for its benefits are essentially identical to those that constitute scientific justifications for demographic diversity. Especially in fields that address political or politicized topics, having people from different political backgrounds available to skeptically vet one another's work is probably essential to making any progress toward truth on many topics. It will also have the side benefit of increasing the credibility of work on politicized topics among policymakers and the lay public. After all, if scientists reach a consensus on some politicized topic but all or most are on one side of the partisan divide, it will be quite difficult for the public to know whether the science is valid or simply a masquerade for political ax-grinding. On the other hand, if scientists from across the political spectrum reach consensus that some conclusion on some politicized topic is actually true, laypeople and policymakers will have a much more difficult time dismissing that as the work of biased researchers.

Of course, embracing different viewpoints may not be necessary *after* science has settled an issue with very high degrees of certainty. For example, we do not need to debate whether evolution occurs; no one's skepticism, theory, demography, or politics is the least bit relevant to that claim. However, there remains a great deal of uncertainty regarding *how* evolution occurs (e.g., Mesoudi, 2015). And in the social and behavioral sciences, uncertainty is the rule rather than the exception. Until our methods are so well honed and the data so compelling that they can conclusively resolve controversies, intellectual diversity, by offering a myriad of ways forward, offers the best opportunity to uncover truths or uncover limitations to our ability to conclusively determine truths.

Specific Practices

Adversarial or Courageous Collaborations

One recommendation we offer is that researchers engage in adversarial or courageous collaborations with those who endorse different theoretical explanations for the phenomenon of interest. Such collaborations may limit the impact of motivated reasoning on the research process (see Stevens et al., 2018) by reducing the likelihood that processes like confirmation bias, desirability bias, or group polarization occur.

Stern and Crawford (2021) recently engaged in such a collaboration that investigated the presence of "symmetry" or "asymmetry" with respect to the views liberals and conservatives hold toward their ideological rivals (see Brandt & Crawford, 2019). The symmetry hypothesis is that liberals and conservatives are similarly biased or hostile toward one another. The asymmetry hypothesis was that conservatives would be more biased or hostile to liberals than liberals to conservatives. Three studies examined the impact of ideological identities on perceived dissimilarity on specific topics (political and nonpolitical), prejudice, and affiliative intentions. Clear hypotheses were presented and while in some instances the authors predicted the same pattern of results, in others they made adversarial predictions (see Stern & Crawford, 2021). Interestingly, although the results were nuanced (see Table 1 in Stern & Crawford, 2021) and not fully consistent with either author's predictions, the main findings (regarding political topics) did find asymmetry—but it was a different type of asymmetry than either had predicted. In brief, they found "liberal asymmetry" dominated perceptions of political topics, which meant that liberals were actually more hostile and biased than were conservatives. Although this result was not predicted by either group, it nonetheless testifies to the values of such collaboration—it was only because research was designed to test for any possible pattern of symmetry and asymmetry that this surprising result was found.

The adversarial nature of Stern and Crawford's (2021) collaboration is encouraging. When their hypotheses conflicted, confirmatory evidence for one hypothesis represents a refutation of the other hypothesis, thereby instantiating a process of falsification—the pervasive lack of which, at least in psychology, may have contributed to the replication crisis (Morey & Lakens, 2017). Popper long ago identified vague predictions as a problem for science, and the social sciences in particular, and offered a series of criteria for theory testing (see Popper, 1963/2002, pp. 47–48):

1. It is easy to obtain confirmations, or verifications, for nearly every theory—if we look for confirmations.
2. Confirmations should count only if they are the result of risky predictions; that is to say, if, unenlightened by the theory in question, we should have expected an event which was incompatible with this theory—an event that would have refuted the theory.
3. Every 'good' scientific theory is a prohibition: it forbids certain things to happen. The more clearly a theory statement identifies what it forbids, the better it is.
4. A theory which is not refutable by any conceivable event is non-scientific. Irrefutability is not a virtue of theory (as people often think) but a vice.
5. Testability is falsifiability; but there are degrees of testability: some theories are more testable, more exposed to refutation, than others; they take as it, were greater risks.

6. Confirming evidence should not count, except when it is the result of a genuine test of the theory; and this means that it can be presented as a serious but unsuccessful attempt to falsify the theory.
7. Some genuinely testable theories, when found to be false, are still upheld by their admirers—for example by introducing ad hoc some auxiliary assumption, or by re-interpreting the theory ad hoc in such a way that it escapes refutation. Such a procedure is always possible, but it rescues the theory from refutation only at the price of destroying, or at least lowering, its scientific status.

Popper (1963/2002) offered these criteria as a way to prevent a researcher from making predictions so vague that they could hardly fail, something he referred to as the "soothsayer's trick." The Stern and Crawford (2021) collaboration provides a clear example of how an adversarial collaboration can help prevent researchers from making vague predictions that lower the evidentiary hurdles their results would need to surmount to lend support to their theory, and avoid mounting a Lakatosian defense (see Meehl, 1990) for results that contradict their preferred theory.

Strong Inference

This is the term used to cover an approach to research that involves identifying opposing predictions generated by alternative theories and then pitting them against one another (Platt, 1964; Washburn & Skitka, 2018). Social psychology articles that pit alternative hypotheses against one another are few and far between. Instead, the typical article develops some theoretical perspective in the introduction, derives one or more hypotheses, and reports one or more studies testing those hypotheses. Although it is fairly common for papers to attempt to rule out artifactual explanations for their findings (e.g., ceiling or floor effects, social desirability), full-throated pitting of predictions generated by competing theories remains rare.

Platt (1964) argued that doing so can rapidly accelerate scientific progress by quickly eliminating false alternatives. He relayed the story of how Francis Bacon proposed resolving whether weight reflected the "inherent nature" of an object, or the pull of gravity from the Earth (a pull that would decrease with distance from the Earth): Bacon proposed that one could compare the time produced by a pendulum clock on the ground versus on a tall steeple (against, say, a spring clock). If the pendulum clock goes slower on the top of the steeple, weight reflects gravity. End of debate.

As a more modern example, Firestone and Scholl (2014) used the method to demonstrate that top-down processes could not possibly explain the results of a study seeming to show that recalling unethical (vs. ethical) actions led participants to see the physical world as darker (less well-lit). The original study used a simple numerical scale to rate lightness (Bannerjee et al., 2012). In contrast, Firestone and Scholl (2014) had participants compare colors by matching the room's brightness to gray-scale patches. If recalling unethical actions makes the world grow darker, then there should be no effect on the matching outcome because everything should look darker (the room, the patches, and everything else), producing no net effect on this outcome. In contrast, if the effect in the Bannerjee et al. (2012) study was produced by a non-perceptual process (e.g., change of standards or explicit use of metaphorical reasoning), one should still obtain participants choosing darker patches. The latter result is what Firestone and Scholl (2014) obtained, indicating that the effect of recalling unethical actions on responses was not a perceptual one.

Strong inference, by pitting alternative hypotheses against one another, ensures some hypothesis is going to be disconfirmed. In contrast, until recently, normal operating procedure in social psychology was to test a single hypothesis or a set of related (rather than competing) hypotheses against a theoretically unspecified null hypothesis; if the null was rejected, publication would follow, but if the null was not rejected, the study rarely saw the light of day. The possibility that the study provided evidence for a different hypothesis or theory was ignored.

We suspect that the very process of considering possible alternatives would improve the research process and consider the Stern and Crawford (2021) project as a prime example. Social judgment biases can be pitted against social perceptual accuracy (West & Kenny, 2011); self-fulfilling prophecies can and have been pitted against self-verification (Swann & Ely, 1984); and top-down perceptual processes can be pitted against bottom-up ones (Firestone & Scholl, 2016). Although alternative theories can sometimes be integrated (Jussim, 1991; Jussim et al., 1987), there will, sometimes, be winners and losers. We not only need to tolerate evidence indicating that a theory has lost but also need to celebrate researchers who take the risk of comparing their pet theory to its rivals (a process that adversarial collaboration also explicitly promotes).

Explicitly Stating How One's Theory or Hypotheses Could Be Falsified

Another option is to strongly encourage researchers to explicitly articulate how the data could disconfirm their theory or hypotheses in the particular study, and what could lead them to conclude that the hypothesis was probably false. It is well known that commonly used null hypothesis significance tests are incapable of disproving the null, which can be viewed as rigging the game in favor of confirmation. Either the result is "significant"—and, by longstanding tradition, such results are usually taken as hypothesis confirmation—or null, which fails to falsify the hypothesis, thereby creating a scientific literature with dubious capacity for falsification.

Philosophy of science perspectives have long embraced some version of falsification as central to science (e.g., Merton, 1973; Mill, 1859; Popper, 1959). Many of those who followed Popper recognized that falsification is often very difficult, and rarely occurs from a single definitive test, but also acknowledged a crucial role for tests disconfirming theoretical predictions (e.g., Kuhn, 1970; Lakatos & Musgrave, 1970; Meehl, 1990). For example, although Kuhn (1970) did not adopt Popper's version of falsificationism, he argued that when there is a sufficient accumulation of findings that cannot be accounted for by an existing theoretical paradigm, a scientific revolution may occur, from which a new paradigm emerges which often can account for the previous anomalous findings. Furthermore, one of the most common defenses of the scientific status of social psychology is that, if we get something wrong, we "self-correct" (e.g., Jost & Andrews, 2011; Markman, 2010). One can only "self-correct" if one acknowledges that, "Well, we used to believe the evidence showed X, but now that we have seen new evidence, we know that X is not the whole story and, possibly, not true at all."

There is a special onus on scientists to embrace falsificationism as one way to combat the powerful tendencies toward confirmation bias in science (Ioannidis, 2005; Jussim et al., 2016b). One of the most effective methods to avoid confirmation bias is to "consider the opposite" (Lord et al., 1984). This idea can be considered a more general form of Platt's (1964) "strong inference" approach that pits conflicting theories against one another. This method implicitly incorporates falsificationism, because if, in the particular study, one finding is confirmed and another disconfirmed, one set of predictions has indeed been falsified. It is also synergistic with adversarial collaborations in which both sides acknowledge that the study may more strongly confirm the other side's views than one's own.

Conclusion

In this chapter, we developed the idea of *questionable interpretive practices*: systematic errors and biases in how scientists reach conclusions based on data. A wealth of research in psychology and other behavioral sciences has identified a host of social, cognitive, and motivational forces that can and, at least sometimes, actually do push scientists to reach invalid or unjustified conclusions. Blind spots, cherry-picking both of results within a study and of studies (based on their results), selective calls for rigor, mythmaking, unjustified claims of "wow" effects, and phantom facts were all identified as ways in which, even if the underlying empirical research is pristine, psychologists can and have reached unjustified conclusions.

We have also argued that the most central problem in psychology (and possibly related disciplines) is not replications, methods, or statistics. Those are all means to an end. The bottom line for any field seeking to uncover new knowledge is *canonization*—what is widely believed to be true based on that field's scholarship. In this context, interpretation can be viewed as crucial to a functional and productive scientific endeavor. No matter how good the studies are, if we get the interpretations wrong, what gets canonized—what we think we have learned from that research—goes wrong (Table 9.3).

In this chapter, we reviewed several areas in which manifestly wrong or unjustified conclusions had been reached, including:

- Decades misspent treating stress as the source of ulcers
- Creation of a "scientific" consensus literature attesting to the effectiveness of antidepression interventions, even though the underlying empirical literature was half ineffective interventions

Table 9.3 Canonization

Research is:	Ignored	Canonized
False or misleading	NO HARM comes from ignoring bad research	REIGN OF ERROR It can take decades to correct bad research that becomes widely accepted
Valid	MISSED OPPORTUNITY Knowledge is impoverished, applications likely ineffective and may be harmful	IDEAL Understanding, theory and applications enhanced by relevant knowledge

- Unjustified allegations of gender discrimination at UC Berkeley and in Dutch grant funding
- Selective calls for rigor when evaluating studies finding opposite patterns of gender bias in STEM hiring
- Stereotype threat and implicit bias as classic examples of mythmaking and "wow" effects
- Two examples of phantom facts: claims that stereotypes are inaccurate and that climate denial is linked to believing bizarre conspiracy theories

There is ample evidence that questionable interpretive practices go well beyond the few examples reviewed here. Work on microaggressions has not been vetted with enough rigor to warrant its widespread use in applications and social programs (Lilienfeld, 2017). Social psychology's longstanding overemphasis on situations as having far more effects on behavior than personality and individual differences is vastly overstated (Funder, 2009). And there is a growing body of literature arguing that researchers' ideology certainly predicts and probably causes different researchers to reach different conclusions about a wide range of politicized topics (e.g., Buss & von Hippel, 2018; Clark & Winegard, 2020; Crawford & Jussim, 2017; Honeycutt & Jussim, 2020). We suggest that one important mechanism by which these sorts of biases occur is through the types of questionable interpretive practices identified here.

We also reviewed strategies for limiting questionable interpretive practices:

- Embrace skepticism and intellectual diversity
- Adversarial/courageous collaborations
- Strong inference
- Inclusion of explicit falsification statements

The widespread and varied manifestations of questionable interpretive practices suggest to us that limiting their influence on psychological science is likely to be difficult. On the other hand, if one wishes for psychological research to live up to its claims to be a scientific field, identifying methods and practices that increase the validity and credibility of its conclusions is worth the effort. Indeed, our view is that improving processes of interpretation and canonization is crucial to doing so.

References

Aarts, A. A., Anderson, J. E., Anderson, C. J., Attridge, P. R., Attwood, A., Axt, J., Babel, M., Bahnik, S., Baranski, E., Barnett-Cown, M., Bartmess, E., Beer, J., Bell, R., Bentley, H., Beyan, L., Binion, G., Borsboom, D., Bosch, A., Bosco, F. A., . . . Zuni, K. (2015). Estimating the reproducibility of psychological science. *Science, 349*(6251), 943.

Albers, C. J. (2015). Dutch research funding, gender bias, and Simpson's paradox. *Proceedings of the National Academy of Sciences USA, 112*(50), E6828–E6829.

Alexander, S. (2014). Beware isolated demands for rigor. https://slatestarcodex.com/2014/08/14/beware-isolated-demands-for-rigor/

American Psychological Association. (2006a). Stereotype threat widens the achievement gap. https://www.apa.org/research/action/stereotype

Appel, M., & Kronberger, N. (2012). Stereotypes and the achievement gap: Stereotype threat prior to test taking. *Educational Psychology Review, 24*, 609–635. https://doi-org.proxy.libraries.rutgers.edu/10.1007/s10648-012-9200-4

Aronson, J., Lustina, M. J., Good, C., Keough, K., Steele, C. M., & Brown, J. (1999). When white men can't do math: Necessary and sufficient factors in stereotype threat. *Journal of Experimental Social Psychology, 35*(1), 29–46.

Bakker, M., van Dijk, A., & Wicherts, J. M. (2012). The rules of the game called psychological science. *Perspectives on Psychological Science, 7*(6), 543–554.

Ballarini, C., & Sloman, S. A. (2017). Reasons and the "motivated numeracy effect." *Proceedings of the 39th Annual Meeting of the Cognitive Science Society*, 1580–1585.

Banerjee, P., Chatterjee, P., & Sinha, J. (2012). Is it light or dark? Recalling moral behavior changes perception of brightness. *Psychological Science, 23*(4), 407–409.

Bargh, J. A., & Chartrand, T. L. (1999). The unbearable automaticity of being. *American Psychologist, 54*(7), 462.

Bargh, J. A., Chen, M., & Burrows, L. (1996). Automaticity of social behavior: Direct effects of trait construct and stereotype activation on action. *Journal of Personality and Social Psychology, 71*(2), 230.

BBC. (2019). Loch Ness Monster may be a giant eel, say scientists. https://www.bbc.com/news/uk-scotland-highlands-islands-49495145

Bem, D. J. (2011). Feeling the future: Experimental evidence for anomalous retroactive influences on cognition and affect. *Journal of Personality and Social Psychology, 100*(3), 407.

Benjamin, D. J., Berger, J. O., Johannesson, M., Nosek, B. A., Wagenmakers, E-J., Berk, R., Bollen, K A., Brembs, B., Brown, L., Camerer, C., Cesarini, D., Chambers, C. D., Clyde, M., Cook, T. D., De Boeck, P., Dienes, Z., Dreber, A., Easwaran, K., Efferson., C., . . . Johnson, V. E. (2017). Redefine statistical significance. *Nature: Human Behavior, 2*, 6–10.

Bickel, P. J., Hammel, E. A., & O'Connell, J. W. (1975). Sex bias in graduate admissions: Data from Berkeley. *Science, 187*(4175), 398–404.

Blanton, H., Jaccard, J., & Burrows, C. N. (2015). Implications of the implicit association test D-transformation for psychological assessment. *Assessment, 22*(4), 429–440.

Blanton, H., Jaccard, J., Strauts, E., Mitchell, G., & Tetlock, P. E. (2015). Toward a meaningful metric of implicit prejudice. *Journal of Applied Psychology, 100*(5), 1468.

Brandt, M. J., & Crawford, J. T. (2019). Studying a heterogeneous array of target groups can help us understand prejudice. *Current Directions in Psychological Science, 28*(3), 292–298.

Brunswik, E. (1952). *The Conceptual Framework of Psychology*. University of Chicago Press.
Buss, D. M., & von Hippel, W. (2018). Psychological barriers to evolutionary psychology: Ideological bias and coalitional adaptations. *Archives of Scientific Psychology*, 6(1), 148.
Clark, C. J., & Winegard, B. M. (2020). Tribalism in war and peace: The nature and evolution of ideological epistemology and its significance for modern social science. *Psychological Inquiry*, 31(1), 1–22.
Crawford, J. T., & Jussim, L. (Eds.). (2017). *Politics of Social Psychology*. Psychology Press.
De Vries, Y. A., Roest, A. M., de Jonge, P., Cuijpers, P., Munafò, M. R., & Bastiaansen, J. A. (2018). The cumulative effect of reporting and citation biases on the apparent efficacy of treatments: The case of depression. *Psychological Medicine*, 48(15), 2453–2455.
Ditto, P. H., & Lopez, D. F. (1992). Motivated skepticism: Use of differential decision criteria for preferred and nonpreferred conclusions. *Journal of Personality and Social Psychology*, 63, 569–584.
Doyen, S., Klein, O., Pichon, C. L., & Cleeremans, A. (2012). Behavioral priming: It's all in the mind, but whose mind? *PloS One*, 7(1), 1–7.
Edwards, K., & Smith, E. E. (1996). A disconfirmation bias in the evaluation of arguments. *Journal of Personality and Social Psychology*, 71, 5–24.
Ellemers, N. (2018). Gender stereotypes. *Annual Review of Psychology*, 69, 275–298.
Fiedler, K. (2009). Voodoo correlations are everywhere—not only in neuroscience. *Perspectives on Psychological Science*, 6(2), 163–171.
Fiedler, K. (2017). What constitutes strong psychological science? The (neglected) role of diagnosticity and a priori theorizing. *Perspectives on Psychological Science*, 12(1), 46–61.
Firestone, C., & Scholl, B. J. (2014). "Top-down" effects where none should be found: The El Greco fallacy in perception research. *Psychological Science*, 25(1), 38–46.
Firestone, C., & Scholl, B. J. (2016). Cognition does not affect perception: Evaluating the evidence for "top-down" effects. *Behavioral and Brain Sciences*, 39, E229. doi: 10.1017/S0140525X15000965
Flake, J. K., & Fried, E. I. (2019, January 17). Measurement schmeasurement: Questionable measurement practices and how to avoid them. https://doi.org/10.31234/osf.io/hs7wm
Funder, D. C. (2009). Persons, behaviors, and situations: An agenda for personality psychology in the postwar era. *Journal of Research in Personality*, 43, 120–126.
Funder, D. C., Levine, J. M., Mackie, D. M., Morf, C. C., Sansone, C., Vazire, S., & West, S. G. (2014). Improving the dependability of research in personality and social psychology: Recommendations for research and educational practice. *Personality and Social Psychology Review*, 18(1), 3–12.
Gelman, A. (2016). What has happened down here is the winds have changed. https://statmodeling.stat.columbia.edu/2016/09/21/what-has-happened-down-here-is-the-winds-have-changed/
Gelman, A., & Stern, H. (2006). The difference between "significant" and "not significant" is not itself statistically significant. *American Statistician*, 60(4), 328–331.
Gilbert, D. T., King, G., Pettigrew, S., & Wilson, T. D. (2016). Comment on "Estimating the reproducibility of psychological science." *Science*, 351(6277), 1037.
Greenwald, A. G., Banaji, M. R., & Nosek, B. A. (2015). Statistically small effects of the Implicit Association Test can have societally large effects. *Journal of Personality and Social Psychology*, 108(4), 553–561. https://doi.org/10.1037/pspa0000016

Greenwald, A. G., McGhee, D. E., & Schwartz, J. L. (1998). Measuring individual differences in implicit cognition: The Implicit Association Test. *Journal of Personality and Social Psychology, 74*(6), 1464.

Fiedler, K. (2009). Voodoo correlations are everywhere—not only in neuroscience. *Perspectives on Psychological Science, 6*, 163–171.

Henrich, J., Heine, S. J., & Norenzayan, A. (2010). The weirdest people in the world? *Behavioral and Brain Sciences, 33*(2–3), 61–83.

Hofstra, B., Kulkarni, V. V., Galvez, S. M. N., He, B., Jurafsky, D., & McFarland, D. A. (2020). The diversity–innovation paradox in science. *Proceedings of the National Academy of Sciences USA, 117*(17), 9284–9291. doi: 10.1073/pnas.1915378117

Honeycutt, N., & Jussim, L. (2020). A model of political bias in social science research. *Psychological Inquiry, 31*(1), 73–85.

Huffington Post. (2013). Loch Ness Monster sighting? Photographer claims 'black object' glided beneath lake's surface. https://www.huffpost.com/entry/loch-ness-monster-sighting-photo_n_3817842

Inbar, Y., & Lammers, J. (2012). Political diversity in social and personality psychology. *Perspectives on Psychological Science, 7*(5), 496–503.

Ioannidis, J. P. (2005). Why most published research findings are false. *PLoS Medicine, 2*(8), e124. https://doi.org/10.1371/journal.pmed.0020124

Ioannidis, J. P. (2008). Why most discovered true associations are inflated. *Epidemiology, 19*, 640–648.

Ioannidis, J. P. (2012). Why science is not necessarily self-correcting. *Perspectives on Psychological Science, 7*(6), 645–654.

Jern, A., Chang, K. K., & Kemp, C. (2014). Belief polarization is not always irrational. *Psychological Review, 121*, 206–224.

John, L. K., Loewenstein, G., & Prelec, D. (2012). Measuring the prevalence of questionable research practices with incentives for truth telling. *Psychological Science, 23*(5), 524–532.

Jost, J. T. (2011). System justification theory as compliment, complement, and corrective to theories of social identification and social dominance. In *Social Motivation* (pp. 223–263). Taylor and Francis. https://doi.org/10.4324/9780203833995

Jost, J. T., and Andrews, R. (2011). System justification theory. In D. J. Christie (Ed.), *Encyclopedia of Peace Psychology*. doi: 10.1002/9780470672532.wbepp273

Jussim, L. (1991). Social perception and social reality: A reflection-construction model. *Psychological Review, 98*(1), 54.

Jussim, L. (2005). Accuracy in social perception: Criticisms, controversies, criteria, components, and cognitive processes. In M. P. Zanna (Ed.), *Advances in Experimental Social Psychology* (Vol., 37, pp. 1–93). Elsevier Academic Press. https://doi.org/10.1016/S0065-2601(05)37001-8

Jussim, L. (2012). *Social Perception and Social Reality: Why Accuracy Dominates Bias and Self-Fulfilling Prophecy*. Oxford University Press, USA.

Jussim, L. (2018, June 5). "Gender stereotypes are inaccurate" if you ignore the data. https://www.psychologytoday.com/blog/rabble-rouser/201806/gender-stereotypes-are-inaccurate-if-you-ignore-the-data

Jussim, L. (2019, June 23). Scientific bias in favor of studies finding gender bias. https://www.psychologytoday.com/us/blog/rabble-rouser/201906/scientific-bias-in-favor-studies-finding-gender-bias

Jussim, L., Cain, T. R., Crawford, J. T., Harber, K., & Cohen, F. (2009). The unbearable accuracy of stereotypes. In T. Nelson (Ed.), *Handbook of Prejudice, Stereotyping, and Discrimination* (pp. 199–227). Erlbaum.

Jussim, L., Careem, A., Goldberg, Z., Honeycutt, N., & Stevens, S. (in press). IAT scores, racial gaps, and scientific gaps. To appear in J. A. Krosnick, T. H. Stark, & A. L. Scott (Eds.), *The Future of Research on Implicit Bias*.

Jussim, L., Coleman, L. M., & Lerch, L. (1987). The nature of stereotypes: A comparison and integration of three theories. *Journal of Personality and Social Psychology*, 52(3), 536.

Jussim, L., Crawford, J. T., Anglin, S. M., Chambers, J., Stevens, S. T., & Cohen, F. (2016a). Stereotype accuracy: One of the largest and most replicable effects in all of social psychology. In T. Nelson (Ed.), *Handbook of Prejudice, Stereotyping, and Discrimination* (2nd ed., pp. 31–63). Erlbaum.

Jussim, L., Crawford, J. T., Anglin, S. M., Stevens, S. T., & Duarte, J. L. (2016b). Interpretations and methods: Towards a more effectively self-correcting social psychology. *Journal of Experimental Social Psychology*, 66, 116–133.

Jussim, L., Crawford, J. T., & Rubinstein, R. S. (2015). Stereotype (in) accuracy in perceptions of groups and individuals. *Current Directions in Psychological Science*, 24(6), 490–497.

Jussim, L., Crawford, J. T., Stevens, S. T., & Anglin, S. M. (2016c). The politics of social psychological science: Distortions in the social psychology of intergroup relations. In P. Valdesolo & J. Graham (Eds.), *Social Psychology of Political Polarization* (pp. 165–196). New York, NY: Routledge.

Jussim, L., Krosnick, J. A., Stevens, S. T., & Anglin, S. M. (2019a). A social psychological model of scientific practices: Explaining research practices and outlining the potential for successful reforms. *Psychologica Belgica*, 59(1), 353–372. http://doi.org/10.5334/pb.496

Jussim, L., Stevens, S. T., Honeycutt, N., Anglin, S. M., & Fox, N. (2019b). Scientific gullibility. In J. Forgas & R. Baumeister (Eds.), *The Social Psychology of Gullibility: Fake News, Conspiracy Theories and Irrational Beliefs*. The Sydney Symposium on Social Psychology (pp. 279–303). Routledge.

Kahan, D. M., Peters, E., Dawson, E. C., & Slovic, P. (2017). Motivated numeracy and enlightened self-government. *Behavioral Public Policy*, 1, 54–86.

Kievit, R., Frankenhuis, W. E., Waldorp, L., & Borsboom, D. (2013). Simpson's paradox in psychological science: A practical guide. *Frontiers in Psychology*, 4, 513.

Klayman, J., & Ha, Y. (1987). Confirmation, disconfirmation, and information in hypothesis testing. *Psychological Review*, 94, 211–228.

Koehler, J. J. (1993). The influence of prior beliefs on scientific judgments of evidence quality. *Organizational Behavior and Human Decision Processes*, 56, 28–55.

Kuhn, T. S. (1970). *Criticism and the Growth of Knowledge: Volume 4: Proceedings of the International Colloquium in the Philosophy of Science, London, 1965*. Cambridge University Press.

Kunda, Z. (1990). The case for motivated reasoning. *Psychological Bulletin*, 108, 480–498.

Lakatos, I., & Musgrave, A. (Eds.). (1970). *Criticism and the Growth of Knowledge: Proceedings of the International Colloquium in the Philosophy of Science, London, 1965*. Cambridge University Press. doi:10.1017/CBO9781139171434

Lakens, D. (2017). Equivalence tests: A practical primer for t tests, correlations, and meta-analysis. *Social Psychological and Personality Science*, 8, 355-362.

Lakens, D. (2021). The practical alternative to the p-value is the correctly used p-value. *Perspectives on Psychological Science, 16*, 639–648.

Lakens, D., Adolfi, F., Albers, C. J., Anvari, F., Apps, M. A. J., Argamon, S. E., Baguley, T., Becker, R. B., Benning, S. D., Bradford, D. E., Buchanan, E. M., Caldwell, A. R., Calster, B., Van, R., Carlsson. S. C., Chen, B., Chung., L. J., Colling, G. S., Collins. Z., . . . Zwaan, R. A. (2018). Justify your alpha. *Nature: Human Behavior, 2*, 168–171.

Ledgerwood, A., Haines, E., & Ratliff, K. (2015). Guest post: Not nutting up or shutting up. https://sometimesimwrong.typepad.com/wrong/2015/03/guest-post-not-nutting-up-or-shutting-up.html

Levitt, S. D., & Dubner, S. J. (2014, September 18). Outsiders by design. https://freakonomics.com/podcast/outsiders-by-design-a-new-freakonomics-radio-podcast-2/

Lewandowsky, S., Oberauer, K., & Gignac, G. E. (2013). NASA faked the moon landing—therefore, (climate) science is a hoax: An anatomy of the motivated rejection of science. *Psychological Science, 24*(5), 622–633.

Lilienfeld, S. O. (2010). Can psychology become a science? *Personality and Individual Differences, 49*, 281–288.

Lilienfeld, S. O. (2017). Microaggressions: Strong claims, inadequate evidence. *Perspectives on Psychological Science, 12*(1), 138–169.

Loeb, A. (2014). Benefits of diversity. *Nature Physics, 10*(9), 616–617.

Lord, C. G., Lepper, M. R., & Preston, E. (1984). Considering the opposite: A corrective strategy for social judgment. *Journal of Personality and Social Psychology, 47*(6), 1231.

Markman, A. (2010). Why science is self-correcting. https://www.psychologytoday.com/us/blog/ulterior-motives/201008/why-science-is-self-correcting

Meehl, P. E. (1990). Appraising and amending theories: The strategy of Lakatosian defense and two principles that warrant it. *Psychological Inquiry, 1*(2), 108–141.

Merton, R. K. (1968). The Matthew effect in science: The reward and communication systems of science are considered. *Science, 159*(3810), 56–63. doi: 10.1126/science.159.3810.56

Merton, R. K. (1973). *The Sociology of Science: Theoretical and Empirical Investigations.* N. W. Storer (Ed.). University of Chicago Press.

Mesoudi, A. (2015). Cultural evolution: A review of theory, findings, and controversies. *Evolutionary Biology, 43*, 481–497.

Mill, J. S. (1859). *On Liberty.* Harper Collins.

Morey, R. D., & Lakens, D. (2017). Why most of psychology is statistically unfalsifiable. https://raw.githubusercontent.com/richarddmorey/psychology_resolution/master/paper/response.pdf

Moss-Racusin, C. A., Dovidio, J. F., Brescoll, V. L., Graham, M. J., & Handelsman, J. (2012). Science faculty's subtle gender biases favor male students. *Proceedings of the National Academy of Sciences USA, 109*(41), 16474–16479.

Munro, G. D., & Ditto, P. H. (1997). Biased assimilation, attitude polarization, and affect in reactions to stereotype-relevant scientific information. *Personality and Social Psychology Bulletin, 23*, 636–653.

Nelson, L. D., Simmons, J., & Simonsohn, U. (2018). Psychology's renaissance. *Annual Review of Psychology, 69*, 511–534.

Nickerson, R. S. (1998). Confirmation bias: A ubiquitous phenomenon in many guises. *Review of General Psychology, 2*, 175–220.

Nosek, B. A., Spies, J. R., & Motyl, M. (2012). Scientific utopia: II. Restructuring incentives and practices to promote truth over publishability. *Perspectives on Psychological Science, 7*(6), 615–631.

Pigliucci, M. (2013). What are we to make of the concept of race? Thoughts of a philosopher–scientist. *Studies in History and Philosophy of Science Part C: Studies in History and Philosophy of Biological and Biomedical Sciences, 44*(3), 272–277.

Platt, J. R. (1964). Strong inference. *Science, 146*(3642), 347–353.

Popper, K. R. (1959). The propensity interpretation of probability. *British Journal for the Philosophy of Science, 10*(37), 25–42.

Popper, K. (1963/2002*)*. *Conjectures and Refutations: The Growth of Scientific Knowledge*. Routledge.

Redding, R. E. (2001). Sociopolitical diversity in psychology. *American Psychologist, 56*, 205–215.

Reyna, C. (2017). Scale creation, use, and misuse: How politics undermines measurement. In J. T. Crawford & L. Jussim (Eds.), *Politics of Social Psychology* (pp. 91–108). Psychology Press.

Richard, F. D., Bond, C. F., & Stokes-Zoota, J. J. (2003). One hundred years of social psychology quantitatively described. *Review of General Psychology, 7*(4), 331–363. https://doi.org/10.1037/1089-2680.7.4.331

Sackett, P. R., Hardison, C. M., & Cullen, M. J. (2004). On interpreting stereotype threat as accounting for African American–White differences on cognitive tests. *American Psychologist, 59*, 7–13. https://doi.org/10.1037/0003-066X.59.1.7

Schimmack, U. (2019). The Implicit Association Test: A method in search of a construct. *Perspectives on Psychological Science*. https://doi.org/10.1177/1745691619863798

Schmader, T., Johns, M., & Forbes, C. (2008). An integrated process model of stereotype threat effects on performance. *Psychological Review, 115*(2), 336.

Schwartz, J. (1998, September 29). Roots of unconscious prejudice affect 90 to 95 percent of people, psychologists demonstrate at press conference. University of Washington News. https://www.washington.edu/news/1998/09/29/roots-of-unconscious-prejudice-affect-90-to-95-percent-of-people-psychologists-demonstrate-at-press-conference/

Shen, H. (2013). Mind the gender gap. *Nature, 495*(7439), 22.

Simmons, J. P., Nelson, L. D., & Simonsohn, U. (2011). False-positive psychology: Undisclosed flexibility in data collection and analysis allows presenting anything as significant. *Psychological Science, 22*(11), 1359–1366.

Simons, D. J. (2014). The value of direct replication. *Perspectives on Psychological Science, 9*, 76–80.

Simpson, E. H. (1951). The interpretation of interaction in contingency tables. *Journal of the Royal Statistical Society: Series B (Methodological), 13*(2), 238–241.

Smaldino, P. (2019). Better methods can't make up for mediocre theory. *Nature, 575*(7781), 9.

Spellman, B. A. (2015). A short (personal) future history of Revolution 2.0. *Perspectives on Psychological Science, 10*(6), 886–899. https://doi.org/10.1177/1745691615609918

Steegen, S., Tuerlinckx, F., Gelman, A., & Vanpaemel, W. (2016). Increasing transparency through a multiverse analysis. *Perspectives on Psychological Science, 11*(5), 702–712.

Steele, C. M., & Aronson, J. (1995). Stereotype threat and the intellectual test performance of African Americans. *Journal of Personality and Social Psychology, 69*(5), 797.

Steele, C. M., & Aronson, J. A. (2004). Stereotype threat does not live by Steele and Aronson (1995) alone. *American Psychologist, 59*(1), 47–48. https://doi.org/10.1037/0003-066X.59.1.47

Stern, C., & Crawford, J. T. (2021). Ideological conflict and prejudice: An adversarial collaboration examining correlates and ideological (a)symmetries. *Social Psychological and Personality Science, 12*(1), 42–53.

Stevens, S. T., Jussim, L., Anglin, S. M., & Honeycutt, N. (2018). Direct and indirect influences of political ideology on perceptions of scientific findings. In B. Rutjens & M. Brandt (Eds.), *Belief Systems and the Perception of Reality* (pp. 115–133). Routledge.

Swann, W. B., & Ely, R. J. (1984). A battle of wills: Self-verification versus behavioral confirmation. *Journal of Personality and Social Psychology, 46*(6), 1287.

Taber, C. S., & Lodge, M. (2006). Motivated skepticism in the evaluation of political beliefs. *American Journal of Political Science, 50*, 755–769.

Tappin, B. M., van der Leer, L., & McKay, R. T. (2017). The heart trumps the head: Desirability bias in political belief revision. *Journal of Experimental Psychology: General, 146*, 1143.

Tomkins, A., Zhang, M., & Heavlin, W. D. (2017). Reviewer bias in single-versus double-blind peer review. *Proceedings of the National Academy of Sciences USA, 114*(48), 12708–12713.

Tversky, A., & Kahneman, D. (1974). Judgment under uncertainty: Heuristics and biases. *Science, 185*, 1124–1131.

Van Bavel, J. J., Reinero, D. A., Harris, E., Robertson, C. E., & Pärnamets, P. (2020). Breaking groupthink: Why scientific identity and norms mitigate ideological epistemology. *Psychological Inquiry, 31*(1), 66–72. doi: 10.1080/1047840X.2020.1722599

Van der Lee, R., & Ellemers, N. (2015). Gender contributes to personal research funding success in the Netherlands. *Proceedings of the National Academy of Sciences USA, 112*(40), 12349–12353.

Vul, E., Harris, C., Winkielman, P., & Pashler, H. (2009). Voodoo correlations in social neuroscience. *Perspectives on Psychological Science, 4*(3), 274–290.

Walton, G. M., & Spencer, S. J. (2009). Latent ability: Grades and test scores systematically underestimate the intellectual ability of negatively stereotyped students. *Psychological Science, 20*(9), 1132–1139.

Walton, G. M., Spencer, S. J., & Erman, S. (2013). Affirmative meritocracy. *Social Issues and Policy Review, 7*(1), 1–35.

Washburn, A. N., & Skitka, L. J. (2018). Strategies for promoting strong inferences in political psychology research. In B T. Rutjens & M. J. Brandt (Eds.), *Belief Systems and the Perception of Reality* (pp. 134–146). Routledge.

Wason, P. C. (1968). Reasoning about a rule. *Quarterly Journal of Experimental Psychology, 20*, 273–281.

Wasserstein, R. L., Schirm, A. L., & Lazar, N. A. (2019) Moving to a world beyond "$p < 0.05$." *American Statistician, 73*(supp. 1), 1–19. doi: 10.1080/00031305.2019.1583913

Weintraub, P. (2010). The doctor who drank infectious broth, gave himself an ulcer, and solved a medical mystery. https://www.discovermagazine.com/health/the-doctor-who-drank-infectious-broth-gave-himself-an-ulcer-and-solved-a-medical-mystery

West, T. V., & Kenny, D. A. (2011). The truth and bias model of judgment. *Psychological Review, 118*(2), 357–378. https://doi.org/10.1037/a0022936

Williams, J. C., & Smith, J. L. (2015, July 8). The myth that academic science isn't biased against women. *Chronicle of Higher Education.* https://www.chronicle.com/article/the-myth-that-academic-science-isnt-biased-against-women/

Williams, W. M., & Ceci, S. J. (2015). National hiring experiments reveal 2:1 faculty preference for women on STEM tenure track. *Proceedings of the National Academy of Sciences USA, 112*(17), 5360–5365.

Wolfe, C. T., & Spencer, S. J. (1996). Stereotypes and prejudice: Their overt and subtle influence in the classroom. *American Behavioral Scientist, 40*(2), 176–185.

10
Questionable Research Practices

Ernest H. O'Boyle and Martin Götz

> What gets us into trouble is not what we don't know. It's what we know for sure that just ain't so.
>
> —Mark Twain

The current crisis in confidence[1] that has plagued a number of subdisciplines in psychology and other scientific fields has in large part been linked to data fabrications by high-profile names, such as Diedrick Stapel, Ulrich Lichtenthaler, and Jan Hendrik Schön (see also Baron et al., 2016; Bhattacharjee, 2013; Simonsohn, 2013). More generally, a review of research articles in the biomedical and life sciences indicated that the vast majority of retractions were attributable to scientific misconduct, such as fraud or suspected fraud, duplicate publication, and plagiarism (e.g., Fang et al., 2012; Grieneisen & Zhang, 2012; Van Noorden, 2011). Undoubtedly, the extent and frequency of such misconduct, the promotions and accolades that the misconduct earned prior to their detection, and the lengthy period these individuals were able to operate in bad faith, are concerning and do warrant handwringing and self-reflection on how we should police ourselves against outright fraudulent behavior.

However, as troublesome as the inability to detect, correct, and deter blatant academic misconduct is, it may not be the most pressing problem facing science. In fact, the most damaging aspect of Stapel and his ilk are that they serve as "red herrings" that take focus away from what may constitute a more significant threat, namely questionable research practices (QRPs; other

---

[1] A variety of terms are used to refer to this perceived crisis, such as replicability, reproducibility, dependability, credibility, confidence, or robustness (De Boeck & Jeon, 2018; see also Chapter 4 in this volume).

researchers have argued for the term "questionable reporting practices" instead; see Wigboldus & Dotsch, 2016). What makes QRPs questionable as opposed to a clear fabrication, falsification, and/or plagiarism (e.g., Fanelli, 2012a, 2012b; Gross, 2016) is that these practices fall into an ethical *gray zone* between acceptable and unacceptable scientific conduct due to a semblance of truth to the research practice or the reporting thereof (e.g., Fanelli, 2012a; Lynøe et al., 1999; Steneck, 2006).[2] These practices can occur before article submission or during the review process and potentially lead to the publication of false-positive "research findings" and ultimately a flawed body of knowledge (Sterling, 1959; Sterling et al., 1995). It stands to reason that QRPs can occur with or without intent or knowledge of their potentially biasing effects and, as such, these practices lie on a continuum between scientific fraud, bias, simple carelessness, and ignorance.

To give an example, suppose a researcher operating under the hypothetico-deductive model of scientific inquiry starts a confirmatory research endeavor with 10 hypotheses but he only reports the five that were supported. Five hypotheses were indeed supported by the data, and he never claimed that these were the only five hypotheses tested. However, the omission of the other hypotheses gives the reader the false impression that the results fully supported *all* a priori hypotheses (for an in-depth discussion, see Rubin, 2017a; Wagenmakers et al., 2012). As another example, consider an experimenter who initially uses four levels of her independent variable. Upon conducting her analysis, she realizes that if she drops one of the levels, her omnibus test achieves statistical significance. In reporting the methodology, the manipulation is described as only having three levels. That statistic and its corresponding p-value do indeed accurately describe the data in their final form. Again, the problem is that by mischaracterizing the methodology, the faith the reader puts in the results exceeds what the faith might be if fully reported.

At this point, the reader may be asking himself or herself why QRPs, such as the two examples described above, should cause more alarm than those unequivocally bad practices like plagiarism or data fabrication. The nefariousness of QRPs is attributable to three related issues. First is their frequency. QRPs appear to be quite common in the published literature (e.g., John et al., 2012; Pashler & Wagenmakers, 2012; Wigboldus & Dotsch, 2016), and it is

---

[2] A humoristic analogy to Dante Alighieri's *Inferno* illustrated the continuum of bad scientific practices as *the nine circles of scientific hell* (Neuroskeptic, 2012).

their collective effect that can be problematic. A QRP in isolation may not seem like a serious threat, but if it were repeated over and over, then one is faced with the tragedy of the commons where the common good being depleted is legitimacy (e.g., meta-analyses, systematic reviews; Gurevitch et al., 2018; Ioannidis, 2016; Siddaway et al., 2019).

Second, many QRPs are quite difficult to detect. A suspected fraudster can be asked to turn over the data for reanalysis and fabricated data can be differentiated from real data in many cases, such as through an inexplicable low frequency of round numbers (Mosimann et al., 1995) or through advanced simulation techniques (Simonsohn, 2013). However, tools and procedures that can identify and deter QRPs are still in their infancy and not widely employed (exemplarily, see discussion sections on the R package statcheck by Hartgerink et al., 2016; Nuijten et al., 2016). The available tools also primarily focus on QRPs related to statistical analysis—specifically null hypothesis significance testing (NHST). For example, without someone having preregistered their study, there is no way to be certain that a hypothesis reported as a priori was indeed developed prior to data analysis and not added afterward or fundamentally altered (e.g., reversed). Often QRP engagement must be inferred based on large-scale trends in the field, and it is challenging to determine if any specific finding is tainted by QRPs.

Third, QRPs are insidiously effective. QRPs get the results researchers want (e.g., publications, tenure) by getting the results researchers want (e.g., statistical significance, theory support). Rather than extensively reviewing the literature to develop a set of hypotheses, identifying the most psychometrically sound instruments to ensure reliable and valid measurement, conducting an a priori power analysis to determine the necessary sample size, and mastering the relevant analytic techniques, all with the *mere hope* of having a good chance (e.g., 80%) of detecting an effect *if* it is truly present, QRPs can be employed. Thus, at the most extreme, a researcher starts with a general idea or hunch and possibly a sense of what theories might be applicable. Selecting measures is about quantity more so than quality as the idea here is to throw everything against the wall and see what sticks. Not to mention, measures can be altered (e.g., items dropped, scaling transformed) to ensure both the appearance of reliability and acceptable results (Flake & Fried, 2020). The desired sample size will be determined once the desired effect is achieved either through continuous data collection or the aforementioned p-hacking. With relative ease, hope is replaced with certainty as QRPs offer a near guarantee of getting the desired results (Simmons et al., 2011).

In sum, their frequency, opaqueness, and effectiveness makes for a troubling cocktail. O'Boyle et al. (2017) labeled this ability of QRPs to transform "ugly" initial results into "beautiful" publications as the chrysalis effect. QRPs have the potential to rose-tint the literature and make it difficult to impossible to determine which findings are built upon the solid foundation of well-conducted and accurately reported research and which are built upon the sand of "white lies" and lies of omission. The injunctive norms the field attempts to impose on what researchers *should do* may very well be superseded by the descriptive norms developed by observing what others *actually do* in their labs, departments, and universities. In this way, QRPs might become normalized, institutionalized, and ingrained (see also Smaldino & McElreath, 2016). Their initial effect of deceiving others soon could give way to self-deception, where researchers would begin to view the research process not as the pursuit of knowledge, but as one of gamesmanship—effectively, this would turn scientists seeking truth into lawyers presenting the most persuasive case (see also Davis, 1971; Hubbard, 2016; Tourish, 2019).

In light of a drastically increased number of retractions (e.g., Cokol et al., 2008; Steen et al., 2013; Van Noorden, 2011) as well as rather disheartening results of large-scale endeavors to replicate psychological findings by the Open Science community and related movements (e.g., Ebersole et al., 2020; Hagger et al., 2016; Open Science Collaboration, 2015), our field—once again—experiences a credibility crisis. It is our contention that if our field is to fall, it will not be from the fatal blow of an outright fraudster, it will be the death of a thousand, self-inflicted cuts delivered by fellow, often well-intentioned researchers skirting the line between best practices and what we argue have unfortunately become common practices. In this chapter we review the extant research of the existence and frequency of QRP engagement. We then transition into the antecedents and outcomes of QRPs, with a focus on the system processes that both encourage and facilitate QRP engagement. We close with a series of steps that might mitigate QRP prevalence in order for research to reflect best scientific practices.

Scope, Prevalence, and Effect of QRPs

A meta-analysis of surveys investigating scientific misconduct by Fanelli (2009) suggests that, on average, only 1% to 2% of scientists have fabricated, falsified, or modified data or results at least once during their careers.

However, up to 34% of the surveyed scientists admitted to engaging in QRPs during their careers. Exemplarily, and consistently across studies, researchers "admitted more frequently to have *modified research results* to improve the outcome than to have reported results they *knew to be untrue*" (Fanelli, 2009, p. 6). Interestingly, when asked about their colleagues' behavior, observation rates for fabrication, falsification, and modification were, on average, up to over 14%, and even up to 72% for QRPs. These high percentages are troubling, but we must first define what exact practices are housed under the QRP umbrella. Thus, we begin with a description of the most commonly studied QRPs and present them in approximate order of where and when they occur during the research process. This is not an exhaustive list of QRPs, and it is important to note that as theories, methods, and analyses change, so too will QRPs.

Unreported Changes to Theory and Hypotheses

A hypothesis can be changed in three ways. First is HARKing (Kerr, 1998) or accommodational hypothesizing (Hitchcock & Sober, 2004). Here, a researcher retroactively (i.e., after knowing the results from the data at hand) presents an unexpected finding as if it were an a priori prediction. Thus, the actual predictive power of a theoretical framework employed to expect a certain pattern of results is essentially compromised (see also Bosco et al., 2016; Murphy & Aguinis, 2019; Rubin, 2017c). Within the currently prevalent NHST framework, our position is that a hypothesis is by its nature a priori: It is a prediction of what might happen, not an explanation of what did happen. The entire logic of NHST requires the hypothesis to be a priori, thus ignorant of the data the hypothesis will eventually be judged in light of. To clarify, Hollenbeck and Wright (2017) aimed for greater conceptual precision and suggested redefining HARKing as SHARKing, namely as "publicly presenting in the Introduction section of an article hypotheses that emerged from post hoc analyses and treating them as if they were a priori" (p. 10). In doing so, these authors demarcated SHARKing from THARKing, which they defined as "clearly and transparently presenting new hypotheses that were derived from post hoc results in the Discussion section of an article" (p. 11). Essentially, Hollenbeck and Wright (2017) emphasized transparency regarding the formulation and testing of hypotheses, and thereby embrace the great value of post hoc exploratory research. However, it needs to be characterized as what it is.

The second QRP is the dropping of hypotheses. The issue is that dropped hypotheses tend to be unsupported hypotheses (see O'Boyle et al., 2017). This gives the reader a false impression about the overall predictive accuracy of a supposedly confirmatory manuscript, and is somewhat analogous to the inflation of the type I error rate under repeated tests (for an in-depth discussion, see Rubin, 2017a; Wagenmakers et al., 2012). Whether right or wrong, a paper that starts with 10 interrelated hypotheses and supports four may be looked at differently than a paper that starts with four and supports all four. There is an additional downside to the dropping of hypotheses in that it whitewashes the manuscript of "failure." Failure is a central part of science. As important as it is to know what works, it is equally important to know what does not. Regardless of how well we mimic the natural sciences with our controlled experiments and extensive statistical tests, the ability to drop hypotheses that are not consistent with our desires invalidates the scientific merit of the research because the work lacks the critical feature of falsification (Popper, 1985).

The third QRP related to hypotheses is fundamental alteration or qualification. In a sense this is a combination of the previous two QRPs as it drops the original hypothesis and adds a new one in its place. For example, an a priori hypothesis predicting a positive relationship is changed to a negative relationship after the results bore out the latter. Or, a hypothesis predicting a positive relationship is changed to a moderation hypothesis after the positive relationship was found to be qualified by certain conditions. Those engaged in this practice often defend it by pointing out that the changes occurred because they became aware of new literature or, after careful consideration, the inconsistent finding with the a priori prediction was in fact consistent with the original theory if viewed through an alternative lens (and subsequently an alternative hypothesis). There is both a philosophical and pragmatic problem with this defense. First, in scientific writing we have an entire section of the paper devoted to *discussing* alternative interpretations and reasons for counterintuitive findings, and this section is not located in the introduction. A hypothesis is a gamble. A thorough literature review, pilot tests, and adequate statistical power increase the probability of success, but it is never a sure thing. Altering a hypothesis based on the findings is like trying to move one's chips from red to black after the roulette wheel stops spinning. From a pragmatic standpoint, academics are creative: Given enough time, we can come up with an explanation of just about any result and find previous research and theory consistent with it. The problem with post hoc revisions to a priori hypotheses is that, like dropped hypotheses, they tend to only occur when the initial results did not support the original prediction (Hollenbeck & Wright, 2017).

Before presenting actual prevalence estimates of QRPs, we would like to repeat Fiedler and Schwarz's (2016) caution that such estimates could accidently set a descriptive norm that QRPs are normal, which could ultimately corrupt the injunctive norm that QRPs are undesirable and should be minimized (see also Cialdini et al., 1991; Fiedler, 2016).[3] Nonetheless, several studies estimated a prevalence rate for HARKing and surveyed a wide array of behavioral researchers (e.g., Agnoli et al., 2017; Banks et al., 2016; Bedeian et al., 2010; Bosco et al., 2016; Fiedler & Schwarz, 2016; John et al., 2012; Kerr, 1998; Motyl et al., 2017).

Averaging estimates across these studies suggests that roughly half of the surveyed researchers admitted engaging in this QRP at least once throughout their career (see also Rubin, 2017c), and the majority of researchers considered this conduct to be defensible (e.g., Agnoli et al., 2017; John et al., 2012; Sacco et al., 2018). However, accurate prevalence estimates of QRP are hard to uncover because most of them rely on self-report survey results that can present a biased estimate due to methodological and sampling issues (e.g., Fanelli, 2009; Fiedler & Schwarz, 2016; Greco et al., 2015). In particular, Fiedler and Schwarz (2016) contested the methodological approach survey researchers generally took and presented updated survey evidence that suggested the actual prevalence of QRPs to be several orders of magnitude smaller than in former surveys. Nonetheless, they concluded that the "most unpleasant result of [the authors'] attempt to disambiguate survey data on scientific norm violations is that their prevalence rate is obviously not zero" (p. 50).

Refraining from survey methodology and comparing actual alterations to hypotheses between dissertations and the resulting journal publications, O'Boyle et al. (2017) found a large majority of projects to have altered hypotheses in the subsequent publication. Specifically, 88.7% of published articles either added or dropped hypotheses from the dissertation. In addition, using

---

[3] By their very covert nature, exact frequencies of QRPs are impossible to pinpoint and estimates and opinions of their frequency range from virtually never (see Chapter 4 in this volume) to ubiquitous (continue reading this chapter).

social network information and a retrospective timeframe of only 1 year, Fox et al. (2020) estimated that 18.80% to 24.40% of American psychologists used QRPs in general. In sum, survey as well as archival data suggest that hypothesis-related QRPs may be far from uncommon.

Unreported Changes to Methods

The various ways that the methodology can be altered are too numerous to discuss individually (for in-depth discussions, see Chambers, 2017; Gelman & Loken, 2013; Wicherts et al., 2016). Central to whether a change in methods is a QRP or not is the motivation and the disclosure. For example, adding and dropping conditions of the independent variable, collecting data beyond the study protocol, and dropping or altering measures can all be done with a clear conscience as long as the motivation was to provide a stronger or more rigorous test of the theory and the behaviors were disclosed to the reader. For example, if it turns out that the confederate went off script and blew the protocol for one condition, there is no reason not to footnote the occurrence in the manuscript and exclude or rerun that condition. On the other hand, if the problem with that condition was that participants did not behave as desired, then rerunning or adding more participants is a QRP.

With regard to methods-related QRPs, initial prevalence estimates by Martinson et al. (2005) suggest that approximately 15% of the 3,247 surveyed researchers admitted to having withheld details of the methodology or results in papers or proposals and/or to have dropped data points from analyses "on a gut feeling that they were inaccurate" (p. 737). Providing a more fine-grained analysis, John et al. (2012) based prevalence estimates on self-admission rates in a large-scale survey and found that 63% of psychology researchers failed to report all of a study's dependent measures, 28% failed to report all of a study's conditions, and 46% selectively reported studies that produced the desired pattern of results. In addition, 56% admitted to having collected more data after having had a peek into the already collected data, while 16% had stopped data collection because the desired result was already visible. Importantly, the majority of researchers considered these behaviors to be somewhat defensible (John et al., 2012). Again, applying a more rigorous survey methodology, Fielder and Schwarz (2016) provided considerably lower prevalence estimates but ultimately corroborated the self-admitted usage of these QRPs.

Unreported Changes to Results

There are a number of behaviors that, depending on the motivation and disclosure, fall squarely into results-related QRPs. What has become the most notorious is p-hacking (Simonsohn et al., 2014a, 2014b), which as described earlier entails repeatedly running analyses, with each iteration making a slight change to the predictors, until desired results are achieved. The "slight changes" include substituting in and out control variables, deleting participants at the tail of one end of the distribution, alternating missing-data techniques (e.g., listwise vs. pairwise), and switching between manifest and latent variable modeling (e.g., Cole & Preacher, 2014; Cortina et al., 2017; Sturman et al., 2021).

O'Boyle et al. (2019) argued that these sorts of changes to data and results explain the paradox of moderated multiple regression tests. It is well known that tests of moderation with ordinary least squares regression are notoriously underpowered and difficult to detect with typical effect sizes and sample sizes in most social sciences (e.g., Edwards, 2008; Holland et al., 2017; Murphy & Russell, 2017). Yet in a 20-year review of top management and applied psychology journals, O'Boyle et al. (2019) found that more than half were not only statistically significant, but also in the hypothesized direction. Further, despite there being no significant changes in sample size over the 20-year timeframe ($r = -=.002$), the percentage of statistically significant moderated multiple regression tests rose from "41% (1995–1999) to 49% (2000–2004), to 60% (2005–2009), and to 69% (2010–2014)." Also, even after controlling for a variety of substantive and methodological features (e.g., level of analysis, reliability of variables, correlations between linear terms and outcomes) and employing a number of different analytical techniques (e.g., meta-regression, multilevel modeling, ordinary least squares regression), the single best predictor of the effect size of an interaction term was sample size. Specifically, the smaller the sample size, the larger the effect size. Based on sampling error theory, the relation between sample size and effect size is zero, ceteris paribus. So why then is there such a strong relation ($r = -0.34$) between the two? There are some possible perfectly legitimate reasons, but O'Boyle et al. (2019) contended that the most likely cause was that when sample sizes are small, effect sizes need to be large in order to achieve statistical significance and that this scenario can encourage unreported changes to results like the ones described earlier (for similar observations regarding statistical tests of mediation, see Götz et al., 2021). There were two other noteworthy findings in this paper. First, a significant spike in p-values just below the 0.05 threshold was clearly visible, indicating likely p-hacking. Second, when exact p-values were recalculated by O'Boyle et al. (2019) and found to be less than 0.05, these results always agreed with the authors' original conclusion of "statistically significant," but when the results were recalculated to be just above the 0.05 threshold (between 0.05 and 0.10; i.e., not statistically significant), agreement between the recalculated values and the original conclusion of statistical significance or not fell to 54%. Rather than just blatantly misrepresenting results, we contend that this low level of agreement indicates that authors may be switching to one-tailed tests but omitting or forgetting to mention the change in the methods and results.

A second form of results-related QRPs is to alter the statistical technique until the desired results are achieved (Gelman & Loken, 2013). This is still a burgeoning area as familiarity of various statistical techniques is increasing. The ability to switch from ordinary least squares regression to structural equation modeling to Bayesian analysis to a host of other analytical techniques with relative ease makes the flexibility in the data analysis somewhat problematic (John et al., 2012). Each technique has its pluses and minuses, and there are multiple judgment calls within each that will alter results (e.g., in Bayes, the prior distribution is at the analyst's discretion). This flexibility is yet another "researcher degree of freedom" (Simmons et al., 2011, p. 1359; Simonsohn et al., 2014a; Simonsohn et al., 2014b) that can limit the generalizability and robustness of results. However, a recent demonstration by 29 research teams analyzing the same dataset to address the same research question vividly illustrated that—even with analysts' honest intentions—significant variation in the results of analyses of complex data arise and may be difficult to avoid (e.g., Silberzahn et al., 2018).

Although likely apocryphal, when a reporter asked Willie Sutton why he robbed banks, his reply was, "because that's where the money is." QRPs are not engaged in equally across all results because not all results are "where the money is." The evidence for QRPs within empirical research disproportionately targets research that incorporates NHST, and this is because "good results" by NHST standards are what get rewarded or at least perceived to be rewarded. Unfortunately, this has potentially resulted in "bad results" disappearing from most disciplines and countries (Fanelli, 2012b). Overall, the frequency of supported research claims has grown by over 22% between 1990 and 2007, with significant differences between disciplines and countries. In a similar vein, meta-analysis evidence suggests that studies with positive results receive more citations, and thus have more impact, than studies without supported hypotheses (Duyx et al., 2017). Exemplarily, Kühberger et al. (2014) investigated the distribution of p-values in a random sample of 1,000 interdisciplinary papers and found a ratio of 3:1 of published studies just reaching the conventional level of significance to those just failing it; the authors deemed this "a highly unlikely result" (p. 4).

However, QRPs are not inextricably or exclusively linked with NHST. There will always be the motivation to alter one's findings in non-ideal ways to increase a paper's chances of publication. If we abandoned NHST, QRPs would persist. If we were all Bayesians, QRPs would persist. If we were all qualitative researchers, QRPs would persist (Banks et al., 2016; O'Boyle et al., 2017). Further, there will always be those who are unfamiliar or untrained and therefore unaware of the effects of QRPs. As will be discussed in a subsequent section, mitigating QRPs is about reducing the motivation to engage in them and the ability to engage in them without detection, as well as properly educating scholars on why they should be avoided.

QRPs in the Review Process

QRPs are not limited to data-related practices. Receiving far less attention are those QRPs that occur during the review and publication process and thus are not necessarily tied to manipulating a specific finding. Rather, QRPs in this vein deal with circumventing the blind peer-review publication process or biasing the reward structures for publication. The blind peer-review process is generally designed to eliminate biased judgments of manuscripts that may result from knowing the identity of authors. Eventually undermining this quality-control mechanism, QRPs can be engaged in by authors, reviewers, and editors, but we note that during the peer-review process, it is the gatekeepers who generally hold the advantage of the power differential, so it is they who must be the most cautious in their communication with authors to discourage QRPs. As with the other sections, this is only a sampling of QRPs in the review process, and many others (e.g., skewing a manuscript to a particular school of thought or political position in order to make "low-quality" results more palatable) fall firmly in the gray area of gamesmanship.

The first review process QRP we will discuss is any attempt by authors to capitalize on their prior success or standing in the field by tipping off the reviewers to their identity (Lee et al., 2013; Rosenblatt & Kirk, 1981). This practice might try to capitalize on the Matthew effect that "consists in the accruing of greater increments of recognition for particular scientific contributions to scientists of considerable repute and the withholding of such recognition from scientists who have not yet made their mark" (Merton, 1968, p. 58). Posting the submitted paper or even the citation online, using letterhead from one's institution when replying to reviewers, and making repeated references to working papers or unpublished datasets in ways that are intended to lead the reviewers to believe that the author would presumably be the only one with access to this work[4] are all QRPs, as are any deliberate attempts to sway the reviewer's opinion with something other than rigor and relevance.

On the other end of trying to disclose one's identity to reviewers are any attempts a reviewer makes to identify the author. Having a general hunch based on the content or writing style is one thing, but going out of one's way to scour conference proceedings and faculty webpages is quite another. This obviously has become a more serious and frequent issue with the internet, but the double-blind review process has served science well for many years, and attempts to violate it out of curiosity or any other motive are undesirable (Lee et al., 2013). Worth repeating, though, is that many researchers operate in fairly close circles, and truly engaged researchers quickly become aware of the style and content of their peers. A reviewer who exerts no effort to identify an author may more or less automatically identify one based on substance, citations, or style. This is not a QRP; this is just an unfortunate artifact of a reviewer's experience and an author's past success.

The other QRP we cover on the author side of the peer-review process relates to gift authorship. Exemplarily, Ioannidis et al. (2018) identified an abundance of interdisciplinary scientific authors who had published more than 72 papers per year between 2000 and 2016—in other words, one paper every 5 days, an output many would consider implausibly prolific (see also Wager et al., 2015). When given without qualification, this is not a QRP

---

[4] This strategy of capitalizing on name recognition is not limited to the one person with the "name." As a graduate student at a relatively new and at the time not highly ranked doctoral program, the lead author of this chapter was informally briefed that reviewers can better see the merits of your paper if they think you are an established name in the field. As such, identify the editor of the journal to which you wish to submit, and cite their conference presentations and working papers. If the reviewers believe the author of the paper is the journal editor, they will be a little more accepting and less contentious in their feedback. There is no way to judge the efficacy of this strategy, but we regard it as a QRP nonetheless.

but outright misconduct. However, the line is somewhat blurred as to what constitutes authorship (e.g., Breet et al., 2018; Helgesson et al., 2018; Ioannidis et al., 2018). Although the American Psychological Association (APA) does set forth standards, there is much room for interpretation on what warrants intellectual contribution to a paper both in terms of author inclusion and authorship order. We refer to this QRP as "fire sale authorship." A researcher did do *something* to advance the paper, so it is not gift authorship, but the contribution was by most standards meager, and authorship is being given at a greatly reduced price. The researcher's inclusion had more to do with loyalty to an advisor or former student, helping an assistant professor with one last tenure push, or superficial quid pro quo exchanges (e.g., "I'll proofread yours if you add me and I'll return the favor with one of my papers").

The problem with fire sale authorship is not the veracity of the findings of any specific paper; rather, it is the long-term effects on the field. If publications are our currency, then we are experiencing hyperinflation. Author chains are lengthening, the number of outlets is increasing, and as a result, expectations are snowballing. In many disciplines, initial placement out of graduate school used to be based on potential; now it is based on the number of "A-hits" and how much grant money they will bring on Day 1.

The next QRP occurs during the publication process and generally falls on the editor and reviewers. First, most gatekeeper-initiated QRPs are the same as those described earlier, such as asking an author to add or drop a hypothesis, but citation coercion is the practice of reviewers or editors promoting certain published works, such as their own papers or those of the journals they represent (Tahamtan & Bornmann, 2018). It is certainly worth noting when relevant literature was missed by the author, but when the work is only tangentially related to the manuscript and has more to do with impact factors and h-indices, this is a QRP. Bruised egos and journal rankings aside, if the existing cited work is sufficient to support the hypothesis, method, or analysis, then cramming in a reviewer's vita or the table of contents of the last issue wastes time and paper, makes the writing more cumbersome, and reduces the amount of original research that can appear in journals. More specifically, this practice directly compromises general scientific guidelines for referencing (Harzing, 2002). For example, the APA urges authors to "cite the work of those individuals whose ideas, theories, or research have directly influenced [their] work" (American Psychological Association, 2020, p. 253).

The final QRP we discuss deals with editorship. Editors have the right to steer the journal they helm in terms of clearly setting out their definition of rigor and relevance. However, when editors favor or disfavor either a perspective or a person, they can bias the process by selecting reviewers they suspect or even know will be favorably or unfavorably predisposed to the paper to be reviewed. Associate editors and reviewers should be assigned based on their knowledge of the content included in the manuscript, not on their predisposition to the topic or their notoriety to wave papers through or vociferously tear them to shreds. Although at present uninvestigated (to our knowledge), we do consider this a QRP.

In order to publish in a specific target outlet, authors might align their cited literature with the target journal's implicit demands (Tahamtan & Bornmann, 2018). Direct prevalence estimates regarding the actual engagement of authors in this practice to increase their chances of publication are currently lacking. However, indirect support for the existence of this conduct comes from a large survey of interdisciplinary researchers showing that approximately 20% of researchers have been coerced to cite and that roughly 50% are aware of this practice (Wilhite & Fong, 2012). Yet another indirect line of support comes from research on identifying so-called citation cartels, namely "groups of authors that cite each other disproportionately more than they do other groups of authors that work on the same subject" (Fister et al., 2016, p. 1).

Recommendations to Reduce QRPs

> An institution under attack must reexamine its foundations, restate its objectives, seek out its rationale. Crisis invites self-appraisal.
> Merton, 1973, p. 267

This chapter thus far has made a case for the damage QRPs may cause to scientific credibility due to their potentially high frequency, difficulty in detection, and efficiency in garnering desired results. Suffice it to say that most QRPs may be attributable to external circumstances and incentives of the current scientific system rather than particular dispositions and intentions of individual researchers (e.g., Chambers, 2017; Edwards & Roy, 2017; Nosek et al., 2012). Although we do not go so far as to equate QRPs with criminal justice violations, the analogy of means, motives, and opportunity fits well. The crime, for lack of a better term, is distortion of research findings. The means are QRPs. The motive is that distorted research can have or at least be perceived to have a better chance of publication. The opportunity is that researchers can engage in most QRPs with little chance of detection.

Extending the criminal justice example further, *ignorantia juris non excusat* (ignorance of the law excuses no one). QRPs can be unintentional, can occur without malice, and can be ordered by powerful co-authors, advisors, reviewers, or editors, but the effect is the same—a lack of replicability and transparency in the published literature. However, this is where the criminal justice analogy must stop. Those engaged in QRPs are colleagues, not criminals. This is a system problem, not a person problem, and pillorying those identified as engaging in QRPs does nothing but satisfy zealots and cowards, and further delay resolution. A system has evolved where authors feel pressure to publish and there is a perception that certain findings foster publication more so than other findings. As such, authors may intentionally or unintentionally alter their manuscripts in non-ideal ways. Reviewers feel pressure to quickly review manuscripts in order to return to their other (often more extrinsically rewarded) duties and thus may use misguided heuristics, such as proxying rigor and relevance with statistical significance. Editors, feeling pressure to preserve and increase their impact factors and journal prestige out of felt responsibility to the journal and building their own reputation as a thought leader, may engage in citation coercion and other QRPs. Publishers feel pressure to maintain journal rankings in order to maximize the attractiveness of their product line to customers (e.g., university libraries) and thus may lay out carrots and sticks that encourage QRPs. In a sense, QRPs are a release valve in that they are a means to deliver the results increasingly demanded by the system—regardless of how impossible it is to meet those demands.

Many actionable steps are under way in psychology and other sciences or have already been implemented or can be implemented/expanded to curb or even eliminate the distortion of research through QRPs. The forms are numerous, but they largely fall into three broad categories: (1) reducing the motivation to engage in QRPs, (2) increasing transparency in reporting, and (3) embracing methodological rigor. All three carry an undertone of the need for education and increased awareness.

Reducing the Motivation to Engage in QRPs

The motivation to get certain results is undeniable and unlikely to change. It is human desire to celebrate the triumph and distance oneself from the defeat (Cialdini et al., 1976; Cialdini & Richardson, 1980), and scientists are no exception to this desire. Nor is this a new phenomenon to academic research. In 1909 the editors of the *Boston Medical and Surgical Journal* stated:

> It is natural that men should be eager to present to the world their successes rather than their failures, and furthermore, that a certain over-enthusiasm should see results where none actually exist. It is not to be questioned, therefore, that many papers are continually appearing written with an entirely conscientious motive, but which present an exaggerated or wholly distorted statement of the actual facts. (Editors, 1909, p. 263)

Ultimately, QRP engagement can be motivated by the rewards researchers can (and essentially have to) achieve in terms of publication, placement, or tenure (see also Giner-Sorolla, 2012; Smaldino & McElreath, 2016). This is not meant to imply that researchers are simply psychopathic utility maximizers. Rather, our *opinion* is that there is a distinct possibility that a researcher, in their last year on the tenure clock and staring at $p = 0.051$ for a key hypothesis, may sub out a control variable or two. To alleviate the pressure on our hypothetical researcher, the rewards must be uncoupled from what is statistically significant, supportive of theory, or consistent with expectations. There is a debate about what effect this pressure has on researchers. Dalton et al. (2012) found similar magnitudes of correlations of those reported in unpublished works, such as dissertations, to those reported in journal articles. However, their conclusion that the "file drawer problem" was not a problem was likely wrong, as it assumes that researchers unilaterally target all values in a correlation matrix for inflation through QRPs or effect suppression. However, what this result does show is that most effect sizes do not undergo inflation via the chrysalis effect. It is only those few, key effects central to a hypothesis test, intervention, or experimental outcome that are prone to manipulation and inflation. These are the effect sizes that are perceived to increase the chances of publication, and here is where we must focus on uncoupling rewards.

Two-Stage Review (Registered Reports)

One approach is the two-step review process (e.g., Benos et al., 2007; Jonas & Cesario, 2016; Kepes & McDaniel, 2013; Liberati, 1992). Essentially, the publication procedure is split into two stages. The first stage requires authors to submit their manuscript, consisting of an introduction, the methods section, and the analysis approach, for review. Here, the editors' and reviewers' focus lies on the originality and necessity of the research question, the soundness of the theoretical background, and the feasibility of the analytical approach; given a promising manuscript, the journal would invite the authors to translate their proposal into action. The second stage of this review process would then require the authors to provide the complete manuscript, including the results and discussion, for a final round of review before publication.[5] One advantage to implementing this approach is that researchers are already familiar with it, as this is what we all did when we proposed and then defended our dissertations.

Publishing Good Research with Bad Results

Another strategy to uncouple the rewards from the results is change the descriptive norms (i.e., what people see and perceive of others' behavior). A central motivation to engage in QRPs may be an attempt to align one's current research efforts with those that they read and cite. In other words, researchers want their manuscripts to look like the papers being published in the journals in which they want to publish. Unfortunately, journals can give a skewed view of how much statistical and theoretical support researchers typically encounter. Even if there was no QRP engagement, it would still be possible, even likely, that due to bias favoring theory-consistent results, novelty, and statistical support, journals might still overrepresent these types of findings at the expense of results not supportive of theory or not statistically significant. Again quoting the 1909 editorial mentioned earlier:

> We have no proper balance to this very natural tendency to publish our successes except through the more frequent publication of the errors and

---

[5] Notably, Hartgerink and van Zelst (2018) suggested an even more modular and real-time system of scientific communication that they refer to as "as-you-go" instead of "after-the-fact." Here, research outputs (e.g., theories, hypotheses, data) were communicated online right after a researcher considered them worthy of communicating and were also linked to each other to form a network of outputs.

failures which likewise mark the path of every successful practitioner. Such papers, written by men of experience and standing, would do much toward overcoming the tendency to over-security and would certainly serve an educational purpose which the ordinary publication so often fails to attain. (Editors, 1909, p. 264)

We echo this advice given more than a century ago (sans sexist language) and urge colleagues to submit good research with bad results. A well-conducted study—especially one authored by one or more leading scholars—where the data did not share the authors' enthusiasm would be such a valuable contribution to the field for many reasons. First, it sends a message that it is okay to be wrong every now and then. Journals filled with only successful interventions and theory-consistent results not only are boring but, we contend, also encourage QRPs. Publishing only that which works signals to researchers that the journal publishes only that which works. When findings are not supportive, researchers may feel pressured to alter their theory, data, or analyses in ways to make their manuscripts align with the *aesthetics* of the publications they read (see also Giner-Sorolla, 2012).

Second, it serves the critical but all-too-often overlooked role of theory pruning (Leavitt et al., 2010). Psychology and related disciplines rely strongly on the hypothetico-deductive model, and we hold theory dear. The great legends in our field, almost to a person, are associated with the introduction of a great theory. We still have much theory to build, but we must also be willing to tear down those structures overburdened by boundary conditions, caveats, and failed replications in order to make way for new theory.

Third and finally, it silences the cynic who claims that publications, like sausages and laws, are created in ways best hidden from the naive, idealistic, and weak-stomached, and that QRPs are a necessary evil. Although it is the defense of a child, "everybody else is doing it" justifies many QRPs. Work that refutes this defense has the potential to contribute to the field in far more reaching ways than yet another successful intervention nestled in between the other successful interventions in that issue, volume, journal, and discipline.

Proper Training and Continuing Education
A final strategy to reduce QRP engagement by reducing the motivation to engage in them is to reinforce the injunctive norms (i.e., what one should

or should not do; Cialdini et al., 1991) regarding QRPs. Because the immediate normative environment of graduate students shapes their research integrity (Mumford et al., 2007), a prudent socialization of graduate students to the desired scientific conduct is fundamental. To that extent, "unrealistic performance standards, extreme publication pressure, unreasonable work demands, excessive peer competition, and ruthless careerism" (Bedeian et al., 2010, p. 721) should be avoided, and policies for scientific conduct should be enacted and publicized (Hofmann et al., 2015).

Increasing Transparency in Reporting

Accompanying methodological rigor, we need a culture of open and reproducible science (e.g., Artner et al., 2020; Banks et al., 2019; Götz et al., 2021; Hesse, 2018; Morey et al., 2016; Munafò et al., 2017; Nosek et al., 2012, 2015; Nosek & Bar-Anan, 2012; Uhlmann et al., 2019). Or, as Feynman put it, "the idea is to try to give all of the information to help others to judge the value of your [scientific] contribution; not just the information that leads to judgement in one particular direction or another" (1985, p. 341). Given the aim of an open research culture, establishing transparent production and communication of research is vital (Miguel et al., 2014). Transparency increases the confidence a reader can have in a result by reducing the researchers' opportunity to engage in undisclosed changes.

Transparency is not meant to constrain researchers from what they study or how they study it, only how they report it. The fluidity and breadth of what to research and how to go about researching it is a hallmark of the profession. However, this fluidity meets strict rigidity when it comes to how we communicate research to peers and practitioners. We are not referring to specific formatting, such as that outlined in the APA's Journal Article Reporting Standards (American Psychological Association, 2020; Appelbaum et al., 2018). Rather, we are referring to the need above all else to be transparent in our reporting. As stated by Walter Massey, the former director of the National Science Foundation,

> [F]ew things are more damaging to the scientific enterprise than falsehoods—be they the result of error, self-deception, sloppiness and haste, or, in the worst case, dishonesty. It is the paradox of research that the reliance on truth is both the source of modern science and engineering's

enduring resilience and its intrinsic fragility. (Cited in Swazey et al., 1993, p. 552)

Given this, we outline two strategies to increase transparency.

Preregistering Studies
Having originated in the medical sciences in the 1960s (Dickersin & Rennie, 2003), a conceptually very similar approach to reduce the opportunity for QRPs is the preregistration of studies on platforms such as the Open Science Framework (Center for Open Science, 2019) or AsPredicted (Simonsohn et al., 2018). This approach requires researchers to state their hypotheses and to define their intended data-collection and the subsequent data-analysis protocol ahead of time (e.g., Gelman & Loken, 2013; Humphreys et al., 2013; Rubin, 2017b). Thus, a time-stamped log file is created that allows readers of future publications to comprehend whether the reported findings truly stem from the data-collection and data-analysis efforts declared in the preregistration. However, just as the 29 analyst teams analyzing the same dataset in light of the same research question came to different conclusions (Silberzahn et al., 2018), preregistering studies per se cannot ensure deriving valid conclusions due to "the garden of forking paths" (e.g., Gelman & Loken, 2013; Oberauer, 2019; Toth et al., 2021).

Data Sharing
General replicability of scientific findings, namely the possibility of replicating another researcher's finding and thereby considering it a basis to build upon, is one vital feature of credible science. The possibility of reproducing a researcher's specific finding with the same dataset in order to verify the feasibility of the data-analysis decisions and subsequent conclusions is another vital feature of open and transparent scientific conduct (e.g., Alter & Gonzalez, 2018; Borgman, 2015; Nosek et al., 2015). In that regard, enabling researchers to share their data in an ethical manner is a fundamental desideratum to allow for a self-aware accumulation of robust knowledge (e.g., Gilmore et al., 2018; Karr, 2016; Martone et al., 2018; Meyer, 2018; Ross et al., 2018). An interesting approach to encourage researchers to share their data and reward them accordingly are "open science" badges that are printed on a qualifying publication (Kidwell et al., 2016). These badges signal the conduct of desirable research practices (Connelly et al., 2011) and also might set a desirable descriptive norm.

Allot Space for Replication Studies

As researchers, we want our findings and conclusions to generate positive attention from peers and practitioners alike. Nonetheless, scientific knowledge is cumulative, and singular findings and conclusions should be understood more as promissory notes than as empirical facts. Ultimately, independent replications of scientific findings are needed to corroborate the progress of knowledge accumulation (e.g., Bollen et al., 2015). In the absence of verification and replication, whether findings are legitimate or bolstered by QRPs generates roughly the same amount of positive attention. If journals began to allot space for replication efforts, then findings colored by QRPs would subject themselves to potential negative attention. Whereas in 1990 authors found a strong editorial bias against publishing replications (Neuliep & Crandall, 1990), we now observe a growing editorial encouragement of this much-needed self-aware stream of research. However, only 3% of the 1,151 reviewed psychology journals explicitly stated that they accept replication studies (Martin & Clarke, 2017).

Embracing Methodological Rigor

Simmons et al. (2011) coined the term *researcher degrees of freedom* to refer to the many decisions researchers have to make in the course of collecting and analyzing data. As such, these degrees of freedom can "blur the lines between what decision is right, what decision produces a desired result, and what decision is most likely to help a finding get published" (Fox et al., 2020, p. 3). As became clear in our review of QRPs, these can occur in essentially any stage of the scientific inquiry; thus, a central aspect to curtailing QRPs is methodological rigor (see also Gelman & Loken, 2013, 2014). Rigor is too broad a topic to cover here with specific methodological improvements, but there is one overarching recommendation we wish to make: Break the NHST monopoly. This is not due to any specific criticism of NHST (although there are many). Rather, the issue is that when all you have is a hammer, everything looks like a nail (e.g., Gigerenzer, 2004, 2018; Gigerenzer & Marewski, 2015). Monopolies cripple ingenuity and give the false impression that there is only one way to do things.

We encourage researchers to embrace alternatives to NHST, such as Bayesian inference. A heated debate has evolved throughout almost all scientific disciplines about the potential superiority of Bayesian statistics.

Exemplarily, Dienes and colleagues (e.g., Dienes, 2008, 2016; Dienes & Mclatchie, 2018) demonstrate the many benefits of testing hypotheses in a Bayesian framework and make informed calls regarding the credibility of statistical models (i.e., hypotheses). However, our advocating for Bayesian statistics should not be taken as a building block for a Bayesian monopoly. Pointedly, Gigerenzer and colleagues (e.g., 2004; 2015) warned the field to not just build another statistical golem. Having multiple ways of considering scientific inferences reduces Gelman's (2016) concerns when he stated that:

> [I]t seems to me that statistics is often sold as a sort of alchemy that transmutes randomness into certainty, an "uncertainty laundering" that begins with data and concludes with success as measured by statistical significance. [. . .] The solution is not to reform *p*-values or to replace them with some other statistical summary or threshold, but rather to move toward a greater acceptance of uncertainty and embracing of variation. (p. 1; see also Gelman & Hennig, 2017)

Lakens et al. (2018) translated these thoughts into practical terms in stating that a cocktail of sound statistical analyses, corroboration of scientific knowledge via the means of replication, validation, and generalization, as well as the already discussed transparency of research workflow, and a self-aware error management culture should help heal the credibility of scientific findings. It is important to keep in mind that a prudent data analysis is a fundamental component of desirable scientific practice, but that embracing methodological rigor also means emphasizing the "principles of good study design and conduct, understanding of the phenomenon under study, interpretation of results in context, complete reporting, and proper logical and quantitative understanding of what data summaries mean" (Wasserstein & Lazar, 2016, p. 132).

Conclusion

> If we want to improve how our scientific culture functions, we must consider not only the individual behaviors we wish to change, but also the social forces that provide affordances and incentives for those behaviors.
> Smaldino & McElreath, 2016, p. 13

Some have argued that the "crisis narrative" is overblown (e.g., Baumeister, 2016; Fanelli, 2018; Chapter 4 in this volume); they argue that the allegedly high frequency of QRPs is due to surveys asking the wrong questions and replication efforts using the wrong thresholds, or that those raising the alarm are witch-hunters, newbies, and disgruntled washouts (i.e., the wrong people). There is no denying that early surveys failed to distinguish scholars who engaged in a single QRP 30 years ago from those who engage in QRPs as a matter of course (i.e., questions framed as "have you ever" versus "how often do you"). Likewise, pure up-or-down votes on whether an effect is robust based on a p-value from a single replication effort misses the nuance and alternative explanations as to why what one researcher found, another did not. Finally, the tone that some of the open science advocates can take in editorials, interviews, anonymous message boards, and even invited book chapters can, at times, match that of any fire-and-brimstone preacher.

The evidence is neither perfect nor definitive, and it is not always delivered by our most revered authorities. However, if, for example, John et al. (2012) had asked the so-called right questions, how many of those XX% of researchers who admitted to HARKing would have said, "just the once" and how many would have said, "once a month"? How many times does a result need to fail to replicate, be it with statistical significance, effect size magnitude, or any other metric, before we conclude that it does not matter whether the original result was a function of QRPs, sampling error, or some other artifact; it simply is not robust? Regardless of how reprehensible we find the messengers or their motives, can we fully discount the message?

Our chapter first outlined how the alleged frequency, difficulty in detection, and effectiveness of QRPs has the very real potential to cause serious harm to scientific accuracy and credibility. Like many others before us, we attribute QRPs to the system of how science is currently done rather than to those doing the science. Ours is a system that puts tremendous pressure on authors, reviewers, editors, and publishers to consistently and increasingly produce desired results. The system offers rewards, such as placement, tenure, accolades, and other extrinsic and intrinsic rewards, but it disproportionately allocates them to the top producers (Pfeffer & Langton, 1993). For our most salient output, publication, even the most staunch defenders of the current model must recognize that getting the "right" results positively impacts the likelihood of publication (Funder et al., 2014). The system also gives near-complete autonomy to researchers to conduct and report their research as they see fit, and reviewers, editors, and readers must accept that what is printed on the page was done in the lab and office with no significant additions, deletions, or alterations.

If we don't have a QRP problem, then we are truly in a Golden Age! Our predictive accuracy as evidenced by hypothesis support is soaring (Fanelli, 2012b). Despite the tremendous influx of scholars into our fields fighting for the same journal space and grants (Stamm et al., 2014), we are immune to the negative consequences that so often accompany increased competition in tournament-style reward systems (Gerhart & Rynes, 2003). Greater access and ease of use of statistical software makes p-hacking as easy as a few keystrokes, and the lack of oversight makes its detection highly unlikely. Nevertheless, unlike those in Major League Baseball, the motion-picture industry, professional cycling, and numerous other institutions, psychology researchers have resisted temptation even when so many of the system's incentives are aligned to have them do the very opposite.

The alternative scenario is that we are in a Gilded Age. What appears in our journals is non-trivially tainted by QRPs in ways that make it impossible to distinguish what is built on rigor and relevance from what is built on QRPs. If so, the system must be reformed. Minimizing the engagement in QRPs will require many significant efforts and reforms in current practices and incentives. We consider it to be imperative that we, as researchers, strive for the betterment of scientific conduct.

Regardless of whether we live in a Golden Age or a Gilded Age, consider the recommendations we have made here. We call for gatekeepers to be more open to research that, despite possessing rigor and relevance, did not achieve desired results, and not to engage in or recommend QRPs. We call for authors to be more transparent in their reporting of findings. Lastly, we call for increased methodological rigor through continuing education and increased awareness. With these recommendations in mind, we ask what harm comes from more openness, greater transparency, and increased rigor? Even those who do not see a current credibility crisis due to ongoing QRP engagement should still recognize its distinct and looming possibility given the increasing pressures and fallibility built into the system. Ultimately, our recommendations help either address a current crisis or prevent a future one.

Acknowledgments

We would like to thank Daniele Fanelli and Lee J. Jussim for their insightful comments on earlier versions of this chapter. Ernest H. O'Boyle's time on this project was partially supported by the Dale M. Coleman Chair of Management.

References

Agnoli, F., Wicherts, J. M., Veldkamp, C. L. S., Albiero, P., & Cubelli, R. (2017). Questionable research practices among Italian research psychologists. *PLoS One*, *12*(3), e0172792. https://doi.org/10.1371/journal.pone.0172792

Alter, G. C., & Gonzalez, R. (2018). Responsible practices for data sharing. *American Psychologist*, *73*(2), 146–156. https://doi.org/10.1037/amp0000258

American Psychological Association. (2020). *Publication Manual of the American Psychological Association: The Official Guide to APA style* (7th ed.). American Psychological Association.

Appelbaum, M., Cooper, H. M., Kline, R. B., Mayo-Wilson, E., Nezu, A. M., & Rao, S. M. (2018). Journal article reporting standards for quantitative research in psychology: The APA Publications and Communications Board task force report. *American Psychologist*, *73*(1), 3–25. https://doi.org/10.1037/amp0000191

Artner, R., Verliefde, T., Steegen, S., Gomes, S., Traets, F., Tuerlinckx, F., & Vanpaemel, W. (2020). The reproducibility of statistical results in psychological research: An investigation using unpublished raw data. *Psychological Methods* (advance online publication). https://doi.org/10.1037/met0000365

Banks, G. C., Field, J. G., Oswald, F. L., O'Boyle, E. H., Landis, R. S., Rupp, D. E., & Rogelberg, S. G. (2019). Answers to 18 questions about open science practices. *Journal of Business and Psychology*, *34*(3), 257–270. https://doi.org/10.1007/s10869-018-9547-8

Banks, G. C., O'Boyle, E. H., Pollack, J. M., White, C. D., Batchelor, J. H., Whelpley, C. E., Abston, K. A., Bennett, A. A., & Adkins, C. L. (2016). Questions about questionable research practices in the field of management: A guest commentary. *Journal of Management*, *42*(1), 5–20. https://doi.org/10.1177/0149206315619011

Baron, J. N., King, M. D., & Sorenson, O. (2016). S/he blinded me with science: The sociology of scientific misconduct. In D. A. Palmer, K. Smith-Crowe, & R. Greenwood (Eds.), *Organizational Wrongdoing: Key Perspectives and New Directions* (pp. 176–202). Cambridge University Press. https://doi.org/10.1017/CBO9781316338827.008

Baumeister, R. F. (2016). Charting the future of social psychology on stormy seas: Winners, losers, and recommendations. *Journal of Experimental Social Psychology*, *66*, 153–158. https://doi.org/10.1016/j.jesp.2016.02.003

Bedeian, A. G., Taylor, S. G., & Miller, A. N. (2010). Management science on the credibility bubble: Cardinal sins and various misdemeanors. *Academy of Management Learning & Education*, *9*(4), 715–725. https://doi.org/10.5465/AMLE.2010.56659889

Benos, D. J., Bashari, E., Chaves, J. M., Gaggar, A., Kapoor, N., LaFrance, M., Mans, R., Mayhew, D., McGowan, S., Polter, A., Qadri, Y., Sarfare, S., Schultz, K., Splittgerber, R.,

Stephenson, J., Tower, C., Walton, R. G., & Zotov, A. (2007). The ups and downs of peer review. *Advances in Physiology Education, 31*(2), 145–152. https://doi.org/10.1152/advan.00104.2006.

Bhattacharjee, Y. (2013, April 26). The mind of a con man. *New York Times*. http://www.nytimes.com/2013/04/28/magazine/diederik-stapels-audacious-academic-fraud.html

Bollen, K. A., Cacioppo, J. T., Kaplan, R. M., Krosnick, J. A., & Olds, J. L. (2015). *Social, Behavioral, and Economic Sciences Perspectives on Robust and Reliable Science: Report of the Subcommittee on Replicability in Science, Advisory Committee to the National Science Foundation Directorate for Social, Behavioral, and Economic Science.* https://www.nsf.gov/sbe/AC_Materials/SBE_Robust_and_Reliable_Research_Report.pdf

Borgman, C. L. (2015). *Big Data, Little Data, No Data: Scholarship in the Networked World.* MIT Press.

Bosco, F. A., Aguinis, H., Field, J. G., Pierce, C. A., & Dalton, D. R. (2016). HARKing's threat to organizational research: Evidence from primary and meta-analytic sources. *Personnel Psychology, 63*(3), 709–750. https://doi.org/10.1111/peps.12111

Botvinik-Nezer, R., Holzmeister, F., Camerer, C. F., Dreber, A., Huber, J., Johannesson, M., Kirchler, M., Iwanir, R., Mumford, J. A., Adcock, R. A., Avesani, P., Baczkowski, B. M., Bajracharya, A., Bakst, L., Ball, S., Barilari, M., Bault, N., Beaton, D., Beitner, J., . . . Schonberg, T. (2020). Variability in the analysis of a single neuroimaging dataset by many teams. *Nature, 582*(7810), 84–88. https://doi.org/10.1038/s41586-020-2314-9

Breet, E., Botha, J., Horn, L., & Swartz, L. (2018). Academic and scientific authorship practices: A survey among South African researchers. *Journal of Empirical Research on Human Research Ethics, 13*(4), 412–420. https://doi.org/10.1177/1556264618789253

Center for Open Science. (2019). *Open Science Framework.* https://osf.io/

Chambers, C. D. (2017). *The Seven Deadly Sins of Psychology: A Manifesto for Reforming the Culture of Scientific Practice.* Princeton University Press. https://doi.org/10.1515/9781400884940

Cialdini, R. B., Borden, R. J., Thorne, A., Walker, M. R., Freeman, S., & Sloan, L. R. (1976). Basking in reflected glory: Three (football) field studies. *Journal of Personality and Social Psychology, 34*(3), 366–375. https://doi.org/10.1037/0022-3514.34.3.366

Cialdini, R. B., Kallgren, C. A., & Reno, R. R. (1991). A focus theory of normative conduct: A theoretical refinement and reevaluation of the role of norms in human behavior. In M. P. Zanna (Ed.), *Advances in Experimental Social Psychology* (Vol. 24, pp. 201–234). Elsevier Academic Press. https://doi.org/10.1016/S0065-2601(08)60330-5

Cialdini, R. B., & Richardson, K. D. (1980). Two indirect tactics of image management: Basking and blasting. *Journal of Personality and Social Psychology, 39*(3), 406–415. https://doi.org/10.1037/0022-3514.39.3.406

Cokol, M., Ozbay, F., & Rodriguez-Esteban, R. (2008). Retraction rates are on the rise. *EMBO Reports, 9*(1), 2–2. https://doi.org/10.1038/sj.embor.7401143

Cole, D. A., & Preacher, K. J. (2014). Manifest variable path analysis: Potentially serious and misleading consequences due to uncorrected measurement error. *Psychological Methods, 19*(2), 300–315. https://doi.org/10.1037/a0033805

Connelly, B. L., Certo, S. T., Ireland, R. D., & Reutzel, C. R. (2011). Signaling theory: A review and assessment. *Journal of Management, 37*(1), 39–67. https://doi.org/10.1177/0149206310388419

Cortina, J. M., Green, J. P., Keeler, K. R., & Vandenberg, R. J. (2017). Degrees of freedom in SEM: Are we testing the models that we claim to test? *Organizational Research Methods, 20*(3), 350–378. https://doi.org/10.1177/1094428116676345

Dalton, D. R., Aguinis, H., Dalton, C. M., Bosco, F. A., & Pierce, C. A. (2012). Revisiting the file drawer problem in meta-analysis: An assessment of published and nonpublished correlation matrices. *Personnel Psychology, 65*(2), 221–249.

Davis, M. S. (1971). That's interesting! Towards a phenomenology of sociology and a sociology of phenomenology. *Philosophy of the Social Sciences, 1*(2), 309–344. https://doi.org/10.1177/004839317100100211

De Boeck, P., & Jeon, M. (2018). Perceived crisis and reforms: Issues, explanations, and remedies. *Psychological Bulletin, 144*(7), 757–777. https://doi.org/10.1037/bul0000154

Dickersin, K., & Rennie, D. (2003). Registering clinical trials. *Journal of the American Medical Association, 290*(4), 516. https://doi.org/10.1001/jama.290.4.516

Dienes, Z. (2008). *Understanding Psychology as a Science: An Introduction to Scientific and Statistical Inference*. Palgrave Macmillan.

Dienes, Z. (2016). How Bayes factors change scientific practice. *Journal of Mathematical Psychology, 72*, 78–89. https://doi.org/10.1016/j.jmp.2015.10.003

Dienes, Z., & Mclatchie, N. (2018). Four reasons to prefer Bayesian analyses over significance testing. *Psychonomic Bulletin & Review, 25*(1), 207–218. https://doi.org/10.3758/s13423-017-1266-z

Duyx, B., Urlings, M. J. E., Swaen, G. M. H., Bouter, L. M., & Zeegers, M. P. (2017). Scientific citations favor positive results: A systematic review and meta-analysis. *Journal of Clinical Epidemiology, 88*, 92–101. https://doi.org/10.1016/j.jclinepi.2017.06.002

Ebersole, C. R., Mathur, M. B., Baranski, E., Bart-Plange, D.-J., Buttrick, N. R., Chartier, C. R., Corker, K. S., Corley, M., Hartshorne, J. K., IJzerman, H., Lazarević, L. B., Rabagliati, H., Ropovik, I., Aczel, B., Aeschbach, L. F., Andrighetto, L., Arnal, J. D., Arrow, H., Babincak, P., . . . Nosek, B. A. (2020). Many Labs 5: Testing pre-data-collection peer review as an intervention to increase replicability. *Advances in Methods and Practices in Psychological Science, 3*(3), 309–331. https://doi.org/10.1177/2515245920958687

Editors. (1909). The reporting of unsuccessful cases. *Boston Medical and Surgical Journal, 161*, 263–264.

Edwards, J. R. (2008). Seven deadly myths of testing moderation in organizational research. In C. E. Lance & R. J. Vandenberg (Eds.), *Statistical and Methodological Myths and Urban Legends: Doctrine, Verity and Fable in the Organizational and Social Sciences* (pp. 143–164). Routledge.

Edwards, M. A., & Roy, S. (2017). Academic research in the 21st century: Maintaining scientific integrity in a climate of perverse incentives and hypercompetition. *Environmental Engineering Science, 34*(1), 51–61. https://doi.org/10.1089/ees.2016.0223

Fanelli, D. (2009). How many scientists fabricate and falsify research? A systematic review and meta-analysis of survey data. *PLoS ONE, 4*(5), e5738. https://doi.org/10.1371/journal.pone.0005738

Fanelli, D. (2012a). The black, the white and the grey areas: Towards an international and interdisciplinary definition of scientific misconduct. In T. Mayer & N. H. Steneck (Eds.), *Promoting Research Integrity in a Global Environment* (pp. 79–90). World Scientific Publishing.

Fanelli, D. (2012b). Negative results are disappearing from most disciplines and countries. *Scientometrics, 90*(3), 891–904. https://doi.org/10.1007/s11192-011-0494-7

Fanelli, D. (2018). Opinion: Is science really facing a reproducibility crisis, and do we need it to? *Proceedings of the National Academy of Sciences USA, 115*(11), 2628–2631. https://doi.org/10.1073/pnas.1708272114

Fang, F. C., Steen, R. G., & Casadevall, A. (2012). Misconduct accounts for the majority of retracted scientific publications. *Proceedings of the National Academy of Sciences USA*, *109*(42), 17028–17033. https://doi.org/10.1073/pnas.1212247109

Feynman, R. P. (1985). *Surely You're Joking, Mr. Feynman!* W.W. Norton.

Fiedler, K. (2016). Ethical norms and moral values among scientists. In J. P. Forgas, L. Jussim, & P. A. M. Van Lange (Eds.), *The Social Psychology of Morality* (pp. 215–235). Routledge.

Fiedler, K., & Schwarz, N. (2016). Questionable research practices revisited. *Social Psychological and Personality Science*, *7*(1), 45–52. https://doi.org/10.1177/1948550615612150

Fister, I. J., Fister, I., & Perc, M. (2016). Toward the discovery of citation cartels in citation networks. *Frontiers in Physics*, *4*(December), 1–5. https://doi.org/10.3389/fphy.2016.00049

Flake, J. K., & Fried, E. I. (2020). Measurement schmeasurement: Questionable measurement practices and how to avoid them. *Advances in Methods and Practices in Psychological Science*, *3*(4), 456–465. https://doi.org/10.1177/2515245920952393

Fox, N. W., Honeycutt, N., & Jussim, L. J. (2020). *Better understanding the population size and stigmatization of psychologists using questionable research practices.* https://doi.org/10.31234/osf.io/3v7hx

Funder, D. C., Levine, J. M., Mackie, D. M., Morf, C. C., Sansone, C., Vazire, S., & West, S. G. (2014). Improving the dependability of research in personality and social psychology. *Personality and Social Psychology Review*, *18*(1), 3–12. https://doi.org/10.1177/1088868313507536

Gelman, A. (2016). The problems with p-values are not just with p-values: Supplemental material to the ASA statement on p-values and statistical significance. *American Statistician*, *70*(2), 129–133. https://doi.org/10.1080/00031305.2016.1154108

Gelman, A., & Hennig, C. (2017). Beyond subjective and objective in statistics. *Journal of the Royal Statistical Society: Series A (Statistics in Society)*, *180*(4), 967–1033. https://doi.org/10.1111/rssa.12276

Gelman, A., & Loken, E. (2013). *The garden of forking paths: Why multiple comparisons can be a problem, even when there is no "fishing expedition" or "p-hacking" and the research hypothesis was posited ahead of time* (pp. 1–17). Department of Statistics, Columbia University. http://www.stat.columbia.edu/~gelman/research/unpublished/p_hacking.pdf

Gelman, A., & Loken, E. (2014). The statistical crisis in science. *American Scientist*, *102*(6), 460. https://doi.org/10.1511/2014.111.460

Gerhart, B., & Rynes, S. L. (2003). *Compensation: Theory, Evidence, and Strategic Implications*. SAGE Publications.

Gigerenzer, G. (2004). Mindless statistics. *Journal of Socio-Economics*, *33*(5), 587–606. https://doi.org/10.1016/j.socec.2004.09.033

Gigerenzer, G. (2018). Statistical rituals: The replication delusion and how we got there. *Advances in Methods and Practices in Psychological Science*, *1*(2), 198–218. https://doi.org/10.1177/2515245918771329

Gigerenzer, G., & Marewski, J. N. (2015). Surrogate science: The idol of a universal method for scientific inference. *Journal of Management*, *41*(2), 421–440. https://doi.org/10.1177/0149206314547522

Gilmore, R. O., Kennedy, J. L., & Adolph, K. E. (2018). Practical solutions for sharing data and materials from psychological research. *Advances in Methods and Practices in Psychological Science*, *1*(1), 121–130. https://doi.org/10.1177/2515245917746500

Giner-Sorolla, R. (2012). Science or art? How aesthetic standards grease the way through the publication bottleneck but undermine science. *Perspectives on Psychological Science*, *7*(6), 562–571. https://doi.org/10.1177/1745691612457576

Götz, M., O'Boyle, E. H., Gonzalez-Mulé, E., Banks, G. C., & Bollmann, S. S. (2021). The "Goldilocks Zone": (Too) many confidence intervals in tests of mediation just exclude zero. *Psychological Bulletin*, *147*(1), 95–114. https://doi.org/10.1037/bul0000315

Greco, L. M., O'Boyle, E. H., & Walter, S. L. (2015). Absence of malice: A meta-analysis of nonresponse bias in counterproductive work behavior research. *Journal of Applied Psychology*, *100*(1), 75–97. https://doi.org/10.1037/a0037495

Grieneisen, M. L., & Zhang, M. (2012). A comprehensive survey of retracted articles from the scholarly literature. *PLoS One*, *7*(10), e44118. https://doi.org/10.1371/journal.pone.0044118

Gross, C. (2016). Scientific misconduct. *Annual Review of Psychology*, *67*(1), 693–711. https://doi.org/10.1146/annurev-psych-122414-033437

Gurevitch, J., Koricheva, J., Nakagawa, S., & Stewart, G. (2018). Meta-analysis and the science of research synthesis. *Nature*, *555*(7695), 175–182. https://doi.org/10.1038/nature25753

Hagger, M. S., Chatzisarantis, N. L. D., Alberts, H., Anggono, C. O., Batailler, C., Birt, A. R., Brand, R., Brandt, M. J., Brewer, G., Bruyneel, S., Calvillo, D. P., Campbell, W. K., Cannon, P. R., Carlucci, M., Carruth, N. P., Cheung, T., Crowell, A., de Ridder, D. T. D., Dewitte, S., . . . Zwienenberg, M. (2016). A multilab preregistered replication of the ego-depletion effect. *Perspectives on Psychological Science*, *11*(4), 546–573. https://doi.org/10.1177/1745691616652873

Hartgerink, C. H. J., van Aert, R. C. M., Nuijten, M. B., Wicherts, J. M., & van Assen, M. A. L. M. (2016). Distributions of p-values smaller than .05 in psychology: What is going on? *PeerJ*, *4*, e1935. https://doi.org/10.7717/peerj.1935

Hartgerink, C. H. J., & van Zelst, M. (2018). "As-you-go" instead of "after-the-fact": A network approach to scholarly communication and evaluation. *Publications*, *6*(2), 21. https://doi.org/10.3390/publications6020021

Harzing, A.-W. (2002). Are our referencing errors undermining our scholarship and credibility? The case of expatriate failure rates. *Journal of Organizational Behavior*, *23*(1), 127–148. https://doi.org/10.1002/job.125

Helgesson, G., Juth, N., Schneider, J., Lövtrup, M., & Lynøe, N. (2018). Misuse of coauthorship in medical theses in Sweden. *Journal of Empirical Research on Human Research Ethics*, *13*(4), 402–411. https://doi.org/10.1177/1556264618784206

Hesse, B. W. (2018). Can psychology walk the walk of open science? *American Psychologist*, *73*(2), 126–137. https://doi.org/10.1037/amp0000197

Hitchcock, C., & Sober, E. (2004). Prediction versus accommodation and the risk of overfitting. *British Journal for the Philosophy of Science*, *55*(1), 1–34. https://doi.org/10.1093/bjps/55.1.1

Hofmann, B., Helgesson, G., Juth, N., & Holm, S. (2015). Scientific dishonesty: A survey of doctoral students at the major medical faculties in Sweden and Norway. *Journal of Empirical Research on Human Research Ethics*, *10*(4), 380–388. https://doi.org/10.1177/1556264615599686

Holland, S. J., Shore, D. B., & Cortina, J. M. (2017). Review and recommendations for integrating mediation and moderation. *Organizational Research Methods, 20*(4), 686–720. https://doi.org/10.1177/1094428116658958

Hollenbeck, J. R., & Wright, P. M. (2017). Harking, sharking, and tharking: Making the case for post hoc analysis of scientific data. *Journal of Management, 43*(1), 5–18. https://doi.org/10.1177/0149206316679487

Hubbard, R. (2016). *Corrupt Research: The Case for Reconceptualizing Empirical Management and Social Science.* SAGE Publications.

Humphreys, M., Sanchez de la Sierra, R., & van der Windt, P. (2013). Fishing, commitment, and communication: A proposal for comprehensive nonbinding research registration. *Political Analysis, 21*(01), 1–20. https://doi.org/10.1093/pan/mps021

Ioannidis, J. P. A. (2016). The mass production of redundant, misleading, and conflicted systematic reviews and meta-analyses. *Milbank Quarterly, 94*(3), 485–514. https://doi.org/10.1111/1468-0009.12210

Ioannidis, J. P. A., Klavans, R., & Boyack, K. W. (2018). Thousands of scientists publish a paper every five days. *Nature, 561*(7722), 167–169. https://doi.org/10.1038/d41586-018-06185-8

John, L. K., Loewenstein, G., & Prelec, D. (2012). Measuring the prevalence of questionable research practices with incentives for truth telling. *Psychological Science, 23*(5), 524–532. https://doi.org/10.1177/0956797611430953

Jonas, K. J., & Cesario, J. (2016). How can preregistration contribute to research in our field? *Comprehensive Results in Social Psychology, 1*(1–3), 1–7. https://doi.org/10.1080/23743603.2015.1070611

Karr, A. F. (2016). Data sharing and access. *Annual Review of Statistics and Its Application, 3*(1), 113–132. https://doi.org/10.1146/annurev-statistics-041715-033438

Kepes, S., & McDaniel, M. A. (2013). How trustworthy is the scientific literature in industrial and organizational psychology? *Industrial and Organizational Psychology, 6*(3), 252–268. https://doi.org/10.1111/iops.12045

Kerr, N. L. (1998). HARKing: Hypothesizing after the results are known. *Personality and Social Psychology Review, 2*(3), 196–217. https://doi.org/10.1207/s15327957pspr0203_4

Kidwell, M. C., Lazarević, L. B., Baranski, E. N., Hardwicke, T. E., Piechowski, S., Falkenberg, L.-S., Kennett, C., Slowik, A., Sonnleitner, C., Hess-Holden, C., Errington, T. M., Fiedler, S., & Nosek, B. A. (2016). Badges to acknowledge open practices: A simple, low-cost, effective method for increasing transparency. *PLOS Biology, 14*(5), e1002456. https://doi.org/10.1371/journal.pbio.1002456

Kühberger, A., Fritz, A., & Scherndl, T. (2014). Publication bias in psychology: A diagnosis based on the correlation between effect size and sample size. *PLoS One, 9*(9), e105825. https://doi.org/10.1371/journal.pone.0105825

Lakens, D., Adolfi, F. G., Albers, C. J., Anvari, F., Apps, M. A. J., Argamon, S. E., Baguley, T., Becker, R. B., Benning, S. D., Bradford, D. E., Buchanan, E. M., Caldwell, A. R., Van Calster, B., Carlsson, R., Chen, S.-C., Chung, B., Colling, L. J., Collins, G. S., Crook, Z., ... Zwaan, R. A. (2018). Justify your alpha. *Nature Human Behaviour, 2*(3), 168–171. https://doi.org/10.1038/s41562-018-0311-x

Leavitt, K., Mitchell, T. R., & Peterson, J. (2010). Theory pruning: Strategies to reduce our dense theoretical landscape. *Organizational Research Methods, 13*(4), 644–667. https://doi.org/10.1177/1094428109345156

Lee, C. J., Sugimoto, C. R., Zhang, G., & Cronin, B. (2013). Bias in peer review. *Journal of the American Society for Information Science and Technology*, 64(1), 2–17. https://doi.org/10.1002/asi.22784

Liberati, A. (1992). Publication bias and the editorial process. *Journal of the American Medical Association*, 267(21), 2891. https://doi.org/10.1001/jama.1992.03480210049017

Lynøe, N., Jacobsson, L., & Lundgren, E. (1999). Fraud, misconduct or normal science in medical research—an empirical study of demarcation. *Journal of Medical Ethics*, 25(6), 501–506. https://doi.org/10.1136/jme.25.6.501

Martin, G. N., & Clarke, R. M. (2017). Are psychology journals anti-replication? A snapshot of editorial practices. *Frontiers in Psychology*, 8(April), 1–6. https://doi.org/10.3389/fpsyg.2017.00523

Martinson, B. C., Anderson, M. S., & De Vries, R. (2005). Scientists behaving badly. *Nature*, 435(7043), 737–738. https://doi.org/10.1038/435737a

Martone, M. E., Garcia-Castro, A., & VandenBos, G. R. (2018). Data sharing in psychology. *American Psychologist*, 73(2), 111–125. https://doi.org/10.1037/amp0000242

Merton, R. K. (1968). The Matthew effect in science: The reward and communication systems of science are considered. *Science*, 159(3810), 56–63. https://doi.org/10.1126/science.159.3810.56

Merton, R. K. (1973). *The Sociology of Science: Theoretical and Empirical Investigations*. University of Chicago Press.

Meyer, M. N. (2018). Practical tips for ethical data sharing. *Advances in Methods and Practices in Psychological Science*, 1(1), 131–144. https://doi.org/10.1177/2515245917747656

Miguel, E., Camerer, C. F., Casey, K., Cohen, J., Esterling, K. M., Gerber, A., Glennerster, R., Green, D. P., Humphreys, M., Imbens, G. W., Laitin, D., Madon, T., Nelson, L. D., Nosek, B. A., Petersen, M., Sedlmayr, R., Simmons, J. P., Simonsohn, U., & Van der Laan, M. (2014). Promoting transparency in social science research. *Science*, 343(6166), 30–31. https://doi.org/10.1126/science.1245317

Morey, R. D., Chambers, C. D., Etchells, P. J., Harris, C. R., Hoekstra, R., Lakens, D., Lewandowsky, S., Morey, C. C., Newman, D. P., Schönbrodt, F. D., Vanpaemel, W., Wagenmakers, E.-J., & Zwaan, R. A. (2016). The peer reviewers' openness initiative: Incentivizing open research practices through peer review. *Royal Society Open Science*, 3(1), 150547. https://doi.org/10.1098/rsos.150547

Mosimann, J. E., Wiseman, C. V., & Edelman, R. E. (1995). Data fabrication: Can people generate random digits? *Accountability in Research*, 4(1), 31–55. https://doi.org/10.1080/08989629508573866

Motyl, M., Demos, A. P., Carsel, T. S., Hanson, B. E., Melton, Z. J., Mueller, A. B., Prims, J. P., Sun, J., Washburn, A. N., Wong, K. M., Yantis, C., & Skitka, L. J. (2017). The state of social and personality science: Rotten to the core, not so bad, getting better, or getting worse? *Journal of Personality and Social Psychology*, 113(1), 34–58. https://doi.org/10.1037/pspa0000084

Mumford, M. D., Murphy, S. T., Connelly, S., Hill, J. H., Antes, A. L., Brown, R. P., & Devenport, L. D. (2007). Environmental influences on ethical decision making: Climate and environmental predictors of research integrity. *Ethics & Behavior*, 17(4), 337–366. https://doi.org/10.1080/10508420701519510

Munafò, M. R., Nosek, B. A., Bishop, D. V. M., Button, K. S., Chambers, C. D., Percie du Sert, N., Simonsohn, U., Wagenmakers, E.-J., Ware, J. J., & Ioannidis, J. P. A. (2017). A manifesto for reproducible science. *Nature Human Behaviour, 1*(1), 0021. https://doi.org/10.1038/s41562-016-0021

Murphy, K. R., & Aguinis, H. (2019). HARKing: How badly can cherry-picking and question trolling produce bias in published results? *Journal of Business and Psychology, 34*(1), 1–17. https://doi.org/10.1007/s10869-017-9524-7

Murphy, K. R., & Russell, C. J. (2017). Mend it or end it: Redirecting the search for interactions in the Organizational Sciences. *Organizational Research Methods, 20*(4), 549–573. https://doi.org/10.1177/1094428115625322

Neuliep, J. W., & Crandall, R. (1990). Editorial bias against replication research. *Journal of Social Behavior & Personality, 5*(4), 85–90.

Neuroskeptic. (2012). The nine circles of scientific hell. *Perspectives on Psychological Science, 7*(6), 643–644. https://doi.org/10.1177/1745691612459519

Nosek, B. A., Alter, G. C., Banks, G. C., Borsboom, D., Bowman, S. D., Breckler, S. J., Buck, S., Chambers, C. D., Chin, G., Christensen, G., Contestabile, M., Dafoe, A., Eich, E., Freese, J., Glennerster, R., Goroff, D., Green, D. P., Hesse, B. W., Humphreys, M., . . . Yarkoni, T. (2015). Promoting an open research culture. *Science, 348*(6242), 1422–1425. https://doi.org/10.1126/science.aab2374

Nosek, B. A., & Bar-Anan, Y. (2012). Scientific utopia: I. Opening scientific communication. *Psychological Inquiry, 23*(3), 217–243. https://doi.org/10.1080/1047840X.2012.692215

Nosek, B. A., Spies, J. R., & Motyl, M. (2012). Scientific utopia: II. Restructuring incentives and practices to promote truth over publishability. *Perspectives on Psychological Science, 7*(6), 615–631. https://doi.org/10.1177/1745691612459058

Nuijten, M. B., Hartgerink, C. H. J., van Assen, M. A. L. M., Epskamp, S., & Wicherts, J. M. (2016). The prevalence of statistical reporting errors in psychology (1985–2013). *Behavior Research Methods, 48*(4), 1205–1226. https://doi.org/10.3758/s13428-015-0664-2

O'Boyle, E. H., Banks, G. C., Carter, K., Walter, S. L., & Yuan, Z. (2019). A 20-year review of outcome reporting bias in moderated multiple regression. *Journal of Business and Psychology, 34*(1), 19–37. https://doi.org/10.1007/s10869-018-9539-8

O'Boyle, E. H., Banks, G. C., & Gonzalez-Mulé, E. (2017). The chrysalis effect: How ugly initial results metamorphosize into beautiful articles. *Journal of Management, 43*(2), 376–399. https://doi.org/10.1177/0149206314527133

Oberauer, K. (2019). *Preregistration of a forking path—What does it add to the garden of evidence?* Psychonomic Society. https://featuredcontent.psychonomic.org/preregistration-of-a-forking-path-what-does-it-add-to-the-garden-of-evidence/

Open Science Collaboration. (2015). Estimating the reproducibility of psychological science. *Science, 349*(6251), aac4716. https://doi.org/10.1126/science.aac4716

Pashler, H., & Wagenmakers, E.-J. (2012). Editors' introduction to the special section on replicability in psychological science. *Perspectives on Psychological Science, 7*(6), 528–530. https://doi.org/10.1177/1745691612465253

Pfeffer, J., & Langton, N. (1993). The effect of wage dispersion on satisfaction, productivity, and working collaboratively: Evidence from college and university faculty. *Administrative Science Quarterly, 38*(3), 382. https://doi.org/10.2307/2393373

Popper, K. R. (1985). *The Logic of Scientific Discovery*. Routledge.

Rosenblatt, A., & Kirk, S. A. (1981). Recognition of authors in blind review of manuscripts. *Journal of Social Service Research, 3*(4), 383–394. https://doi.org/10.1300/J079v03n04_04

Ross, M. W., Iguchi, M. Y., & Panicker, S. (2018). Ethical aspects of data sharing and research participant protections. *American Psychologist, 73*(2), 138–145. https://doi.org/10.1037/amp0000240

Rubin, M. (2017a). Do p values lose their meaning in exploratory analyses? It depends how you define the familywise error rate. *Review of General Psychology, 21*(3), 269–275. https://doi.org/10.1037/gpr0000123

Rubin, M. (2017b). An evaluation of four solutions to the forking paths problem: Adjusted alpha, preregistration, sensitivity analyses, and abandoning the Neyman-Pearson approach. *Review of General Psychology, 21*(4), 321–329. https://doi.org/10.1037/gpr0000135

Rubin, M. (2017c). When does HARKing hurt? Identifying when different types of undisclosed post hoc hypothesizing harm scientific progress. *Review of General Psychology, 21*(4), 308–320. https://doi.org/10.1037/gpr0000128

Sacco, D. F., Bruton, S. V., & Brown, M. (2018). In defense of the questionable: Defining the basis of research scientists' engagement in questionable research practices. *Journal of Empirical Research on Human Research Ethics, 13*(1), 101–110. https://doi.org/10.1177/1556264617743834

Siddaway, A. P., Wood, A. M., & Hedges, L. V. (2019). How to do a systematic review: A best practice guide for conducting and reporting narrative reviews, meta-analyses, and meta-syntheses. *Annual Review of Psychology, 70*(1), 747–770. https://doi.org/10.1146/annurev-psych-010418-102803

Silberzahn, R., & Uhlmann, E. L. (2015). Crowdsourced research: Many hands make tight work. *Nature, 526*(7572), 189–191. https://doi.org/10.1038/526189a

Silberzahn, R., Uhlmann, E. L., Martin, D. P., Anselmi, P., Aust, F., Awtrey, E., Bahník, Š., Bai, F., Bannard, C., Bonnier, E., Carlsson, R., Cheung, F., Christensen, G., Clay, R., Craig, M. A., Dalla Rosa, A., Dam, L., Evans, M. H., Flores Cervantes, I., . . . Nosek, B. A. (2018). Many analysts, one data set: Making transparent how variations in analytic choices affect results. *Advances in Methods and Practices in Psychological Science, 1*(3), 337–356. https://doi.org/10.1177/2515245917747646

Simmons, J. P., Nelson, L. D., & Simonsohn, U. (2011). False-positive psychology: Undisclosed flexibility in data collection and analysis allows presenting anything as significant. *Psychological Science, 22*(11), 1359–1366. https://doi.org/10.1177/0956797611417632

Simonsohn, U. (2013). Just post it: The lesson from two cases of fabricated data detected by statistics alone. *Psychological Science, 24*(10), 1875–1888. https://doi.org/10.1177/0956797613480366

Simonsohn, U., Nelson, L. D., & Simmons, J. P. (2014a). P-curve: A key to the file-drawer. *Journal of Experimental Psychology: General, 143*(2), 534–547. https://doi.org/10.1037/a0033242

Simonsohn, U., Nelson, L. D., & Simmons, J. P. (2014b). P-curve and effect size: Correcting for publication bias using only significant results. *Perspectives on Psychological Science, 9*(6), 666–681. https://doi.org/10.1177/1745691614553988

Simonsohn, U., Simmons, J. P., & Nelson, L. D. (2018). *AsPredicted*. https://aspredicted.org/

Smaldino, P. E., & McElreath, R. (2016). The natural selection of bad science. *Royal Society Open Science, 3*(9), 160384. https://doi.org/10.1098/rsos.160384

Stamm, K., Christidis, P., Hamp, A., & Nigrinis, A. (2014). *How many psychology doctorates are awarded by U.S. institutions? News from APA's Center for Workforce Studies.* APA's Center for Workforce Studies. https://www.apa.org/monitor/2014/07-08/datapoint.aspx

Steen, R. G., Casadevall, A., & Fang, F. C. (2013). Why has the number of scientific retractions increased? *PLoS One, 8*(7), e68397. https://doi.org/10.1371/journal.pone.0068397

Steneck, N. H. (2006). Fostering integrity in research: Definitions, current knowledge, and future directions. *Science and Engineering Ethics, 12*(1), 53–74. https://doi.org/10.1007/PL00022268

Sterling, T. D. (1959). Publication decisions and their possible effects on inferences drawn from tests of significance—or vice versa. *Journal of the American Statistical Association, 54*(285), 30. https://doi.org/10.2307/2282137

Sterling, T. D., Rosenbaum, W. L., & Weinkam, J. J. (1995). Publication decisions revisited: The effect of the outcome of statistical tests on the decision to publish and vice versa. *American Statistician, 49*(1), 108–112. https://doi.org/10.1080/00031305.1995.10476125

Sturman, M. C., Sturman, A. J., & Sturman, C. J. (2021). Uncontrolled control variables: The extent that a researcher's degrees of freedom with control variables increases various types of statistical errors. *Journal of Applied Psychology* (advance online publication). https://doi.org/10.1037/apl0000849

Swazey, J. P., Anderson, M. S., & Louis, K. S. (1993). Ethical problems in academic research. *American Scientist, 81*(6), 542–553.

Tahamtan, I., & Bornmann, L. (2018). Core elements in the process of citing publications: Conceptual overview of the literature. *Journal of Informetrics, 12*(1), 203–216. https://doi.org/10.1016/j.joi.2018.01.002

Toth, A. A., Banks, G. C., Mellor, D. T., O'Boyle, E. H., Dickson, A., Davis, D. J., DeHaven, A., Bochantin, J. E., & Borns, J. (2021). Study preregistration: An evaluation of a method for transparent reporting. *Journal of Business and Psychology, 36*, 553–571. https://doi.org/10.1007/s10869-020-09695-3

Tourish, D. (2019). *Management Studies in Crisis: Fraud, Deception and Meaningless Research.* Cambridge University Press.

Uhlmann, E. L., Ebersole, C. R., Chartier, C. R., Errington, T. M., Kidwell, M. C., Lai, C. K., McCarthy, R. J., Riegelman, A., Silberzahn, R., & Nosek, B. A. (2019). Scientific utopia III: Crowdsourcing science. *Perspectives on Psychological Science, 14*(5), 711–733. https://doi.org/10.1177/1745691619850561

Van Noorden, R. (2011). Science publishing: The trouble with retractions. *Nature, 478*(7367), 26–28. https://doi.org/10.1038/478026a

Wagenmakers, E.-J., Wetzels, R., Borsboom, D., van der Maas, H. L. J., & Kievit, R. A. (2012). An agenda for purely confirmatory research. *Perspectives on Psychological Science, 7*(6), 632–638. https://doi.org/10.1177/1745691612463078

Wager, E., Singhvi, S., & Kleinert, S. (2015). Too much of a good thing? An observational study of prolific authors. *PeerJ, 3*, e1154. https://doi.org/10.7717/peerj.1154

Wasserstein, R. L., & Lazar, N. A. (2016). The ASA's statement on p-values: Context, process, and purpose. *American Statistician, 70*(2), 129–133. https://doi.org/10.1080/00031305.2016.1154108

Wicherts, J. M., Veldkamp, C. L. S., Augusteijn, H. E. M., Bakker, M., van Aert, R. C. M., & van Assen, M. A. L. M. (2016). Degrees of freedom in planning, running, analyzing, and reporting psychological studies: A checklist to avoid p-hacking. *Frontiers in Psychology, 7*(November), 1–12. https://doi.org/10.3389/fpsyg.2016.01832

Wigboldus, D. H. J., & Dotsch, R. (2016). Encourage playing with data and discourage questionable reporting practices. *Psychometrika, 81*(1), 27–32. https://doi.org/10.1007/s11336-015-9445-1

Wilhite, A. W., & Fong, E. A. (2012). Coercive citation in academic publishing. *Science, 335*(6068), 542–543. https://doi.org/10.1126/science.1212540

11
P-hacking

A Strategic Analysis

Robert J. MacCoun

The phenomenon of p-hacking occurs when researchers engage in questionable practices that enable them to report findings as being statistically significant. I offer four models of p-hacking behavior—unconditional, strategic, greedy, and restrained—and explore the implications of each model. I then discuss the implications of recent reforms (routine replication, preregistration, and blinded data analysis) for each model, under the assumption that the model is valid.

The term *p-hacking* was introduced by Simonsohn et al. (2013) as an apt and pithy label for a class of behaviors that are surely as old as the practice of null hypothesis statistical testing (NHST):[1]

> While collecting and analyzing data, researchers have many decisions to make, including whether to collect more data, which outliers to exclude, which measure(s) to analyze, which covariates to use, and so on. If these decisions are not made in advance but rather are made as the data are being analyzed, then researchers may make them in ways that self-servingly increase their odds of publishing. We refer to such behavior as p-hacking. (p. 534)[2]

Thus, p-hacking joins a growing taxonomy for describing the myriad ways in which "cold cognitive" and "hot motivational" biases can creep into the interpretation and use of research findings (see John et al., 2012; MacCoun, 1998;

---

[1] In 1978, Theodore X. Barber described the same concept with the less pithy "investigator data analysis effect."
[2] For a clever interactive demonstration of p-hacking, see https://projects.fivethirtyeight.com/p-hacking/.

Nuzzo, 2015; Pashler & Wagenmakers, 2012; Yong, 2012). While my focus is on p-hacking, in Table 11.1 I distinguish it from some related concepts–which is difficult because they surely overlap. First, some biases involve the selective search for evidence that will either confirm or discredit a hypothesis (confirmation bias and disconfirmation bias, respectively). Data dredging ("fishing," "hunting") involves the capitalization on chance that occurs when researchers spot statistically significant features in their data that were not specifically predicted a priori. This is most likely to happen when researchers conduct very large numbers of tests, as can happen in genetic research, neuroimaging, and psychometrics. HARKing ("hypothesizing after the results are known"; Kerr, 1998) involves the way we present and explain the results of these practices. In contrast, I take p-hacking to mostly involve analytical decisions in response to a failure to obtain statistical significance in a test of an a priori hypothesis. Finally, p-hacking overlaps with the category of publication bias in cases where authors, editors, and/or reviewers choose to selectively report results—usually by filtering out nonsignificant tests.

Table 11.1 Varieties of Investigator Bias in Empirical Research

Phenomenon	Definition
Confirmation bias	"[T]he seeking or interpreting of evidence in ways that are partial to existing beliefs, expectations, or a hypothesis in hand" (Nickerson, 1998, p. 175)
Disconfirmation bias	Occurs when "arguments incompatible with prior beliefs are scrutinized longer, subjected to more extensive refutational analyses, and consequently are judged to be weaker than arguments compatible with prior beliefs" (Edwards & Smith, 1996, p. 5)
Data dredging, fishing, capitalization on chance	"[S]earching through a body of data and examining many relations in order to find some worth testing" (Selvin & Stuart, 1966, p. 22)
HARKing	"Hypothesizing after the results are known"; defined as "presenting a post hoc hypothesis (i.e., one based on or informed by one's results) . . . as if it were, in fact, an a priori hypothesis" (Kerr, 1998, p. 196)
p-hacking	Unplanned analytical decisions made in an attempt to maximize the chance of having a significant (and hence publishable) result
Publication bias	Selective publication of only those manuscripts reporting a statistically significant test of the primary hypothesis of interest

The phenomenon of p-hacking is of great concern because it threatens the validity and perceived legitimacy of empirical research and evidence-based interventions in the social, natural, and medical sciences. But it is also of interest because NHST is an exemplar of a larger class of "criterial control systems" where quantitative thresholds or benchmarks are established to establish accountability and incentives (Darley, 2001). In many such domains, participants have been found to "game the system" by distorting performance measures (McCrary, 2008). There are many well-documented examples involving management (Degeorge et al., 1999), finance (Carhart et al., 2002), school performance (de Wolf & Janssens, 2007), food safety regulation (Ho, 2012), and environmental regulation (Chen et al., 2012). "Campbell's Law" (Campbell, 1979, p. 85; also see Darley, 2001) suggests that "[t]he more any quantitative performance measure is used to determine a group or an individual's rewards and punishments, the more subject it will be to corruption pressures and the more apt it will be to distort and corrupt the action patterns and thoughts of the group or individual it is intended to monitor."

An emerging literature attempts to infer the presence and magnitude of the p-hacking problem by working backwards from a comparison of observed distributions of p-values or test statistics to what one would expect in the absence of p-hacking or publication bias (e.g., Bishop & Thompson, 2016; Brunner & Schimmack, 2018; Gerber & Malhotra, 2008; Hartgerink et al., 2016; Head et al., 2015; Ho, 2012; Lakens, 2015b, 2015c; Simonsohn et al., 2013). That approach has its strengths, but also some drawbacks. For example, it is difficult to assess reported p-values without knowing the underlying distribution of true p-values from which they were drawn. There are different views about how to appropriately sample p-values, and how to weigh multiple p-values from a single source. And because published distributions of p-values reflect choices made by reviewers and editors, they reflect a broader set of publications biases than just statistical p-hacking.

Here, I approach the question from the opposite direction, proposing four different models of p-hacking behavior and examining what kinds of aggregate patterns they might be expected to produce. I emphasize strategy rather than tactics; that is, the models differ with respect to what the analyst is attempting to accomplish rather than how he or she does so. I show that the models predict different behavioral signatures, and while I do not offer direct evidence to validate the models, I do explore their implications for the interpretation of samples of published research. I argue that two of the three models converge on an upper bound on the amount of p-hacking that is possible without outright fraudulent data fabrication. I end with an assessment of solutions to p-hacking in light of these models.

The word "strategic" may seem to imply that p-hacking is always an intentional and/or conscious process. It can be, but not necessarily. With respect to intent, I developed the models by adopting Dennett's (1971) "intentional stance," asking what we would expect to see if a rational actor had the goal of achieving statistical significance and various means of achieving that. But with respect to consciousness, the models require only the most minimal assumption: The actor must be able to detect (through whatever statistical cues) whether the analysis is producing a p-value that crosses the 0.05 threshold, both before and after applying a "questionable research practice" like discarding or transforming some of the data. Thus, the models could easily describe the behavior of someone who wants to do careful, responsible science but has plenty of "researcher degrees of freedom"—different analytical choices together with off-the-shelf rationales for using them.

Two caveats before proceeding. First, this essay is framed in terms of NHST as it is practiced in the behavioral and social sciences, but there are compelling arguments for other normative approaches to statistical inference, including Gelman and Carlin's (2014) call for a focus on Type S (sign) and Type M (magnitude) errors, Cumming's (2014) call for prioritizing estimation over inference, Mayo's (1996) severe-testing account, and an assortment of different Bayesian perspectives (see Gelman & Shalizi, 2012; Wagenmakers et al., 2018). These perspectives are sometimes as different from each other as each is from NHST in practice, and it not yet clear which of these boats researchers will climb in if we abandon the leaky ship NHST.

Second, it is important to state at the outset that I find concerns about p-hacking so plausible because I know I have transformed data, engaged in subgroup analyses, and pooled items into composites, often in contexts where I was also pondering why the data were obscuring what I was sure was the actual result—a disconfirmation bias. I can only ask new generations of scholars, trained in an era of preregistration and meta-science, to look on their elders with compassion or at least pity. Our understanding of these issues has grown by leaps and bounds in a short period of time, and much that may now seem obvious was not understood by generations of smart people who entered science with a genuine passion for finding truth.

Types of P-hackers

Assume that an investigator is conducting a simple experiment with treatment mean m_1, control mean m_0, and test statistic t, and will conduct a two-tailed t-test of a directional hypothesis that $m_1 > m_0$. For simplicity, we can ignore any detailed cost–benefit calculations for the investigator other than the assumption that statistically significant results are desired. (For more comprehensive analyses of researcher incentives, see Bakker et al., 2012; Miller & Ulrich, 2016.)

In keeping with the "intentional stance" noted earlier, assume a world in which all investigators are willing to engage in p-hacking, either out of ignorance or disregard for normative arguments against doing so. If the models describe that world, they probably provide upper-bound estimates on p-hacking. I hope this is unrealistically pessimistic, but it may not be far from the truth. A meta-analysis of surveys of scientists suggests that only about 2% self-report fabricating or falsifying data, but up to 34% admitted to various other dubious research practices (Fanelli, 2009). But when asked about their colleagues, 14% of respondents reported some falsification and nearly three-fourths reported other problematic practices. John et al. (2012) asked similar questions of over 2,000 academic psychologists, some of whom were assigned to respond under a clever system that provided incentives for honesty. Under that condition, nearly all respondents appeared to have engaged in at least some questionable research practices (e.g., "failing to report all dependent measures," "collecting more data after seeing whether results were statistically significant," "selectively reporting studies that 'worked,'" "excluding data after looking at the impact of doing so"). But Fiedler and Schwarz (2016, p. 50) note that the question wording in this survey "suffers from ambiguities that prohibit the damning conclusions drawn."

Let $\pi(p)$ indicate the probability of p-hacking and let $\phi(p)$ indicate the expected value (probability × magnitude) of the p-hack. Note that the maximum possible magnitude of a p-hack for a given test is in fact the p-value; that is, if p = 0.22, the p-value cannot be hacked down any lower than 0.22 − 0.22 = 0. I ignore (for now) the possibility that p-hacking becomes more difficult as $p \to 0$, as suggested by simulations by Simonsohn et al. (2015).

I distinguish four types of p-hackers, differing solely in the function that determines $\pi(p)$ (top panel of Figure 11.1). Informally, people who are going to p-hack can do so without paying attention to p-values (e.g., they simply

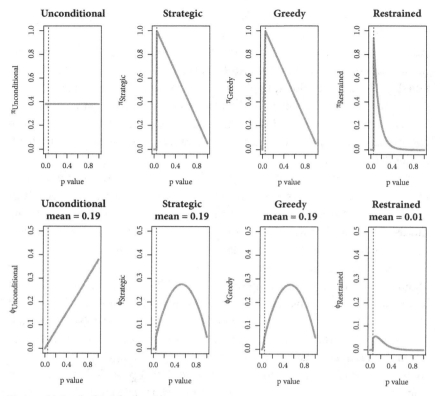

Figure 11.1. Styles of p-hacking.

have a policy of throwing out all outliers irrespective of the effect on their results), or they can do so until they cross the 0.05 threshold, or they can push even harder to push p closer to 0.

The first type is the *unconditional* p-hacker. This type has a constant probability of p-hacking, ranging from 0 (never p-hack) to 1 (p-hack at every opportunity). Formally, $\pi(p)_{Unconditional} = h$, where h is a constant. This is the least strategic type of p-hacking, but it is not random. Unconditional p-hacking is directional—always striving to reduce the p-value—but with a probability that is independent of the observed p-values. This style is useful as a baseline, but it might also be plausible in some situations (preregistration and blinded data analysis), as I discuss later.

In contrast, for *strategic* p-hackers, the probability of p-hacking varies as a function of the obtained (pre-hacked) p-value. Formally,

$$\pi(p)_{Strategic} = \begin{cases} 1-p+\alpha, & p > \alpha \\ 0, & p \leq \alpha \end{cases}$$

where $\pi(p)$ is the probability of p-hacking, p and α have their conventional interpretation, and the rules in the left column are applicable when the conditions in the right column are met.

A third model is a *greedy* variant of the strategic model, with the added assumption that p-hackers will continue to p-hack when $p < \alpha$, but at an amount that tapers off linearly as $p \to 0$. Formally,

$$\pi(p)_{Greedy} = \begin{cases} 1-p+\alpha, & p > \alpha \\ p/\alpha, & p \leq \alpha \end{cases}$$

The strategic and greedy models of p-hacking share the same (to two decimal places) average $\phi = .19$; thus they make nearly identical predictions on average. In the analyses that follow, I set the constant for the *unconditional* model to $\pi = .38$ because this is the value that yields the same mean $\phi = .19$ as the strategic and greedy models (viz., $.38 * mean(p) = .38 * .5 = .19$). Thus, the comparison across models focuses on the shapes of the functions rather than their average height. Trivially, π could be raised to predict more p-hacking in the *unconditional* model, but the other two models, if valid, predict at most an average of $\phi = .19$ given a uniform distribution of true p-values. In any given setting, the average amount of p-hacking under each model will depend on the distribution of pre-hacked p-values, as shown in what follows.

Readers who are familiar with the publication bias literature might well be surprised by the shape of the strategic and greedy functions in the bottom row of Figure 11.1. Many scholars have inferred publication bias and/or p-hacking from a conspicuous "bump" in histograms of published p-values, right below the p < 0.05 threshold. To detect this bump, Gerber and Malhotra (2008) proposed a binomial "caliper" test comparing the frequency of p-values in adjacent bins (viz., 0.04 to 0.045 vs. 0.045 to 0.05).

In contrast, the strategic and greedy functions show a "ramp" rather than a bump (top panel, for the predicted probability of p-hacking). (The bumps in the bottom panel of Figure 11.1 describe the expected magnitude of p-hacking, not its probability.) The comparisons are not straightforward because Figure 11.1 (top panel) shows probabilities conditional on the raw p-value rather than unconditional probabilities. Analyses by Bishop and Thompson (2016), Hartgerink et al. (2016), and Krawcyzk (2015) demonstrate that the "bump" is neither necessary nor sufficient to indicate p-hacking. Nevertheless, the "bump" suggests a fourth model that is a more *restrained* variant of the strategic model; it assumes that the propensity to p-hack falls off exponentially with the distance between the obtained p-value and α. Specifically,

$$\pi(p)_{Restrained} = \begin{cases} g^*exp(k(\alpha-p)), & p > \alpha \\ 0, & p \leq \alpha \end{cases}$$

where the g parameter controls the peak of the function and the k parameter controls the steepness of the decay. I set $g = 0.94$ because that is the percentage of respondents who admitted to at least one questionable research practice in the John et al. (2012) survey, and I set $k = 10$ to produce a low $\pi(p)$ for p > 0.2 or so.

As noted earlier, for each model, we can obtain an index of the expected amount a p-value will be hacked, $\phi(p) = p\pi(p)$, yielding a post-hacked p-value of $p - p\phi(p)$.

Predicted Effects of P-hacking Styles

Under a wide range of conditions (Hung et al., 1997; Murdoch et al., 2008), p-values will be uniformly distributed under the null hypothesis, whereas their distribution has a strong positive skew under an alternative hypothesis that $\mu_0 < \mu_1$.

Using R code adapted from Lakens (2015a), here are simulated distributions of 100,000 p-values under two scenarios: Cohen's d = 0 (null hypothesis), and d = 0.4, which was the mean effect size in the 100 psychology experiments sampled for replication by the Open Science Collaboration (2015), and very close to the median Cohen's d = 0.36 in Richard et al.'s (2003) synthesis of 322 different meta-analyses in social psychology.[3]

The baseline cell size of each experiment is n = 49, which provides 0.50 power for d = 0.40 in the scenario modeled here—sadly, not atypical in psychology experiments (Marszalek et al., 2011). For each simulated p-value, I computed an expected magnitude of p-hacking under each model, and plotted the kernel densities to show the distribution of p-values both before

---

[3] Cohen's $d = (M_1 - M_0)/sd$

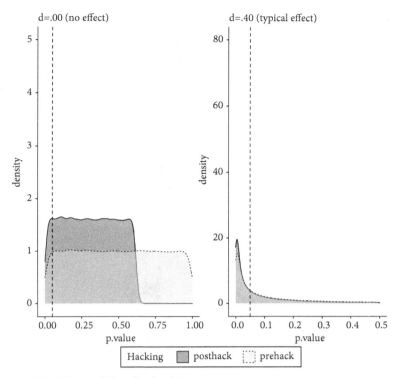

Figure 11.2. Unconditional p-hacking.

and after p-hacking.[4] Significance rates for each scenario, for both 0.50 and 0.80 power, appear in the Appendix.

Figure 11.2 shows the results for "unconditional" p-hackers, with the constant hack rate of h = 0.38 (see earlier).

In reading these plots, note that I've allowed the y-axis to vary to call attention to the qualitative patterns. Thus, what may look like a dramatic effect of unconditional p-hacking (with a hack rate of 0.38) under the null distribution is only a 3-percentage-point gain over the expected null significance rate of 5%. In actuality, the unconditional style actually reduces more false negatives (right panel) than it produces false positives (left panel).

In marked contrast, strategic hacking (Figure 11.3) increases the significance rate from 0.05 to 0.25 under the null distribution, and from 0.50 to

---

[4] Kernel density algorithms are smoothing methods for visualizing the shape of a probability distribution function given a finite sample of data points. Despite the name, probability distribution functions do not directly produce probability estimates; for instance, density values are bounded at zero but can exceed one.

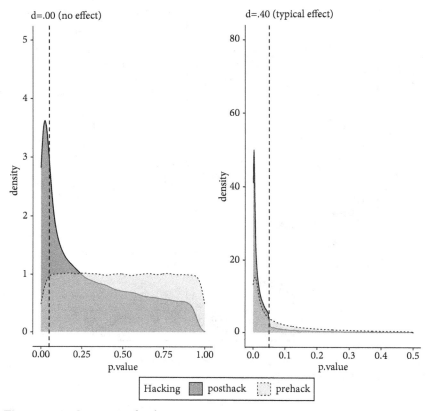

Figure 11.3. Strategic p-hacking.

0.80 under the alternative distribution. That research biases can reduce false negatives as well as false positives has been recognized at least since Ioannidis (2005), but it is still startling to find that when an effect is "real" (d = 0.40), strategic p-hacking can produce an effect equivalent to a rise in statistical power from 0.50 to 0.80.

The "greedy" variant (Figure 11.4) is conceptually distinct, and produces a larger spike. But because the greed occurs for p-values less than 0.05, most of the distortion occurs for p-values that were already statistically significant, so in a qualitative sense, the greedy model is very similar to the strategic model. And there is reason to believe that in practice, the greedy variant is even closer to the strategic model. Simulations conducted by Simonsohn et al. (2015) suggest that p-hacking becomes increasingly difficult below p = 0.05. In the Appendix to this chapter, I examine a "constrained greed"

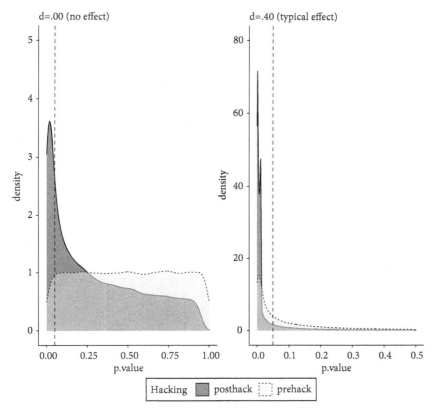

Figure 11.4. Greedy p-hacking.

model. For these reasons, I drop the greedy variant from the analyses that follow.

Finally, Figure 11.5 shows the predicted effects of the "restrained" model with $g = 0.94$ and $k = 10$. This model is less dramatic than the strategic model but has a similar signature. This is a psychologically plausible model, but with two free parameters it is also the most speculative in the absence of direct evidence.

Susceptibility to P-hacking Across Empirical Literatures

The "unconditional" model of p-hacking suggests that the practice is mostly a consequence of researchers' general analytical practices, irrespective of the

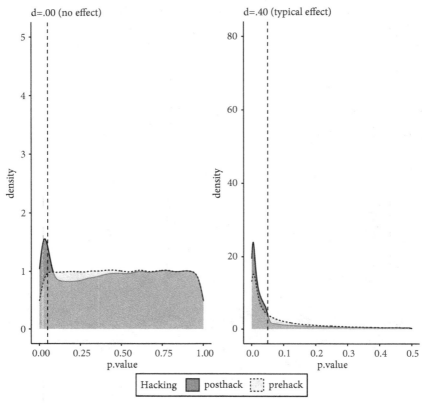

Figure 11.5. Restrained p-hacking.

strength of their findings. But the strategic, greedy, and restrained models suggest that p-hacking should be most prevalent in datasets with weak effects. Though it is difficult to retrospectively determine whether authors have p-hacked data, we can examine literatures and see which ones appear to be most vulnerable.

In Figure 11.6, I plot the distributions of p-values between 0 and 0.15 for two sets of studies. The top panel is drawn from a study by Wetzels et al. (2011), who assembled Cohen's d effect-size values for 166 two-sample t-tests assembled from articles in the 2007 issues of *Psychonomic Bulletin & Review* and *Journal of Experimental Psychology: Learning, Memory, and Cognition*. This is a heterogenous collection of articles on many topics in experimental psychology; they were assembled to be representative of these journals and not because of any controversy about their claims. For the bottom panel,

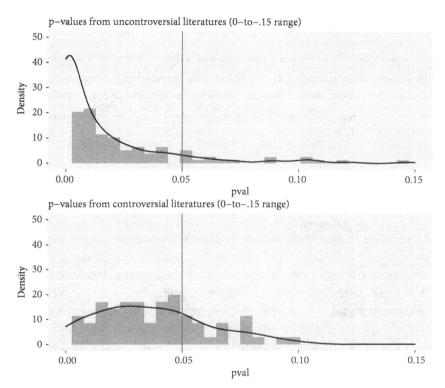

Figure 11.6. Comparing uncontroversial and controversial literatures.

I pooled p-values that have been assembled from various recently controversial research programs—social priming research (Schimmack et al., 2017), the "power of the pen" literature (Schimmack & Chen, 2017), the "power pose" literature (Simmons & Simonsohn, 2017), and the "ego depletion" literature (Schimmack, 2016). Because I have pooled these, the reader should draw no conclusions about any single paradigm, much less the results of any single lab. This is a very heterogeneous set with respect to research topics, but it forms a meaningful sample of "the set of controversial statistical claims" in recent psychology.

Inspection of the top panel suggests that there probably isn't a lot of strategic p-hacking in these studies. If we were to "reverse engineer" these published p-values under the extreme assumption that each one had been p-hacked (strategic model), we would be likely to find that most of the tests that were significant in the published articles were also significant prior to p-hacking—at least according to the strategic and restrained models presented here.[5]

Inspection of the bottom panel suggests a different story: The p-values in these controversial studies are more likely to be found in the region near 0.05 than in the region near 0.01. This does not constitute proof of p-hacking, but it does suggest that p-hacking is harder to rule out in these research programs.

Discussion

I know of no existing data that might directly validate these models as descriptions of how data analysts actually behave. In principle, one could ask a sample of social scientists to analyze a simulated dataset (i.e., with effect sizes and other parameters that are known to the simulator but not to the analysts) while varying instructions and incentives to enhance the motivation to p-hack, or one could closely track the keystrokes of data analysts. But the challenge would be to validly capture true p-hacking, as it occurs "in the wild," while somehow overcoming the likelihood of social desirability biases, so a complementary approach might compare p-values in initial versus final reports of analyses, as in a clever paper by O'Boyle et al. (2014) comparing journal articles with the doctoral dissertations that spawned them.

These p-hacking models depart from the p-curve logic by including data from nonsignificant p-values. A priori, even nonsignificant p-values might contain clues about questionable research practices. As one example, if a researcher selectively publishes some studies but not others (on the basis of a significant result), or chooses a subgrouping of the cases that favors a hypothesis, this will have implications for various ancillary tests that will then get reported, even if they are nonsignificant. Note also that the well-known McCrary (2008) procedure, used to test for "gaming the threshold" in regression discontinuity designs, also relies on data both above and below the cutoff point. In any case, the simulations presented here suggest that most of the "action" of p-hacking is observed near the α threshold. Also, any increase

---

[5] I conducted a p-curve analysis of these data using p-curve app 4.06 (http://www.p-curve.com/app4/), and it concurs with this conclusion; the continuous test for right skew based on Stouffer's method was significant for both the full and half p-curves, with $Z = -23$, $p < 0.0001$ and $Z = 21.63$, $p < 0.0001$, respectively. Note that even if there is little p-hacking here, Wetzels et al. (2011) argue that by Bayesian norms, these studies provide fairly weak evidentiary strength for their claims.

in probability mass below threshold is necessarily accompanied by a reduction in probability mass above threshold, so the p > 0.05 effects are partially redundant.

I believe this modeling has potential implications for the active discussion of reforms to reduce p-hacking (see Benjamin et al., 2018; Funder et al., 2014; MacCoun & Perlmutter, 2015, 2017; Miguel et al., 2014). As I have argued, these models involve only the most minimal requirements of intent and awareness—just a desire to achieve statistical significance, data that fall just short of that goal, and an arsenal of seemingly reasonable analytical options. Reforms needn't change researchers' motives to change their behavior. Two such proposals are preregistration (Miguel et al., 2014) and blinded data analysis (see MacCoun & Perlmutter, 2015, 2017). Both reforms are intended to make strategic p-hacking very difficult: preregistration by committing to an analysis plan before seeing the obtained p-values, and data blinding by making it difficult to know the side of α on which those obtained p-values lie. Their ability to prevent unconditional p-hacking is less certain. In either situation, some researchers might be tempted to embark on "unguided" p-hacking on a gamble that it will favor $H_{alternative}$, but they would face the risk of committing to an analysis that ends up obscuring the predicted effect or favoring some other theory.

Two other reforms involve statistical benchmarks—encouraging researchers to increase their statistical power, and adopting a more stringent α level. The former approach fared quite well here (see "Effects of Raising Statistical Power" in the Appendix), but calls for increased sample size have been made for decades with surprisingly little effect (Cohen, 1994; Marszalek et al., 2011). There are many good arguments for reducing α from 0.05 to 0.005 (Benjamin et al., 2018), but the idea is not without risk: A smaller α combined with inadequate power is a recipe for false negatives, and the latter can't get corrected if a field abandons hypotheses prematurely. Moreover, the simulations of Simonsohn et al. (2015), supplemented by new simulations here, raise a question of whether we might get roughly the same purported benefits of α = 0.005 at lower risk by adopting α = 0.01 as the new standard.

In fairness, some (but not all) of the emerging evidence for p-hacking also indicates that many psychologists are studying more subtle (and hence difficult to detect) phenomena. As Harvard social scientist Gary King eloquently argued on Twitter (September 19, 2018),

> Worried about all journal t-tests being 1.96? No problem! What would you do with a new telescope? Set it on low and see only what you already know?

No, you'd set it to 10, stand on your toes, squint, and write about the farthest, most surprising thing you can just barely see.

Of course, there are drawbacks to that strategy. Observational errors by early telescope users are legion. In 1647, Johannes Hevelius reported seeing active volcanos on the moon; his misinterpretation of craters took over two centuries to correct (Wood, 2019).

It seems clear that the set of behaviors that constitute p-hacking are quite consequential for the validity of our research and the perceived legitimacy of our authority as empirical researchers. The models of p-hacking presented here are speculative, but hopefully help shine light on some of the shadier aspects of empirical social science.

Acknowledgments

I thank Dan Ho and E. J. Wagenmakers for helpful comments on an earlier draft.

References

Bakker, M., van Dijk, A., & Wicherts, J. M. (2012). The rules of the game called psychological science. *Perspectives on Psychological Science, 7,* 543–554.

Barber, T. X. (1978). *Pitfalls in Human Research.* Pergamon General Psychology Series.

Benjamin, D. J., Berger, J. O., Johannesson, M., Nosek, B. A., Wagenmakers, E-J., Berk, R., Bollen, K. A., Brembs, B., Brown, L., Camerer, C., Cesarini, D., Chambers, C. D., Clyde, M., Cook, T. D., De Boeck, P., Dienes, Z., Dreber, A., Easwaran, K, Efferson, C., . . . Johnson, V. E. (2018). Redefine statistical significance. *Nature Human Behaviour, 2*(1), 6–10.

Bishop, D. V. M., & Thompson, P. A. (2016). Problems in using p-curve analysis and text-mining to detect rate of p-hacking and evidential value. *PeerJ, 4,* e1715. doi: 10.7717/peerj.1715

Brunner, J., & Schimmack, U. (2018). *Estimating population mean power under conditions of heterogeneity and selection for significance.* Unpublished manuscript.

Campbell, D. T. (1979). Assessing the impact of planned social change. *Evaluation and Program Planning, 2*(1), 67–90.

Carhart, M. M., Kaniel, R., Musto, D. K., & Reed, A. V. (2002). Leaning for the tape: Evidence of gaming behavior in equity mutual funds. *Journal of Finance, 82,* 661–693.

Chen, Y., Jin, G. Z., Kumar, N., & Shi, G. (2012). Gaming in air pollution data? Lessons from China. *B.E. Journal of Economic Analysis & Policy, 13*(3), Article 2.

Cohen, J. (1994). The earth is round (p < .05). *American Psychologist, 49,* 997–1003.

Cumming, G. (2014). The new statistics: Why and how. *Perspectives in Psychological Science, 25,* 7–29.

Darley, J. M. (2001). The dynamics of authority influence in organizations and the unintended action consequences. In J. M. Darley, D. M. Messick, & T. R. Tyler (Eds.), *Social Influences on Ethical Behavior in Organizations* (pp. 37–52). Lawrence Erlbaum Associates Publishers.

Degeorge, F., Patel, J., & Zeckhauser, R. (1999). Earnings management to exceed thresholds. *Journal of Business, 72,* 1–33.

Dennett, D. C. (1971). Intentional systems. *Journal of Philosophy, 68,* 87–106.

de Wolf, I. F., & Janssens, F. J. G. (2007). Effects and side effects of inspections and accountability in education: An overview of empirical studies. *Oxford Review of Education, 33,* 379–396.

Edwards, K., & Smith, E. E. (1996). A disconfirmation bias in the evaluation of arguments. *Journal of Personality and Social Psychology, 71,* 5–24.

Fanelli, D. (2009). How many scientists fabricate and falsify research? A systematic review and meta-analysis of survey data. *PLoS One, 4,* e5738.

Fiedler, K., & Schwarz, N. (2016). Questionable research practices revisited. *Social Psychology and Personality Science, 7,* 45–52.

Funder, D. C, Levine, J. M., Mackie, D. M., Morf, C. C., Sansone, C., Vazier, S., & West, S. G. (2014). Improving the dependability of research in personality and social psychology: Recommendations for research and educational practice. *Personality and Social Psychology Review, 18,* 3–12.

Gelman, A., & Carlin, J. (2014). Beyond power calculations: Assessing Type S (sign) and Type M (magnitude) errors. *Perspectives on Psychological Science, 9,* 641–651.

Gelman, A., & Shalizi, C. R. (2012). Philosophy and the practice of Bayesian statistics. *British Journal of Mathematical and Statistical Psychology, 66,* 8–38.

Gerber, A., & Malhotra, N. (2008). Do statistical reporting standards affect what is published? Publication bias in two leading political science journals. *Quarterly Journal of Political Science, 3,* 313–326.

Hartgerink, C. H. J., van Aert, R. C. M., Nuijten, M. B., Wicherts, J. M., & van Assen, M. A. L. M. (2016). Distributions of p values in psychology: What is going on? *PeerJ, 4,* e1935. doi: 10.7717/peerj.1935

Head, M. L., Holman, L., Lanfear, R., Kahn, A. T., & Jennions, M. D. (2015). The extent and consequences of p-hacking in science. *PLoS Biology, 13,* e1002106. doi: 10.1371/journal.pbio.1002106

Ho, D. E. (2012). Fudging the nudge: Information disclosure and restaurant grading. *Yale Law Journal, 122,* 574–688.

Hung, H. M. J., O'Neill, R. T., Bauer, P., & Kohne, K. (1997). The behavior of the p-value when the alternative hypothesis is true. *Biometrics, 53,* 11–22.

Ioannidis, J. (2005). Why most published research findings are false. *PLoS Medicine, 2,* e124. doi: 10.1371/journal.pmed.0020124

John, L. K., Loewenstein, G., & Prelec, D. (2012). Measuring the prevalence of questionable research practices with incentives for truth telling. *Psychological Science, 23,* 524–532.

Kerr, N. L. (1998). HARKing: Hypothesizing after the results are known. *Personality and Social Psychology Review, 2*, 196–217.

Krawcyzk, M. (2015). The search for significance: A few peculiarities in the distribution of p values in experimental psychology literature. *PLoS One, 10*, e0127872.

Lakens, D. (2015a, March 20). How a p-value between 0.04-0.05 equals a p-value between 0.16-017. The 20% Statistician. http://daniellakens.blogspot.nl/2015/03/how-p-value-between-004-005-equals-p.html

Lakens, D. (2015b). What p-hacking really looks like: A comment on Masicampo and LaLande (2012). *Quarterly Journal of Experimental Psychology, 68*, 829–832.

Lakens, D. (2015c). On the challenges of drawing conclusions from p-values just below 0.05. *PeerJ, 3*, e 1142. doi: 10.7717/peerj.1142

MacCoun, R. J. (1998). Biases in the interpretation and use of research results. *Annual Review of Psychology, 49*, 259–287.

MacCoun, R. J., & Perlmutter, S. (2015). Hide results to seek the truth. *Nature, 526*, 187–189.

MacCoun, R. J., & Perlmutter, S. (2017). Blind analysis as a correction for confirmatory bias in physics and in psychology. In S. O. Lilienfeld & I. Waldman (Eds.), *Psychological Science Under Scrutiny: Recent Challenges and Proposed Solutions* (pp. 297–322). John Wiley and Sons.

Marszalek, J. M., Barber, C., Kohlhart, J., & Holmes, C. B. (2011). Sample size in psychological research over the past 30 years. *Perceptual and Motor Skills, 112*, 331–348.

Mayo, D. G. (1996). *Error and the Growth of Experimental Knowledge.* University of Chicago Press.

McCrary, J. (2008). Manipulation of the running variable in the regression discontinuity design: A density test. *Journal of Econometrics, 142*, 698–714.

Miguel, E., Camerer, C., Casey, K., Cohen, J., Esterling, K. M., Gerber, A., Glennerster, R., Green, D. P., Humphreys, M., Imbens, G., Laitin, D., Madon, T., Nelson, L., Nosek, B. A., Peterson, M., Sedlmayr, R., Simmons, J. P., Simonsohn, U., & Van der Laan, M. (2014). Promoting transparency in social science research. *Science, 343*, 30–31.

Miller, J., & Ulrich, R. (2016). Optimizing research payoff. *Perspectives on Psychological Science, 11*, 664–691.

Murdoch, D. J., Tsai, Y. L., & Adcock, J. (2008). P-values are random variables. *American Statistician, 62*, 242–245.

Nickerson, R. S. (1998). Confirmation bias: A ubiquitous phenomenon in many guises. *Review of General Psychology, 2*, 175–220.

Nuzzo, R. (2015). Fooling ourselves. *Nature, 526*, 182–185.

O'Boyle, E. H., Banks, G. C., & Gonzalez-Mulé, E. (2014). The chrysalis effect: How ugly initial results metamorphize into beautiful articles. *Journal of Management, 43*, 376–399.

Open Science Collaboration. (2015). Estimating the reproducibility of psychological science. *Science, 349*, 943.

Pashler, H., & Wagenmakers, E. J. (2012). Editors' introduction to the special section on replicability in psychological science: A crisis of confidence? *Perspectives on Psychological Science, 7*, 528–530.

Richard, F. D., Bond, C. F., & Stokes-Zoota, J. J. (2003). One hundred years of social psychology quantitatively described. *Review of General Psychology, 7*, 331–363.

Schimmack, U. (2016, April 18). Replicability report no. 1: Is ego-depletion a replicable effect? https://replicationindex.wordpress.com/2016/04/18/is-replicability-report-ego-depletionreplicability-report-of-165-ego-depletion-articles/

Schimmack, U., & Chen, Y. (2017, September 4). The power of the pen paradigm: A replicability analysis. https://replicationindex.wordpress.com

Schimmack, U., Heene, M., & Kesavan, K. (2017, February 2). Reconstruction of a train wreck: How priming research went off the rails. https://replicationindex.wordpress.comSelvin, H. C., & Stuart, A. (1966). Data dredging procedures in survey analysis. *American Statistician, 20*, 20–23.

Simmons, J. P., & Simonsohn, U. (2017). Power posing: P-curving the evidence. *Psychological Science, 28*, 678–693.

Simonsohn, U., Nelson, L. D., & Simmons, J. P. (2013). P-curve: A key to the file-drawer. *Journal of Experimental Psychology: General, 143*, 534–547. doi: 10.1037/a0 033242

Simonsohn, U., Simmons, J. P., & Nelson, L. D. (2015). Better p-curves: Making p-curve analysis more robust to errors, fraud, and ambitious p-hacking, a reply to Ulrich and Miller. *Journal of Experimental Psychology: General, 144*, 1146–1152.

Wagenmakers, E. J., Marsman, M., Jamil, T., Ly, A., Verhagen, J., Love, J., Selker, R., Gronau, Q. F., Smira, M., Epskamp, S., Matzke, D., Rouder, J. N., & Morey, R. D. (2018). Bayesian inference for psychology, Part I: Theoretical advantages and practical ramifications. *Psychonomic Bulletin and Review, 25*, 35–57.

Wetzels, S. R., Matzke, D., Lee, M. D., Rouder, J. N., Iverson, G. I., & Wagenmakers, E. J. (2011). Statistical evidence in experimental psychology: An empirical comparison using 855 t-tests. *Perspectives on Psychological Science, 6*, 291–298.

Wood, C. A. (2010, July 9). Before Apollo: The scientists who discovered the moon. *Sky & Telescope.* https://www.skyandtelescope.com/astronomy-resources/before-apollo-scientists-who-discovered-moon/

Yong, E. (2012). Bad copy. *Nature, 485*, 298–300.

Appendix

Effects of Raising Statistical Power

Table 11.A shows significance rates under 0.50 power (for d = 0.4, cell n = 49) and 0.80 power (cell n = 99). P-hacking under either strategy is unaffected by the increase in power when the null hypothesis is true. Unconditional p-hacking is reduced more than 50% by the increased power (viz., from (0.59 − 0.50)/0.5 = 0.18 down to (0.86 − 0.8)/0.8 = 0.08). Strategic hacking is reduced by about two-thirds (viz., (0.80 − 0.5)/0.5 = 0.6 down to (0.95 − 0.8)/0.8 = 0.2). Note that raising power is more effective than either type of p-hacking as way to reduce false negatives.

Table 11.A Proportion Significant by Scenario

	Alpha	Power	Pre (d = 0)	Post (d = 0)	Pre (d = 0.40)	Post (d = 0.40)
Unconditional	0.05	0.5	0.050	0.079	0.502	0.587
Strategic	0.05	0.5	0.052	0.250	0.498	0.795
Greedy	0.05	0.5	0.049	0.249	0.500	0.794
Restrained	0.05	0.5	0.050	0.107	0.498	0.637
Unconditional	0.05	0.8	0.049	0.080	0.799	0.855
Strategic	0.05	0.8	0.050	0.252	0.800	0.953
Greedy	0.05	0.8	0.049	0.249	0.801	0.952
Restrained	0.05	0.8	0.050	0.107	0.799	0.884

Constrained Greedy P-hacking

Simonsohn et al. (2015) report a series of simulations of p-hacking tactics. The left panel in Figure 11.A shows my attempt to model their estimate of the number of different p-hack tactics needed to try to achieve a given p-value. A reasonable approximation is $y = exp(6 - 90p)$. I assume that the maximum probability of successfully p-hacking for a given p-value is inversely related to this function, with a suitable scaling constant (0.2) in the numerator, yielding a revised greed function for p-values below α (right panel):

$$\phi_{p<\alpha} = \frac{.2}{exp(6-90p)}$$

When I simulated this "constrained" greedy function, the results were nearly indistinguishable from those of the strategic model. Thus, I concur with Simonsohn et al. that p-hacking is probably inconsequential once one gets below p = 0.03 or so.

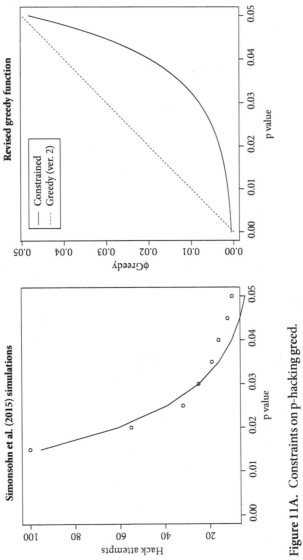

Figure 11A. Constraints on p-hacking greed.

12
The Importance of Type III and Type IV Epistemic Errors for Improving Empirical Science

Charlotte Ursula Tate

Introduction

This chapter has two major goals. One goal is to introduce the reader to another class of knowledge or epistemic errors that can be made in the conduct of empirical science, in addition to the familiar type I and type II errors (see definitions and descriptions in the next paragraph). This other class of epistemic errors focuses on the activity or process of analyzing data at a broad level, rather than at the specific level of making decisions about whether a phenomenon is more or less frequent in a null distribution or, separately, whether new data are consistent or inconsistent with a distribution of prior probabilities. To achieve the goal of introduction, I must define the previous well-known type I and II errors; introduce the historical existence of a third type of error; define that third type of error in its historical context and juxtapose it with the current understandings of data analysis; make clear what I believe to be the underlying issues at play; provide the other specific meanings of errors of this third kind and proposed fourth kinds; consolidate the previous meanings into generic type III and type IV errors; and provide examples of each class of error, focusing specifically on behavioral science (which is my specialty). The second goal is to consolidate the various meanings and terms previously associated with these two epistemic errors into a cumulative knowledge understanding of what is present in all the empirical sciences (not just the ones that focus on human behavior). In order to achieve the second goal, I must first collect the major terms and meanings of the previous literatures and then argue for their consolidation into one of the two larger epistemic errors—namely, as either a type III or a type IV error.

Charlotte Ursula Tate, *The Importance of Type III and Type IV Epistemic Errors for Improving Empirical Science* In: *Research Integrity.* Edited by: Lee J. Jussim, Jon A. Krosnick, and Sean T. Stevens, Oxford University Press. © Oxford University Press 2022. DOI: 10.1093/oso/9780190938550.003.0012

Importantly, the success of each individual goal is not dependent on the other. A reader may be convinced that two broad classes of epistemic errors exist, but may be unconvinced of the specific organization of previous literature statements into the locations I specify. Likewise, a reader may be convinced of the specific organization of previous literature that I provide, but may believe that there are more than two broad classes of epistemic errors relevant to data analysis. In any case, the chapter is presented as a starting point for a longer and more detailed conversation about these issues.

Types of Decision and Epistemic Errors in Data Analysis

Statisticians and researchers are most familiar with two types of decision errors that can occur in empirical research using null hypothesis statistical testing (NHST): the false positive (type I error) and the false negative (type II error). These two errors are based on the Neyman–Pearson (1933) lemma and extensions of this reasoning (viz., Cohen, 1977). In psychology, type I error rate has been traditionally set at 5% (or $p \leq 0.05$). Also in psychology, type II error has been traditionally set at 20% (or $\beta = 0.20$) based on Cohen's idea that type I error be considered four times more serious than type II error (Cohen, 1977). Type I and II errors have garnered much attention over the years, and most recently in terms of replication and reproducibility (e.g., Ioannidis, 2005; Simmons et al., 2011). There has also been a recent debate about whether to lower the type I error threshold to $p \leq 0.005$ (or 0.5%), with proponents (Benjamin et al., 2018), opponents (Lakens et al., 2018), and neutral commenters (Ioannidis, 2018). In any case, these two errors are firmly situated within the NHST based on the Neyman–Pearson original formulation and the initial Cohen extension to power analysis.

In the meanwhile, statisticians have also identified another class of epistemic decision errors that also have some (yet-to-be formalized) probability of occurring. This class of errors was collected under a single referent, being called *errors of the third kind*, by statistician A. W. Kimball in 1957. We can update Kimball's original phrase as *type III error*. Kimball (1957) defined type III error as "giving the right answer to the wrong problem" (p. 134). What is more, Kimball (1957) suggested that this third type of error was relevant to all of statistical thinking, not simply NHST decisions. In the 1957 article, Kimball details a variety of ways in which the right answer to the wrong problem can be given based on the match between theory, research methods, and statistical evaluation of either the theory or the methods. Kimball's (1957) examples included (a) running a test for independent correlation coefficients on a matched-samples design and (b) making statistical transformations to raw data without understanding the experimental method used (which, in one of the cases presented, resulted in transformed values that were outside of the measured range of known particle sizes)—both of which provide the right answer to a separate question not being asked in the design of each example study (hence the "wrong problem"). The take-home point of Kimball's discussion is that those engaged in statistical consulting need to be aware of at least three pieces of information: (a) the theory being tested, (b) the research design, and (c) the underlying assumptions of the statistical tests used. It is the connection among these three information pieces—and any pairwise combination thereof—that defines the existence of a type III error. Stated differently, for Kimball, errors of the third kind result from any mismatch between theory, research design, and statistical assumptions.

However, a number of applied statisticians, particularly those working in the science of human behavior, might have some difficulty in truly appreciating the arguments of Kimball because they rely on a characterization of *data analysis* that is not well used these days. During the time of Kimball's writings, statistician J. W. Tukey (1962) was also writing about data analysis in a manner that closely resembles what Kimball might have also been tacitly referencing. Tukey (1962) defined *data analysis* as "procedures for analyzing data, techniques for interpreting the results of such procedures, ways of planning the gathering of data to make its analysis easier, more precise and more accurate, and all the machinery and results of (mathematical) statistics which apply to analyzing data" (p. 64). In the same section, Tukey continues by describing that statistical procedures are only part of what data analysis involves. In addition, "some parts of data analysis . . . guide us in the distribution of effort and other valuable considerations in observation, experimentation, or analysis. Data analysis is a larger and more varied field than inference" (Tukey, 1962, p. 64).

One way to interpret Tukey's description of the capaciousness of data analysis is to understand it in connection to another of his phrases, "data analysis is detective work" (Tukey, 1969/1986, p. 736). This phrase is popularly understood to reference *exploratory data analysis* as in inspecting the actual patterns in the data collected to determine whether and how they can be subjected to *confirmatory data analysis*, the latter in the sense of hypothesis testing (see, e.g., Behrens, 1997). Yet, focusing on the totality of Tukey's writings and connecting these writings to the other discussions of that time (viz., Kimball's), we might also describe exploratory data analysis as a set of procedures or activities that a researcher enacts—some of which are focusing on statistical properties, but some of which (as noted in the foregoing paragraph) will be larger than the application of the mathematics as such, and move into the "distribution of effort" (as Tukey described it) and the somewhat opaquely described "other valuable considerations."

To make these abstract considerations more tangible, imagine a scientist who is trying to determine whether there are any metals in a pile of material. (I use a physical science example because it lessens the focus on null hypothesis testing or other forms of inferential statistics well known to behavioral scientists. The point of the imagined scenario is to illustrate the procedures and activities [rather than statistical decisions] at play.) To do detective work well in this metal-detecting case, it seems that there are two broad aspects of the procedures or activities that the scientist needs to enact correctly. One aspect is that the scientist needs to obtain and apply a correct understanding of the relevant properties of all metals. Notice that this understanding is not necessarily statistical but has to do with how the construct "metal" is operationalized in the field of study. The other aspect is that the scientist needs to have adequate tools to detect any metal that are, additionally, used in the proper manner.

In the language of behavioral and social scientists, for the first aspect, the fictitious metal-detecting scientist has to have the correct understanding of both the operationalization of and the construct validity associated with all metals. As a simple and direct example of the foregoing, the scientist needs to understand that "metals" include both magnetic and non-magnetic materials. Further, the scientist needs to then correctly apply this understanding (that metals feature both types of materials) to any detection of metals. Accordingly, for data analysis to even commence, the scientist has to begin with a consideration that is outside of what instruments will eventually be applied to the problem and how. This is one way to make tangible Tukey's "other valuable considerations"—namely, a scientist has to approach the process of thinking about how to analyze data in a useful and correct manner based on the theoretical, methodological, and non-statistical considerations. If the fictitious scientist tries to detect metals in the pile of material only using a magnetic metal detector, for instance, that would be *an error in the process of doing the detective work*—what we might call a theoretical or methodological error. Notice further that this error is on only one aspect of the two aspects described earlier. In this fictitious scenario, the scientist could operate the magnetic metal detector properly—and it is one of (but not the exhaustive list of) the correct tools to be used—and this scientist would still be in error. Thus, the locus of the error is not in the tool (or instrument) used or even how the tool (or instrument) was applied, but rather in the fact that the detecting process was incomplete for the task, based on knowledge about the phenomenon. It is an error of the procedure used in the detective work.

Separately, in terms of stated conclusions, if under the conditions described earlier, this fictitious scientist claimed that "there is no metal in this pile," then this conclusion is also an error. Notice further that this conclusion maps closely to the general meaning of type II error (as a false negative). Nevertheless, the procedural error described earlier (viz., incorrectly characterizing what counts as metal) leads to a decision error (type II error), but these are not the same errors. Notice that if the scientist makes no claim about whether metal was found, the procedural error of data analysis still exists. Moreover, this procedural error occurs irrespective of whether one of the correct tools (as an instrument of data analysis) was chosen to provide evidence. In short, how the "theory" of data analysis is implemented can itself be an error—and this is irrespective of stated conclusions and how tools or instruments were actually applied.

The other side of this discussion is the second aspect of doing good detective work—namely, applying the correct tool in the correct way (for the successful operation of the tool itself). This error may be very clear to many scientists because it is comparatively less abstract than the procedure of applying knowledge correctly. The instrument has known and stated parameters of correct use; these parameters need to be followed for correct use; and the relevant scientists are trained in the use of that instrument. Nevertheless, it is worth stating explicitly the two general ways by which instruments are used incorrectly as procedures. Now imagine that another fictitious metal-detecting scientist remembered that there were both magnetic and non-magnetic metals but forgot to calibrate their magnetic detector properly. Even before (or without) making any conclusions from the use of the instrument, it is clear that an error has been made. Failing to properly calibrate the detector is an error of instrumentation—and notably a procedural one. Consequently, any conclusions about magnetic metals will be in error in this case. Yet, notice that this error is separate from the prior procedural error of applying the relevant construct knowledge. In this new fictitious example case, the "theory" of data analysis was correct (viz., the second fictitious scientist remembered and intended to find both magnetic and non-magnetic metals), but the use of the tool was incorrect. Moreover, notice that the proper tool was chosen (a magnetic detector to detect magnetic metals), but operated incorrectly. This shows that the use of the tools has to be correct in two ways: (a) the correct tool must be chosen and (b) the correct tool must be operated correctly. Either or both of the errors creates an incorrect analysis of the data—as a process or an activity. As noted earlier, any conclusions made or communicated to the public are separate from (but ultimately connected to) the procedural error. To make this separation of conclusions and procedures clear, if using the improperly calibrated metal detector, this second fictitious scientist claimed that "there is metal in this pile," then that claim may be a type I error (a false positive). Nonetheless, even if no claim were made, this second procedural error of data analysis still exists. Thus, this procedural error of incorrect instrumentation use can occur irrespective of stated conclusions and whether the construct validity actually holds in the specific case.

Bringing this all together, my interpretation of Tukey's detective work metaphor is that there are two salient aspects to detective work as a procedure or activity—pithily stated, correct understanding and correct execution—to properly conduct science. To foreshadow the main argument of this chapter, these two aspects will become, generically, the two types of epistemic data-analysis errors that can be committed in empirical science. Now that the reader is sufficiently positioned to understand my specific use of the concept of data analysis (in line with the Tukey meaning), in the next section, I detail the other existing uses of the terms type III and type IV errors in order to then propose a consolidation of these various meanings—one that is consistent with the detective work metaphor.

Other Definitions of Type III Error

Kimball (1957) was neither the first nor the only statistician to provide a definition of a type III error. In fact, type III error has several definitions, with none appearing to enjoy wide acceptance. Mosteller (1948) described type III error with respect to the NHST as "correctly rejecting the null hypothesis for the wrong reason" (p. 61). Kaiser (1960) argued that a type III error is an incorrect decision of the direction of rejection in a two-tailed NHST. (More recently, Gelman and Carlin, 2014, have described Kaiser's version of type III error as a *type S error* or a sign error.) Additionally, Schwartz and Carpenter (1999) defined type III error as a discrepancy between the causal components of a theory and how they are operationalized. To use one of Schwartz and Carpenter's examples, the rate of homelessness in any country is structural—based on policies related to housing and poverty. Understanding the "true cause" of homelessness will help epidemiologists and other behavioral scientists correctly model how homelessness is produced and reproduced. However, an error (specifically a type III error) can occur when researchers focus only on the demographics of homeless individuals (e.g., the ethnicity, gender, or sexual orientation of these individuals). Counting homeless individuals by demographic variables can recover important information—such as certain ethnicity groups in a country being more likely than others to experience homelessness. However, as Schwartz and Carpenter argue, by focusing only on the demographic variables, the researchers would miss the structural component of homelessness—governmental policies—and, worse yet (according to those authors), possibly believe that individual differences themselves might contribute to or control the phenomenon. In this manner, researchers have failed to appropriately operationalize the phenomenon under study in terms of its actual causes. (To fully appreciate this argument, remember the meaning of data analysis as detective work in the foregoing section.)

Similarly, Schwartz and Carpenter (1999) argued that obesity is a result of gene and environment interplays—as the focal causal mechanisms. Yet, alignable to the homelessness example, researchers who focus on individual-difference contributions to obesity (e.g., gender, age) without even modeling the environments in which these individual differences exist might routinely miss or underplay the environmental factors. Here again, Schwartz and Carpenter argue that a type III error has occurred insofar as the "true cause" is not being modeled by only focusing on half of a two-part causal model. Whether the reader agrees with the specific presented argument from Schwartz and Carpenter, the larger point is that their argumentation can be aligned with (my interpretation of) Tukey's data analysis as detective work metaphor. Much like the first fictitious metal-detecting scientist (in the previous section), the incomplete focus from a theoretical or methodological standpoint on one part of a larger phenomenon is an error of process in deriving and evaluating scientific knowledge.

A Commonality Among the Type III Error Definitions

Although disparately focused, I argue that each of the definitions of type III error provided earlier can be reasonably subsumed under Kimball's axiom of *giving the right answer to the wrong problem*. The misspecification errors of Mosteller, Kaiser, and Schwartz and Carpenter can be viewed as correctly answering another question—just the wrong problem for the investigation at hand. To draw this out explicitly, for Mosteller (1948), the null should be rejected, just not for the reason provided by the researchers; for Kaiser, the direction of the two-tailed test was misspecified, so the right answer (rejecting the null) was given to the wrong problem (incorrect direction specified); for Schwartz and Carpenter, focusing on individual differences answers the right question (there really are individual-difference contributors or aspects to certain phenomena) but these were discovered for the wrong problem, insofar as the "right problem" is the full causal structure of homelessness politically determined in part, or obesity as environmentally determined in part.

From this perspective, type III errors appear to be focused on how theories become operationalized or implemented for empirical research. Considering the interplay among theory, research methods, and statistical assumptions, type III errors focus on methodological implementation errors, specifically focused on the connection between theory and method. By implication, it would seem that a commonality among all the type III error definitions listed is that they do *not* concern statistical assumptions. This lack of focus on statistical assumptions can be most directly observed in the Schwartz and Carpenter (1999) definition of type III error, in which the connection between the theory-level causal structure and what is being incompletely or inadequately implemented in the research methods by measuring only half of the causal structure. Yet, even the direction or sign errors in NHST formulations of type III error (Mosteller, Kaiser, and Gelman and Carlin) are not actually focusing on the assumptions of the statistical tests being used. A researcher could easily mis-predict the direction of an effect using the correct statistical procedures. In fact, while focusing on probabilities to demonstrate the potential frequencies of type S (sign) and type M (magnitude) errors, Gelman and Carlin (2014) assume that the statistical test run is correct—at least in terms of meeting the assumptions of the test to make it applicable to the research design. Notice that while taking Kanazawa's (2007) beauty and sex-ratio study to task to illustrate type S errors, Gelman and Carlin (2014) are moot about whether the analysis used by Kanazawa was correct. Instead, Gelman and Carlin (2014) tacitly assume the analysis was correct by focusing on the fact that one predicted direction is more common probabilistically than the other using the same statistical test as Kanazawa (2007) did, thereby illustrating their type S error.

If it is true that the potential commonality across many of the previous versions of the type III error in the foregoing section does not include a focus on statistical assumptions, then what of Kimball's (1957) other examples of errors of the third kind—the ones focused on violating statistical assumptions? Can these be easily integrated into the larger type III error framework? I would argue no, for the reason stated earlier: It is entirely possible to misspecify theory to methods implementations while still conducting the correct statistical procedure for the design that was implemented.

The Need for a Fourth Type of Error

Recalling that Kimball also noted that the error of statistical assumptions violations also exists, it might be useful to consider this a unique error—not the same as an implementation error. If it is possible for a researcher to make an implementation error of sign or magnitude even while meeting all the assumptions for the correct statistical test used (cf., Gelman & Carlin, 2014), this may show *by implication* that using the incorrect statistical procedure for the research design or theory should also be possible *even when the error of theory-to-research methods implementation is not present*. Another way to consider this situation is to further unpack Kimball's (1957) pithy statement. If one can argue for *giving the right answer to the wrong problem* (as Kimball described it), then it is worth asking: Can one argue for a logical counterpart: *giving the wrong answer to the right problem*? And, if so, could this be considered a type IV error? Interestingly enough, such a consideration already exists in the literature—albeit narrow in scope.

An Existing Definition of Type IV Error

The existing research literature has already called this incorrect use of statistical procedures a *type IV error*, but with a very narrow focus. The earliest version of the type IV error was provided by Marascuilo and Levin (1970) and then extended by Umesh et al. (1996); both focused on incorrectly interpreting a statistical interaction term (also called a moderation analysis). While the particulars of each argument are interesting (and can be reviewed in the Umesh et al., 1996, paper), the way that Umesh et al. described a type IV error as focusing on cell means to understand the interaction term rather than the cell residuals, the latter of which is endorsed by Rosnow and Rosenthal (1989, 1991). The reason that focusing on cell means could be considered an error of statistical assumptions is because the interaction effect is, mathematically, the difference (or residual) between the main effects model's expectation about the values of the cell means and the observed cell values, as Rosnow and Rosenthal demonstrate. While apparently a minute distinction, Umesh et al. (1996) argue that phenomena can be fundamentally misrepresented by focusing on the cell means (rather than residuals) during simple effects analysis because these, by definition, carry information about the main effects too.

Generalizing Type IV Error to All Cases of Errors of Statistical Assumptions

While some principled replies to the Umesh et al. (1996) argumentation can be made (thereby softening the force of that critique), it is more important to consider the larger context. Incorrectly interpreting one kind of statistical effect might simply be an exemplar for the general phenomenon of misspecifying any statistical effect by violating the underlying assumptions of the test. In fact, all statistical tests that have been developed have assumptions about their application. Some statistical assumptions were ones of convenience (e.g., the normality assumption in the t-tests) and the tests themselves have been shown to be robust against certain violations. Yet, other assumptions are integral, and violating these assumptions produces either an inaccurate or incorrect result. Take, for instance, the homogeneity of variance assumption in the two-sample t-test (and between-groups analysis of variance by extension). If the variances differ at too large a ratio, then the traditional Student t-test (which assumes approximately equal variances between the groups) is biased in its estimate of whether the groups differ from each other (Welch, 1938). To rectify this situation, Welch developed the t' (t-prime) correction to control type I error inflation and also to "even out" the variance estimates inside the standard error calculation (see Welch, 1938). Thus, if a researcher conducts the Student t-test (equal variances assumed) when approximately equal variances do not exist between the two groups, then, I would argue, another specific instance of the generalized type IV error has been committed. To assess whether a type IV error exists (or would exist) in this two-sample t-test case, all the researcher needs to do is check the assumption of homogeneity of variance using either Hartley's *F*-max test (Hartley, 1950) or Levene's test (Levene, 1960). In this way, generalized type IV errors can be ascertained by understanding the assumptions of specific statistical techniques and then testing or screening for the violations of those assumptions.

But, let us return to the example at hand—a researcher running the Student t-test when that person should have run the Welch correction. In this case, the researcher can be described as *giving the wrong answer to the right problem* insofar as the setup is correct (i.e., the between-groups means-based analysis is the right problem [as in correct tool]), but the wrong or incorrect answer was provided because the assumptions of the statistical technique were violated and thus the specific analysis does not apply to that setup. Materially, whatever the researcher's conclusion (e.g., to either retain or to reject the null hypothesis; to describe the Bayes factor), it is incorrect (the wrong answer) in that moment because the statistical evaluation was erroneous.

To see other exemplars of the generalized type IV error, consider the series of assumptions that characterize ordinary least squares (OLS) multiple regression analysis—a very common technique in psychological science. In OLS multiple regression, the core statistical assumptions include (a) sufficient ratio of variables to cases; (b) absence of outliers on the predictors and the outcome; (c) absence of collinearity among the predictors; (d) linearity of outcome prediction; and (e) homoscedasticity of the residuals (see Tabachnick & Fidell, 2013, pp. 122–128). Focusing on just one of these OLS assumptions, it is known that collinearity of the predictors (i.e., high and/or symmetrical inter-predictor correlations) reduces one's ability to interpret the influence of either predictor (in addition to reducing overall model fit; see also Cohen et al., 2003). Thus, if one has severe collinearity between predictors and still proceeds with analysis, this can be viewed as *giving the wrong answer to the right problem*—whatever that answer appears to be. Yet, as a statistical assumption, collinearity can be diagnosed before analyses are conducted using either a zero-order correlation matrix (to check for size and symmetry) or the calculation of a variance inflation factor or its reciprocal expression, tolerance (Tabachnick & Fidell, 2013). If collinearity is observed, then there are alternative statistical techniques available (e.g., partial least squares regression; Wold et al., 1984) or methods to handle the collinearity (e.g., collapse highly correlated predictors, remove one of the highly correlated predictors, statistically separate the correlated predictors using partial correlation; cf., Tabachnick & Fidell, 2013).

In sum, each statistical test used in behavioral science (and beyond) has statistical assumptions about the data structure that must be respected and demonstrated before the use of the technique can be considered valid in that instance. And, further notice that these assumptions are separable from the probabilities of making type I and type II errors because these mathematical assumptions exist even if one does not use the tests as NHSTs. Of course, even when the statistical technique is used when all relevant assumptions are met, there is still a type I error probability associated with it, as well as a type II error probability (indexed via power analysis) using the NHST logic. Finally, even when all statistical assumptions are met for the technique being used, this does not guarantee the absence of type III errors as defined earlier as errors of theory or method implementation.

Bringing it All Together: Examples of the Implementation (Type III) and Evaluation (Type IV) Errors in Psychological Science

To make these considerations meaningful for improving science, in this section, I detail empirical examples of type III and type IV errors in the psychology literature. All will be examples using the same overarching theoretical framework to show how different versions of the type III and IV errors are possible within the same literature. Providing illustrations from different literatures might seem fairer and more generalizable, but it might also be viewed as associating certain errors with certain literatures. Thus, by showing type III and IV errors within one literature, a reader can use the formal structure of the errors and apply them to any specific literature. The literature chosen for the examples is evolutionary psychology. Relevantly, I am both a theorist and researcher in this literature—so this set of examples is not meant to be seen as an outsider critiquing evolutionary psychology; instead, it is meant to be viewed as an insider critique. Additionally, I nominate one of my own studies as an example involving one of these two generalized errors.

Specific Examples of Type III Errors as Theory or Method Implementation Errors in Evolutionary Psychology Literature

Given that I have defined a generalized type III error as an implementation error, I provide two examples of errors of implementation—one that deals with misspecified or unknown construct validity (Example 1) and another that deals with misspecified operationalization of a theory's implications (Example 2). Together the examples showcase how implementation of theories into methods is a central consideration for type III error.

Example 1: Masculinity and Femininity Predicting Desired Number of Sexual Partners?

Tate (2011) conducted a conceptual replication of the Buss and Schmitt (1993) study in which college student participants were asked to provide their desired number of sexual partners over their lifetime. Buss and Schmitt (1993) had claimed that men desire more sexual partners over the lifetime as compared to women for reasons related to their version of evolutionary psychology, in which sexual reproduction is the main goal of human sexual behavior.[1] In any case, Tate (2011) was interested in whether there was an alternative explanation for the original gender differences reported in the Buss and Schmitt (1993) study, using existing literature in gender roles at that time. Tate (2011) reasoned that participants' endorsement of either masculinity or femininity gender-typed behavior as measured by the Bem Sex-Role Inventory (BSRI; Bem, 1974) could recover these findings in the following manner. Because sexual promiscuousness was not seen as compatible with feminine gender roles in the United States, at least at that time (e.g., Marks & Fraley, 2005), then it is entirely possible that what Buss and Schmitt believed to be a group-level difference (based on gender approximating genetic differences between men and women) is really a spurious correlation between the feminine traits being more likely to be endorsed by women than men. As Tate reasoned, if a researcher allowed both women and men to endorse their personal agreement with both feminine and masculine gender-typed traits, then a researcher could see that either (or both) drive the reports for desired number of sexual partners *within each gender group*. This is

---

[1] There are alternative views to the function of human sexual behavior that cast reproduction as a consequence, not a goal (see Tate, 2013).

exactly what Tate (2011) found: Within each gender group, participants' endorsement of femininity traits was negatively predictive of desired number of sexual partners (such that increasing femininity trait endorsement was associated with reporting fewer sexual partners over the lifetime), at very similar effect sizes for both groups: $sr_{Men} = -0.396$, $sr_{Women} = -0.338$. In addition, Tate (2011) also showed an average difference between the gender groups on femininity trait endorsement, such that women reported substantially more femininity trait endorsement, $d = 0.57$. Thus, a reason for the original Buss and Schmitt findings was offered: spurious correlation of gender group with gender-typed trait endorsement.

Yet, the Tate (2011) results likely show a type III error related to construct validity of the BSRI itself—the measurement instrument used to assess femininity and masculinity trait endorsement. There has been much debate since its original development as to whether the BSRI actually measures femininity and masculinity or whether it measures agency and communion personality traits (e.g., Bem, 1981). In fact, recently, my own research group found a near-zero correlation between a face-valid measure of self–other similarity based on gender (viz., gender typicality) and BSRI-femininity for women and BSRI-masculinity for men (Tate, Bettergarcia, & Brent, 2015)—even while Bem's (1974, 1981) theory argues for a positive relationship for both comparisons. Thus, whether the BSRI is actually measuring personal endorsement of femininity and masculinity gender stereotypes is unknown at present. Why does this matter, and why is it a type III error? It matters because if the construct validity is in question, then reasonable extensions of the phenomenon based on apparently similar constructs would not necessarily replicate.

For instance, if a researcher tried to extend the Tate (2011) findings using a measure of conformity to feminine gender roles—such as one developed by Mahalik et al. (2005)—then the expected pattern of more conformity correlating with fewer desired sexual partners may not emerge. While a type I error in the original Tate (2011) investigation is possible (based on using an NHST), it seems more likely that the lack of a conceptual replication could result from the feminine gender-role conformity scale actually measuring something like gender roles and the BSRI-femininity subscale measuring something closer to communal trait endorsement, or even a facet of agreeableness. In that case, only other communal trait endorsement measures would likely replicate the Tate (2011) findings. Accordingly, I hope it is clear that unknown (or incorrect) construct validity can lead to apparently contradictory findings because of a type III error. However, the findings would not be truly contradictory; instead, they would come from an implementation error in which it is believed that construct A is related to outcome Y, but it is really construct B that is related to outcome Y. In effect, Tate (2011) could have offered the right answer to the wrong problem: The right answer is that a BSRI dimension truly is related to mate preferences ("right answer"), but that same BSRI dimension may have nothing to do with gender roles ("wrong problem").

Example 2: Cross-Cultural Differences in Mate Preferences as Statistical Moderation?
Example 2 focuses on construct validity likely being acceptable, but the type III error occurs as an implementation error *of incorrectly or incompletely operationalizing the standard for an observable effect*. Some readers may be familiar with the Buss et al. (1990) "many cultures" or "37 cultures" dataset, in which Buss et al. collected data from 37 different nation-states around the world on questions of gender and mate preference. The details of the methodology and major results can be found in the Buss et al. (1990) citation. What I call attention to for Example 2 is how Buss et al. argued for the lack of influence of national culture on their obtained results. Specifically, those authors argued that culture was not a statistical moderator of the gender differences that they obtained across the cultures. Without additional information, we can—and will for the present discussion—assume that the statistical assumptions for testing moderation (i.e., a statistical interaction effect) were all met—precluding a type IV error. Yet, relevant to type III error, we can ask the pertinent question: Was the moderation of gender by culture the *only* appropriate manner by which to address the question of national-culture influence on mate preferences?

In terms of forms, interaction effects are either synergistic, buffering, or antagonistic (for technical descriptions of each in regression, see Cohen et al., 2003). All of this is to say that any moderation tests whether there is a more-than-additive combination of two predictor variables on an outcome variable. Yet, the underlying logical and statistical comparison for the moderation effect is that the two predictor variables are purely additive in their influence on the outcome variable. To claim that there is an interaction effect of two variables, one rejects the purely additive model and determines which form of moderation is present. Why is this important for the Buss et al. 37 cultures data? Because there are two ways to argue for national-culture influence on gender for mate preferences, and Buss et al. (1990) only provided empirical evidence for one of the two ways. In this case, Buss et al. (1990) committed a type III error by not fully specifying the operationalizations that count as falsification or support for their theory. It may be true that national culture does not statistically moderate mate-preference differences, but, with this result in hand, one should *not* make the argument that culture does not importantly influence mate preferences as Buss et al. (1990) did. Instead, those authors should have checked the purely additive influence results before making this claim.

When the purely additive model is tested, it shows that national culture is significantly related to mate-preference differences between women and men. As Kasser and Sharma (1999) showed using the original Buss et al. (1990) data, when objective indicators of the equality between women and men in each society were included, mate-preference differences tracked linearly (and additively) with gender equality. That is, Kasser and Sharma (1999) basically found that in cultures where women had fewer resources than men, these women desired men with resources. However, in cultures where women and men had near-equal resources, women did not desire men with resources above chance levels. Thus, culture has a linear or additive (rather than moderating) influence on gender for mate preference. Similarly, Zenter and Mitura (2012) show that when national cultures are measured on the size of their respective gender gaps as measured by the Global Gender Gap Index (Hausmann et al., 2010), presumed-to-be universal evolutionary mate preferences are linearly related to the gender parity across countries—such that they appear most strongly in the cultures with the lowest levels of gender parity (and virtually disappear in the countries with the highest levels of gender parity).

In this example, we see shades of Schwartz and Carpenter's (1999) warnings about conceiving of the phenomenon appropriately to implement methods correctly. Consequently, Buss et al. (1990) provided the right answer to the wrong problem: The influence of culture on gendered mate preferences is not a statistical moderation ("right answer"), but this is only one meaning of the influence of culture on gendered mate preference ("wrong problem" as in an "incomplete statement of the problem").

Specific Examples of Type IV Errors as Statistical Evaluation Errors in Evolutionary Psychology

Example 3: Outliers Influencing the Desired Number of Sexual Partners
This example focuses on a type IV error made by Buss and Schmitt (1993) in their analysis of their original data to apparently demonstrate that men desire more sexual partners than women over the lifetime. As Pedersen et al. (2002) showed, a replication of the Buss and Schmitt (1993) methodology produced both outliers and extreme skewness even after the outliers were pseudo-Winsorized (i.e., setting all values past an arbitrary upper limit value to that value). This is a type IV error because the assumption of homogeneity of variance within the two-sample test was violated even with the pseudo-Winsorizing procedure, such that women's and men's responses were still heterogeneous after this procedure. This violation of the assumption renders the Student t-test prone to returning false positives. While the Welch t-test could be used to help lower the false-positive rate (by correcting degrees of freedom downward, thereby making it more difficult to reject the null hypothesis), it is also possible and better given the distributional properties of these data to conduct a Mann–Whitney U-test or some other median-based non-parametric test. When Pedersen at el. (2002) conducted the non-parametric test, the median values differed between women and men at only chance levels—providing no support for the gender-difference claim of Buss and Schmitt (1993).

In this case, it is easy to see that a type IV error has been committed by offering the wrong answer to the right problem. The "right problem" is the correctness of the setup: Is there a between-groups gender difference between women and men on desired number of sexual partners over the lifetime? The "wrong answer" is provided by Buss and Schmitt (1993) by not using the correct statistical procedure for the circumstances. The Pedersen et al. (2002) analysis avoided a type IV error by using the correct statistical procedure for the circumstance.

Example 4: Aggregation Bias Influencing Ovulation and Imagined Political Behavior
This example showcases another violation of statistical assumptions, this one within a between-groups design. Durante et al. (2013) examined the influence of ovulation on imagined political behavior using women who were both single and in partnered relationships as one of the main comparison

variables—reasoning that relationship status would interact with ovulation status (ovulating or not) to influence their imagined political behavior outcome variables. It is worth noting that for such a comparison of relationship status to work statistically, the two groups should be equivalent with respect to other non-focal variables, such as child status (viz., having children or not having children). An easy way to examine similarity across the non-focal variables is to compare descriptives and/or run an NHST on those non-focal variables. To their credit, Durante et al. (2013) did this and found that women in partnered relationships were significantly more likely to have children than single women (pp. 1010–1011). This is a sensible result given U.S. cultural dynamics. However, it is also sensible to suggest from a reproduction-centered evolutionary psychology perspective that women who have children would engage in different political actions as compared to women without children. As a result, the difference between the groups on relationship status is confounded with child status, and this creates a statistical phenomenon called aggregation bias, in which confounding, non-focal differences between groupings influence the results in addition to (or in place of) the putative focal variable effect. While Durante et al. (2013) show that the aggregation bias existed in both their studies, they did not correct for this bias in any way. When the bias is modeled statistically and corrected, there is no effect of relationship status moderating ovulation status.[2]

A material consequence of not correcting for or otherwise handling aggregation bias is that when another group tries to replicate the results of this study, they may not find the same level of aggregation bias—in this particular case because it is a natural groups variable that cannot be manipulated. Accordingly, when Harris and Mickes (2014) tried to replicate the Durante et al. results at a similar level of power, they could not do so. Although Harris and Mickes did not report all the details of the demographic characteristics of their participants, it would not be surprising to find that they had a different dispersion of child status to relationship status that created a different effect—in this case, no effect of relationship status moderating ovulation status.

In this example, it is also easy to see that a type IV error has been committed by offering the wrong answer to the right problem. The "right problem" is the correctness of the setup: Is there a between-groups relationship status

---

[2] You may contact the chapter author for a research report showing disaggregation of the original Durante et al. (2013) data and the null findings.

difference between single and partnered women that moderates ovulation status in its effect on imagined behavior? The "wrong answer" is provided by Durante et al. (2013) by not using the correct statistical procedure for the circumstances.

Moving Forward with Type III and IV Errors to Improve Science

The importance of considering whether epistemic errors occur on the side of theory or method implementation (type III error) or statistical evaluation (type IV error) for empirical research is that attention can be focused on two sources of errors in addition to false positive (type I error) and false negative (type II error). In fact, with this organization of information and from the breadth of examples provided, one can see that either type III or IV errors could lead to either type I or II errors. For example, not noticing and not addressing outliers in a variance-based test (a type IV error) can provide either a false-positive effect (type I error) or a false-negative effect (type II error)—depending on outlier location across the comparisons. Likewise, focusing on obesity as gene-based only—when it is also influenced by the environment (Schwartz & Carpenter, 1999; a type III error)—can produce either type I or type II errors on the genetic influence itself across studies because the influence of the moderating variable (the environment) sometimes appears within the measured gene-only effect (type I error) and sometimes appears mostly in the error term for the gene-only effect (type II error).

In the end, type III and IV errors provide researchers and statisticians with relevant language and conceptual tools to understand the many sources of influence on statistical inference with or without relying on the NHST. Those moving toward Bayesian statistical techniques will still have to contend with the errors of implementation (type III) and errors of statistical evaluation (type IV). In this case, it may simply be that type IV error in the Bayesian context will focus intensively on meaningful priors for new phenomena.

Understanding and utilizing the generalized type III and IV errors will improve science in fundamental ways. One of the ways will be facilitating the conduct of more sound science. By recognizing that researchers must pay attention to type III errors, implementation errors can be identified and reduced over time. By recognizing that type IV errors are indispensable for understanding the quality of inferences from statistical tests, and that they can be easily avoided by respecting the underlying statistical assumptions of the tests, researchers will create even better inferences by using the techniques as they were originally intended. Working toward the reduction of both errors will increase the reproducibility of methods in science. Research methods will be more uniform because of trying to avoid type III errors; statistical methods will be more consistent because of knowing how to avoid type IV errors.

References

Behrens, J. T. (1997). Principles and procedures for exploratory data analysis. *Psychological Methods, 2*, 131–160.

Bem, S. L. (1974). The measurement of psychological androgyny. *Journal of Counseling and Clinical Psychology, 42*, 155–162.

Bem, S. L. (1981). Gender schema theory: A cognitive account of sex typing. *Psychological Review, 88*, 354–364.

Benjamin, D. J., Berger, J. O., Johannesson, M., Nosek, B. A., Wagenmakers, E-J., Berk, R., Bollen, K. A., Brembs, B., Brown, L., Camerer, C., Cesarini, D., Chambers, C. D., Clyde, M., Cook, T. D., De Boeck, P., Dienes, Z., Dreber, A., Easwaran, K, Efferson, C., . . . Johnson V. E. (2018). Redefine statistical significance. *Nature Human Behaviour, 2*(1), 6–10.

Buss, D. M., Abbott, M., Angleitner, A., Asherian, A., Biaggio, A., Blanco-Villasenor, A., Bruchon-Schweitzer, M., Ch'U, H.-Y., Czapinski, J., Deraad, B., Ekehammar, B., El Lohamy, N., Fioravanti, M., Georgas, J., Gjerde, P., Guttman, R., Hazan, F., Iwawaki, S., Janakiramaiah, N., . . . Yang, K.-S. (1990). International preferences in selecting mates: A study of 37 cultures. *Journal of Cross-Cultural Psychology, 21*(1), 5–47.

Buss, D. M., & Schmitt, D. P. (1993). Sexual strategies theory: An evolutionary perspective on human mating. *Psychological Review, 100*, 204–232.

Cohen, J. (1977). *Statistical Power Analysis for the Behavioral Sciences*. Academic Press.

Cohen, J., Cohen, P., West, S. G., & Aiken, L. S. (2003). *Applied Multiple Regression/Correlation Analysis for the Behavioral Sciences* (3rd ed.). Erlbaum.

Durante, K. M., Rae, A., & Griskevicius, V. (2013). The fluctuating female vote: Politics, religion, and the ovulatory cycle. *Psychological Science, 24*, 1007–1016.

Gelman, A., & Carlin, J. (2014). Beyond power calculations: Assessing type S (sign) and type M (magnitude) errors. *Perpsectives on Psychological Science, 9*, 641–651.

Harris, C. R., & Mickes, L. (2014). Women can keep the vote: No evidence that hormonal changes during the menstrual cycle impact political and religious beliefs. *Psychological Science, 25*, 1147–1149.

Hartley, H. O. (1950). The maximum F-ratio as a short-cut test for heterogeneity of variances. *Biometrika, 37*, 308–312.

Hausmann, R., Tyson, L. D., & Zahidi, S. (2010). *The Global Gender Gap Report 2010*. World Economic Forum.

Ioannides, J. P. A. (2005). Why most published findings are false. *PLoS Medicine*, *2*(8), e124.

Ioannides, J. P. A. (2018). The proposal to lower *p* value thresholds to .005. *Journal of the American Medical Association, 319*(14), 1429–1430.

Kaiser, H. F. (1960). Directional statistical decisions. *Psychological Review, 67*, 160–167.

Kanazawa, S. (2007). Beautiful parents have more daughters: A further implication of the generalized Trivers-Willard hypothesis. *Journal of Theoretical Biology, 244*, 133–140.

Kasser, T., & Sharma, Y. S. (1999). Reproductive freedom, education equality, and females' preference for resource-acquisition characteristics in mates. *Psychological Science, 10*, 374–377.

Kimball, A. W. (1957). Errors of the third kind in statistical consulting. *Journal of the American Statistical Association, 52*(278), 133–142.

Lakens, D., Adolfi, F. G., Albers, C. J., Anvari, F., Apps, M. A. J., Argamon, S. E., Baguley, T., Becker, R. B., Benning, S. D., Bradford, D. E., Buchanan, E. M., Caldwell, A. R., Van Calster, B., Carlsson, R., Chen, S.-C., Chung, B., Colling, L. J., Collins, G. S., Crook, Z., ... Zwaan, R. A. (2018). Justify your alpha. *Nature Human Behaviour, 2*(3), 168–171. https://doi.org/10.1038/s41562-018-0311-x

Levene, H. (1960). Robust tests for equality of variances. In I. Olkin (Ed.), *Contributions to Probability and Statistics* (pp. 278–292). Stanford University Press.

Mahalik, J. R., Morray, E. B., Coonerty-Femiano, A., Ludlow, L. H., Slattery, S. M., & Smiler, A. (2005). Development of the conformity to feminine norms inventory. *Sex Roles, 52*, 417–435.

Marascuilo, L. A., & Levin, J. R. (1970). Appropriate post-hoc comparisons for interaction terms and nested hypotheses in the analysis of variance designs: The elimination of type IV errors. *American Educational Research Journal, 7*, 397–421.

Marks, M. J., & Fraley, R. C. (2005). Sexual double-standard: Fact or fiction? *Sex Roles, 52*, 175–186.

Mosteller, F. (1948). A *k*-sample slippage test for an extreme population. *Annals of Mathematical Statistics, 19*, 58–65.

Neyman, J., & Pearson, E. S. (1933). On the problem of the most efficient tests of statistical hypotheses. *Philosophical Transactions of the Royal Society of London. Series A, Containing Papers of a Mathematical or Physical Character, 231*, 289–337.

Pedersen, W. C., Miller, L. C., & Putcha-Bhagavatula, A.D., & Yang, Y. (2002). Evolved sex differences in desired number of sexual partners? The long and the short of it. *Psychological Science, 13*, 157–161.

Rosnow, R. L., & Rosenthal, R. (1989). Definition and interpretation of interaction effects. *Psychological Bulletin, 105*, 143–146.

Rosnow, R. L., & Rosenthal, R. (1991). If you're looking at the cell means, you're not looking at *only* the interaction (unless all main effects are zero). *Psychological Bulletin, 110*, 574–576.

Schwartz, S. & Carpenter, K. M. (1999). The right answer for the wrong question: Consequences of type III errors for public health research. *American Journal of Public Health, 89*, 1175–1180.

Simmons, J. P., Nelson, L. D., & Simonsohn, U. (2011). False-positive psychology: Undisclosed flexibility in data collection and analysis allows presenting anything as significant. *Psychological Science, 22*, 1359–1366.

Tabachnick, B. A., & Fidell, L. S. (2013). *Using Multivariate Statistics* (6th ed.). Pearson.

Tate, C. (2011). The "problem of number" revisited: The relative contributions of psychosocial, experiential and evolutionary factors to the desired number of sexual partners. *Sex Roles, 64*, 644–657.

Tate, C. C. (2013). Another meaning of Darwinian feminism: Toward inclusive evolutionary accounts of sexual orientations. *Journal of Social, Cultural, and Evolutionary Psychology, 7*, 344–353.

Tate, C. C., Bettergarcia, J. N., & Brent, L. M. (2015). Re-assessing the role of gender-related cognitions for self-esteem: The importance of gender typicality for cisgender adults. *Sex Roles, 72*, 221–236.

Tukey, J. W. (1962). The future of data analysis. *Annals of Mathematical Statistics, 33*, 1–67.

Tukey, J. W. (1969/1986). Analyzing data: Sanctification or detective work? In L.V. Jones (Ed.), *The Collected Writings of John Tukey: Vol. IV: Philosophy and Principles of Data Analysis 1965–1986* (pp. 721–740). Wadsworth.

Umesh, U. N., Peterson, R. A., McCann-Nelson, M., & Vaidyananthan, R. (1996). Type IV error in marketing research: The investigations of ANOVA interactions. *Journal of the Academy of Marketing Science, 24*, 17–26.

Welch, B. L. (1938). The significance of the difference between two means when the population variances are unequal. *Biometrika, 29*, 350–362.

Wold, S., Ruhe, A., Wold, H., & Dunn, W. J. (1984). The collinearity problem in linear regression. The partial-least squares (PLS) approach to generalized inverses. *SIAM Journal of Scientific and Statistical Computing, 5*, 735–743.

Zenter, M., & Mitura, K. (2012). Stepping out of the caveman's shadow: Nation's gender gap predicts degree of sex differentiation in mate preferences. *Psychological Science, 23*, 1176–1185.

13

Publication Bias in the Social Sciences

A Threat to Scientific Integrity

Neil Malhotra and L. J. Zigerell

A key goal of scientific research is the accumulation of knowledge, or what Isaac Newton referred to as "standing on the shoulders of giants." An individual social science study is typically conducted in one place at one time in one context with a limited number of cases, and thus lacks full generalizability. Yet the hope is that synthesizing the collective efforts of numerous researchers working on the same research question will generate more valid inferences and more accurate effect-size estimates than a single study alone. This synthetization can be done informally through literature reviews or formally through statistical meta-analytic procedures. The synthetization process is threatened by publication bias in which conducted studies are not published and, most consequentially, when published studies are not representative of conducted studies (Begg & Berlin, 1988; Dickersin, 1990). Publication bias is essentially a form of selection bias. If published studies are a non-random and systematically biased sample of the population of conducted studies, then meta-analyses will not be able to recover true population parameters of social phenomena. This chapter discusses two types of publication bias, provides evidence that such publication bias has occurred, and discusses procedures that can be adopted to limit the pernicious effects of publication bias.

Two Types of Publication Bias

One form of publication bias is *selection for statistical significance*. Social scientists often report a statistic called the p-value, which is the probability of finding a result at least as extreme as the observed result when the null hypothesis is true. Low p-values indicate that the data are unlikely under a

Neil Malhotra and L. J. Zigerell, *Publication Bias in the Social Sciences* In: *Research Integrity*. Edited by: Lee J. Jussim, Jon A. Krosnick, and Sean T. Stevens, Oxford University Press. © Oxford University Press 2022.
DOI: 10.1093/oso/9780190938550.003.0013

true null. Social scientists have conventionally used 0.05 as the threshold for separating "statistically significant" associations (for which there is strong evidence) from "statistically insignificant" associations (for which the evidence is weaker and more ambiguous) (Gill, 1999).[1] Given the inferential ambiguity about statistically insignificant associations, statistically significant associations have in practice been more likely to be published than statistically insignificant associations, even holding fixed research quality (Franco et al., 2014).[2] This higher likelihood of publication of statistically significant associations can arise at various stages in the research process. During manuscript review, editors and peer reviewers might be more likely to reject manuscripts reporting statistically insignificant associations or to recommend dropping statistically insignificant results from a manuscript. If researchers anticipate rejection of these manuscripts at peer-reviewed journals, researchers might also be less likely to write up and submit reports of studies that produced statistically insignificant associations. Finally, researchers may manipulate results so as to include only statistically significant findings in papers (Simmons et al., 2011).

The second major type of publication bias is *selection on inference*, which occurs when data-analysis reporting choices or the submission or acceptance of manuscripts are influenced by the inferences and effect-size estimates produced by a study. For instance, researchers might prefer inferences that are the opposite of the inferences produced by a set of data and therefore fail to report on these data or, in the case of data that permit multiple inferences, to report on these data in a way that does not reflect the full set of inferences that the data can support. Like with selection for statistical significance, selection on inference can be exacerbated by editor and peer-reviewer actions that condition the rigor and outcomes of the peer-review process on the inferences produced by the analyses.

Figure 13.1 illustrates these two types of publication bias and the problems that can be caused by the particular type of publication bias, using the funnel plot method introduced by Light and Pillemer (1984). Each panel of Figure 13.1 presents a funnel plot that depicts a set of hypothetical studies testing

---

[1] There is less consensus on whether hypothesis testing should be one-tailed or two-tailed, and the appropriate conditions for selecting one test over another. This should be decided before observing the data, but in practice tail selection has likely often been post hoc (Gerber et al., 2010). Moreover, there has been discussion about whether 0.05 should remain the default p-value threshold for new discoveries (Benjamin et al., 2018).

[2] Research quality is an important conditioning factor, which we discuss in further detail later in the chapter.

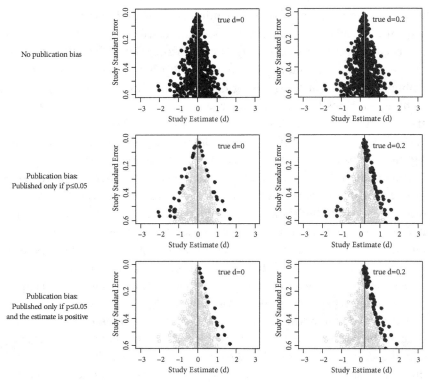

Figure 13.1. Simulations to illustrate different forms of publication bias

Figure panels report results from a simulation of hypothetical studies of different sample sizes testing the same research question. The left panels are for a simulation in which all studies test a research question for which the true effect size is d = 0, and the right panels are for the same simulation but in which all studies test a research question for which the true effect size is d = 0.2. Black dots indicate published studies, and gray open dots indicate unpublished studies. The top left graph illustrates the expected funnel plot shape if the studies are testing for an effect that is null and all studies are published. The middle left graph illustrates the hollowing out expected to occur if the studies are testing for an effect that is null and only studies with a p-value of 0.05 or lower are published; in this case, the pooled estimate from the published studies is expected to fall at or near the true value of zero for the null effect, creating little or no bias in the pooled estimate. The bottom left graph illustrates the hollowing out expected to occur if the studies are testing for an effect that is null and only studies with a positive effect and a p-value of 0.05 or lower are published; in this case, the pooled estimate from the published studies is biased higher than true value of zero for the null effect. The top right graph illustrates the expected funnel plot shape if the studies are testing for an effect that has a size of 0.2 and all studies are published. The middle right graph illustrates the hollowing out expected to occur if the studies are testing for an effect that has a size of 0.2 and studies are published only if the studies have a p-value of 0.05 or lower; in this case, the pooled estimate from the published studies is biased above the true value of 0.2. The bottom right graph illustrates the hollowing out expected to occur if the studies are testing for an effect that has a size of 0.2 and studies are published only if the studies have a p-value of 0.05 or lower and a positive effect; in this case, the pooled estimate from the published studies is biased above the true value of 0.2 and the bias is even greater than if the publication bias were based on only the p-value.

the same research question using the same research design but with different sample sizes and thus different levels of precision. Panels on the left side of the figure indicate the set of studies from a simulation in which the true effect size is zero, and panels on the right side of the figure indicate the set of studies from the same simulation but for which the true effect size is a small effect size of d = 0.2. The x-axis indicates the estimated effect size from a given study; the y-axis indicates the precision of a study, represented by the study's standard error, in which higher values along the y-axis indicate more precise studies with lower standard errors. For a research question in which study precision varies among studies and all studies are available in the field's literature, the shape of the funnel plot for studies testing that research question should be an upside-down filled-in funnel, as in the top panels of Figure 13.1, in which all perfectly precise studies should have the same effect-size estimate, and, for less-precise studies, random variation in experimental randomizations or sampling imperfections should cause the set of studies for a given level of precision to be symmetric about the estimate from the perfectly precise studies, with more variation in effect-size estimates for the less-precise studies.

The middle row of panels in Figure 13.1 illustrates publication bias due to selection for statistical significance. If, as in the left panel in the middle row of Figure 13.1, the true effect size for the research question is zero and studies are published only if they had a statistically significant result, the funnel plot of published studies is hollowed out where the statistically insignificant results are. In this case, the effect-size estimate for a synthetization of the studies on this research question is unbiased even though the literature exhibited publication bias due to selection for statistical significance. However, as in the right panel in the middle row of Figure 13.1, if the true effect size for the research question is nonzero and studies are published only if they had a statistically significant result, the hollowing out of the funnel plot due to non-publication of statistically insignificant studies produces an effect-size estimate that is biased toward a larger effect-size estimate. For an estimate of the bias that can be caused by publication bias due to selection for statistical significance, Franco et al. (2016) found that effect-size estimates for unreported outcome variables were roughly half as large as effect-size estimates for outcome variables reported on in the published results.

The bottom row of panels in Figure 13.1 illustrates publication bias due to selection for statistical significance coupled with selection on inference and, in particular, selection in favor of studies with a positive estimated effect and against studies with a negative estimated effect. The right panel in the bottom row illustrates how, like with selection for statistical significance, selection on inference can bias research syntheses when the true effect size is nonzero. However, the left panel in the bottom row illustrates that, in contrast to publication bias due to selection for statistical significance, publication bias due to selection on inference can bias synthetizations even when the true effect size is zero.

Evidence for Publication Bias: Selection for Statistical Significance

A well-known method for detecting the presence of publication bias is testing for a relationship between effect size and sample size for a given research question, based on the idea that, if there is no selection bias in published studies based on statistical significance, there should be no relationship between effect size and sample size (see, e.g., Gerber et al., 2001). Studies with small samples should on average have similar effect sizes as studies with larger samples, with the smaller-sample studies exhibiting more variance. However, if studies for which results reach statistical significance are more likely to be published than studies for which results do not reach statistical significance, then lower-powered studies will exhibit on average larger effect sizes than higher-powered studies for a given research question. This is because lower-powered studies require larger effect sizes to exceed the statistical significance threshold.

Often the funnel plot methodology is not useful in the social sciences because there are not many similar studies on a particular research question. Consequently, several other methods have been used to test for the presence of publication bias due to a selection for statistical significance. Gerber and Malhotra (2008a, 2008b) analyzed studies in two prominent political science journals and three prominent sociology journals, finding that articles across these journals were substantially more likely to report p-values just under the conventional 0.05 threshold for statistical significance than to report p-values just over the 0.05 threshold, a disparity that would have been highly unlikely to have occurred due to chance under reasonable estimates of the distribution of p-values. Brodeur et al. (2016) conducted a similar study in economics and reached similar results. Moreover, Ioannidis and Trikalinos (2007) proposed and applied a test for excess statistical significance in a set of studies; the logic of the test is to compare the percentage of reported studies that found statistically significant associations with the percentage of reported studies that would have been expected to find statistically significant associations given the characteristics of the studies. Francis (2014) applied this test to a set of articles published in the journal *Psychological Science* that had at least four studies with sufficient data available to produce an estimate for the test. Francis's application of this test produced an estimate of reporting bias in 82% of the 44 articles that met inclusion criteria.[3] More direct evidence of publication bias due to selection for statistical significance is provided by surveys that ask researchers about their research practices. For example, John et al. (2012) reported on a survey of psychology faculty at U.S. universities with a psychology doctoral program and found that roughly half of respondents admitted to selectively reporting studies that "worked" and roughly two-thirds of respondents admitted to selectively reporting dependent variable measures. These plausibly represent lower bounds on the prevalence of such practices, given social desirability bias in admitting to these practices.

Omission of statistically insignificant associations might be at least partially justified based on the fact that studies with insignificant results are more likely to have low-quality research designs. Addressing this potential explanation, Franco et al. (2014) leveraged a program sponsored by the National Science Foundation called TESS (Time-sharing Experiments for the Social Sciences), in which researchers propose survey-based experiments. Substantial non-publication of these TESS studies cannot reasonably be attributed to the studies having low-quality research designs, because TESS studies have had their proposed research designs reviewed in a stringent peer-review process and have had their data collected by competent third parties such as GfK/Knowledge Networks or the Indiana University Center for Survey Research. TESS policy is to place online the data and documentation from conducted studies 1 year after the proposal authors have had exclusive access to the data. In an analysis of data from TESS studies, Franco et al. (2014) found that the strength of results strongly predicted whether a study was published, with about 60% of studies with strong results published, compared to 20% of those with statistically insignificant results. This difference

---

[3] For critiques of this method and its applications, see Simonsohn (2012) and the *Journal of Mathematical Psychology* special issue on publication bias and the test for excess significance (Volume 57, Issue 5).

is mainly due to researchers not submitting statistically insignificant results, possibly because they anticipate rejection or because they have a preference themselves for statistically significant results. Around 65% of studies with statistically insignificant results had not even been written up, compared to only 4% of studies with strong results.

Publication bias due to selection for statistical significance makes it more likely that published findings reflect false positives (Humphreys et al., 2013), so that researchers trying to understand the state of knowledge in a field might be misled because statistically insignificant results from conducted-but-unpublished studies are unobserved. However, publication bias also affects the incentives of researchers. If researchers perceive or experience that statistically insignificant results are substantially less likely to be accepted for publication, then scientific integrity may be compromised in many ways. Researchers might selectively report experimental conditions and outcome variables or subset the data in ways to achieve statistically significant results, not reporting the full set of analyses that were conducted (Simmons et al., 2011). Additionally, researchers might not report entire studies that were conducted but failed, reporting only the studies that yielded statistically significant results, perhaps by chance. For example, further analysis of the TESS archive in Franco et al. (2015) indicated substantial underreporting of TESS studies published in peer-reviewed political science journals, with roughly 80% of published reports for these TESS studies not reporting the full set of experimental conditions or the full set of outcome variables.

Evidence for Publication Bias: Selection on Inference

Publication bias can also occur due to selection on inference. In many cases, a set of data can be analyzed in different ways to produce different effect-size estimates or even different inferences. For example, Silberzahn et al. (2018) reported on the work of 29 research teams using the same dataset to investigate the research question of whether soccer players with darker skin tone were more likely to receive a red card from a referee, relative to soccer players with lighter skin tone. Roughly two-thirds of research teams reported a statistically significant finding, and roughly one-third of teams reported a statistically insignificant finding, with effect-size estimates in odds ratios ranging from a statistically insignificant 0.89 to a statistically significant 2.93. Researchers with a preference for finding skin-color discrimination against players with darker skin and researchers with a preference for not finding skin-color discrimination had the flexibility to analyze and re-analyze the data until the analysis produced their preferred inference. Publication bias due to selection on inference might also occur due to decisions at the manuscript-review stage: Journal editor preference for initial results on a research question might be biased toward statistical significance, but incentives for publishing novel and newsworthy research that overturns past findings might cause the "overturn bias" detected in the Galiani et al. (2017) survey of editors of leading economics journals.

Publication bias due to selection on inference might not produce incorrect inferences and biased effect-size estimates in research synthetizations if numeric representation, funding, resources, and propensity to select on inference were balanced between researchers with conflicting inferential preferences so that, for instance, results producing an inference preferable to political liberals are as equally likely to be unreported as results producing an inference preferable to political conservatives. But the large imbalance in political ideology within and across social science fields makes such balance in results reporting unlikely. For example, the Gross and Simmons (2014) survey of 1,416 American professors indicated that 44% of respondents self-identified as liberal or extremely liberal and 9% of respondents self-identified as conservative or extremely conservative (p. 25), with respective percentages of 58% and 5% in the social sciences, a roughly 11-to-1 ratio.

To address whether it is reasonable to expect publication bias due to selection on inference, we start by reviewing evidence from a survey reported on in Honeycutt and Freberg (2017) of a convenience sample of 618 faculty across 76 disciplines at the Humboldt, Monterey Bay, San Luis Obispo, and Stanislaus campuses of the California State University system. Survey results indicated a positive correlation between respondent's reported liberalism and willingness to discriminate against conservatives and a positive correlation between respondent's reported conservatism and willingness to discriminate against liberals regarding decisions on grant applications, decisions on papers, inviting of colleagues to a symposium, and votes on who to hire for an opening in one's department. There was a rough symmetry between the percentage of liberals with an anti-conservative bias and the percentage of conservatives with an anti-liberal bias, which—if liberals and conservatives were equally represented—might produce little to no net bias in decisions on papers, grants, and hiring and therefore produce little to no bias in research output due to selection on inference. However, as in social science as a whole, the Honeycutt and Freberg (2017) sample had a large disparity between the percentage of liberals and the percentage of conservatives, which were, respectively, 71% and 14%, a roughly 5-to-1 ratio.[4]

If the rough symmetry in left/right political discrimination in peer review detected in the Honeycutt and Freberg (2017) survey and the ideological imbalance among social scientists reported in Gross and Simmons (2014) indicate true patterns in social science, then it is reasonable to expect peer review to bias the literature toward findings with politically liberal inferences, relative to the full set of studies that have been conducted or the full set of studies that would have been conducted if there were no political bias in hiring and in the funding of grant applications. Banks et al. (2016, p. 330) noted that most research on questionable research practices has investigated activities that impact statistical significance. However, it seems reasonable to expect researchers who use questionable research practices to use these practices to produce preferred inferences as well.

In many cases, the cost of selecting studies and analyses on inference is negligible, involving only the underreporting of outcome variables or the testing of a few additional analyses with various combinations of control variables. Even excluding entire studies can have a negligible cost for manuscripts that report multiple studies and are still publishable—or perhaps more publishable—after excluding studies with politically undesired results. Selection on inference can even lower research costs, such as in cases in which a researcher decides to not collect more or better data for a correlational study in which the association in uncontrolled or under-controlled analyses is in the researcher's preferred direction. And it might even be rational for researchers to forgo pursuit of publication of a statistically significant but politically undesired result in a manuscript with only one study if the researcher has sufficient work in the pipeline to substitute with little to no opportunity cost a new project in place of the project with politically undesired results.

Like with detection of publication bias due to selection for statistical significance, detecting publication bias due to selection on inference is difficult, compounded by the fact that in many cases selection on inference is observationally equivalent to selection for statistical significance. For example, a researcher may decline to report a study that detected a small to nil effect size

---

[4] Honeycutt and Freberg (2017) replicated and extended research reported on in Inbar and Lammers (2012), but Skitka (2012) raised several important concerns about the sampling and research design in Inbar and Lammers (2012).

for sex discrimination with a p-value above p = 0.05 either because (1) the researcher perceives it to be difficult to publish statistically insignificant results or (2) the researcher fears that the small to nil effect-size estimate indicates little to no real-world discrimination and would undercut support for policies to combat discrimination against women. However, one phenomenon that is inconsistent with selection for statistical significance but is consistent with selection on inference is when a report of research omits a statistically significant result that conflicts with reported results or claims.

One such example can be found in a published report on the 2006 Lovaglia and Rogalin TESS survey experiment. Participants received four items, with the manipulation that participants were randomly assigned to receive items about male targets or items about female targets. The items were as follows, with square brackets indicating the text that varied between experimental conditions:

- Suppose you needed advice on an important problem and had the choice of asking one of two [male/female] coworkers of quite different ages. Ideally, how old or young would the [man/woman] be who you asked for advice?
- Now that [men/women] are staying on the job longer, at what age do you think the contributions of [male/female] workers start to decline?
- In your opinion, at what age do [male/female] executives make the best bosses?
- Ideally, how many years of work experience should a [man/woman] have before being promoted to run a major company?

Responses for all four items indicated higher values for male targets than for female targets, as indicated in Table 13.1. Lovaglia et al. (2017) reported on this survey experiment, but, of the four items, mentioned only the third item in which participants reported a lower mean "ideal" age for women than for men for the age at which executives make the best bosses. The authors suggested that "'ideal age' estimates for men and women executives likely disadvantage women competing for top leadership positions against equally qualified men" (pp. 91–92). However, the inference that women executives are disadvantaged in the competition for leadership positions is complicated by results for the fourth item, which indicated that participants perceived men to need more than 2 years more work experience than women before being promoted to run a major company. The absence of this finding

Table 13.1 Results from the Lovaglia and Rogalin (2006) TESS Survey Experiment

	Unweighted analyses			Weighted analyses			
	Male target	Female target	p-value	Male target	Female target	p-value	N
Ideal age of a coworker for asking advice	45.1	43.1	<0.001	44.7	42.6	<0.001	2,002
Age at which workers start to decline	63.5	61.9	0.007	62.4	61.3	0.121	2,006
Age at which executives make the best bosses	47.6	43.5	<0.001	47.0	42.9	<0.001	2,003
Years of work experience before being promoted to run a major company	17.6	15.3	<0.001	17.2	14.6	<0.001	2,007

Note: The table reports mean values of responses to the four Lovaglia and Rogalin (2006) items in the male target condition and the female target condition, plus the p-value for the difference in means for unweighted and weighted analyses. See the main text for full item wording. There were 2,020 dataset cases, but the 13 participants who did not provide a substantive response to at least two of the four items did not have a dataset weight and were excluded from the analysis.

indicating a clear disadvantage for male workers cannot be attributed to a lack of statistical significance or to redundancy in inferences with the included item. Rather, the results from the fourth item appear inconsistent with Lovaglia et al.'s (2017) statement that "gender is a status characteristic that advantages men" (p. 88).

Patterns consistent with selection on inference also appear in research synthetizations, such as in Figure 1 in the Zigerell (2017) re-analysis of the Nguyen and Ryan (2008) meta-analysis of stereotype threat studies. Stereotype threat is the idea that negative stereotypes can negatively influence the performance of members of negatively stereotyped groups (see, for example, Steele & Aronson, 1995, and Spencer et al., 1999). Evidence for stereotype threat can be used to support interventions that favor negatively stereotyped groups, so the traditional liberal concern for underprivileged groups and for equality of outcome is reasonably expected to positively correlate with a desire to find evidence of stereotype threat. Statistical analyses reported in Zigerell (2017) indicated that the funnel plot of stereotype threat effect-size estimates is asymmetric, with the asymmetry—especially regarding outlier effect sizes—consistent with underreporting of studies that detected statistically significant evidence that negative stereotypes *improve* the performance of negatively stereotyped groups, a finding that would undercut liberal policy preferences based on the idea that negatively stereotyped groups should have assistance to overcome the effects of negative stereotypes.[5]

For another example, Figure 1 in Roth et al. (2015) presents funnel plots from a meta-analysis of the correlation between scores on intelligence tests and school grades. As suggested by Kirkegaard (2016), in this case, the funnel plot asymmetry is consistent with the non-publication of conducted studies that detected a *large* association between scores on intelligence tests and school grades. This large correlation between IQ and school grades would presumably have been a finding that is more inconvenient for persons on the political left, who are more likely than persons on the political right to emphasize structural factors for educational disparities such as inequalities in school funding, and less likely to emphasize individual-level explanations such as intelligence.

Procedures for Reducing Publication Bias

Publication bias involving selection for statistical significance can produce excess false positives that lead to wasted time if researchers try to build on phenomena that do not exist and can lead to wasted spending on useless interventions. Publication bias due to selection on inference involving research with policy implications can also lead to unfair interventions that privilege the preferences of researchers. What can be done to reverse these patterns? Most immediately, the research community needs to be made aware of research that has been conducted but not published, so that published results can be placed in proper context. Researchers should be encouraged to report on results in their file drawer or at least to post data and documentation in public outlets such as the Open Science Framework so that other researchers can analyze and report on the data. For instance,

---

[5] Zigerell (2017) and Ryan and Nguyen (2017) noted that funnel plot asymmetry can be caused by phenomena other than publication bias, and Simonsohn (2017) reported results from simulations indicating that funnel plot asymmetry can be caused by researchers correctly estimating the effect size for a study and then setting the sample size for their studies accordingly. For example, applied to the stereotype threat meta-analysis, it could be that the most-precise studies are testing for stereotype threat in a context in which stereotype threat is relatively small, so that the estimated effect size is small and the sample is large; correspondingly, it could be that the least-precise studies are testing for stereotype threat in a context in which stereotype threat is relatively large, so that the estimated effect size is large and the sample is small. This would produce an asymmetric funnel plot even if all studies were published.

the TESS archives contain many survey experiments that have not yet been reported on in the literature; researchers uninvolved with the proposal for an unpublished TESS study could nonetheless draft a report on that study, in isolation or in a group of studies, and then submit the report for publication or post the report to a repository that can be searched by researchers conducting meta-analyses.

Encouragement to researchers to make file drawer data public or to release descriptions of results for unpublished studies can take several forms, such as disciplinary norms or funding agency requirements, and researchers who release data from their file drawer or describe these file drawer results can serve as role models for other researchers, especially if the research community signals the high value of such disclosures. Going forward, publication bias could be reduced or eliminated by studies being preregistered before being conducted, as is often the case with medical clinical trials. Such preregistration could be done voluntarily by researchers themselves or be required or encouraged by funders or publication outlets. Researchers performing meta-analyses could then consult the registries to potentially include studies that were conducted but never published. Interestingly, the TESS archives represent such a registry for social science survey experiments, but this archive has not been used extensively in this fashion. Would researchers agree to this extra preregistration step prior to pursuing research? After the publication of the Belmont Report (National Commission for the Protection of Human Subjects of Biomedical and Behavioral Research, 1978), researchers conducting human subjects research have regularly been required to gain approval from institutional review boards. Moreover, there is evidence that researchers respond to acknowledgments of their transparency practices: Kidwell et al. (2016) reported that open data practices increased substantially in *Psychological Science* relative to comparison journals after *Psychological Science* began using badges to identify articles that had open data or open materials. Given the crisis in the reproducibility of social science, preregistration could be an additional required step that could become ingrained in the process of doing research.

Researchers can also be encouraged or required to file pre-analysis plans (PAPs) in advance of publication (Casey et al., 2012). PAPs bind researchers to analyze the data in a prespecified way, thereby curtailing researcher ability to selectively analyze and report the data in such a manner as to produce findings that comport with pre hoc theoretical predictions. One criticism is that PAPs might stifle creativity in the research process. However, the use of a PAP does not preclude a researcher from conducting more exploratory, inductive analyses. All the PAP does is make clear to the reader which analyses were specified in advance and which ones are post hoc. This then provides the research community the information to assess which results are more likely to be valid, and which interesting results might need more scrutiny via replication. This seems to be more honest than a status quo that permits researchers to observe the data and then construct theoretical hypotheses after the fact to justify the observed relationships in the data.

Regarding ways to avoid selection on inference occurring in the peer-review process, journals can engage in results-blind review of research in which researchers submit their theoretical hypotheses and research designs for review but peer reviewers and editors do not have access to the results, which would encourage peer reviewers and editors to judge the papers on the strength of the theory and research design, regardless of how the data ultimately turned out (see Findley et al., 2016). This would likely increase the number of published statistically insignificant results, but these statistically insignificant results would have relatively high levels of information about the research question, given that results-blind peer review selects on the quality of theory and research design. Moreover, results-blind review could be used to conceal politically unpopular results from peer reviewers, which would lessen potential publication bias due to selection on inference. Of course, results-blind review might preclude the publication of certain types of findings, if, for instance, reviewers reject proposals that have research hypotheses that are so counterintuitive as to be perceived to be implausible. However, an argument can be made that the initial questions social science disciplines should be addressing are results independent. Only once a strong, replicable empirical foundation is built should the social sciences move into more exotic territory where only a positive finding would be interesting.

The Registered Report method combats publication bias using a two-stage peer-review process that combines the benefits of preregistration and results-blind review. In a typical process for a Registered Report, peer review is conducted on a proposed method before data collection and then, if the proposal is provisionally accepted, the data are collected and the analysis is written, with the resulting manuscript undergoing another round of peer review.

One other way to help better avoid selection for statistical significance and selection on inference occurring in the peer-review process is for peer reviewers and editors to be more active in requiring researchers to report—in a paper, a supplemental appendix, or a memo to the peer reviewers—robustness checks for analyses that the researcher did not report in the initial submission of a non-preregistered report. Moreover, journals can require researchers to make declarations that provide the reader information about the potential for selective reporting; for example, the journal *Psychological Science* currently requires submitting authors to make declarations about the fullness of the reporting of dependent variables, independent variables, and case deletions.[6]

Of course, one argument that can be leveled at the concerns outlined in this chapter is that papers produce statistically insignificant findings because they are poorly theorized and poorly designed. In other words, we would not want a proliferation of useless statistically insignificant findings that clutter the literature. Instead of the "file drawer," imagine the metaphor of the "cluttered desk." There is a clear response to this concern. Publication bias is defined as the increased likelihood of the publication of statistically significant results, conditional on research quality. Hence, the theoretical concern of this chapter is a counterfactual where two equally high-quality projects are conducted but only the one producing positive results–perhaps by chance alone–is published. Even if papers with statistically insignificant findings are of lower quality, the innovation of results-blind review addresses this issue. It allows papers to be evaluated on the quality of the underlying theory and research design. Consequently, a reviewer will be able to assess ex ante whether a given theory or research design is sufficiently weak and thus unlikely to produce informative findings because of the design itself. In the status quo, a reviewer's assessment of design quality is likely biased by observing the results alongside the design.

There does exist a legitimate concern that papers published based on a results-blind review format may be more obvious and less "splashy" than papers published under more traditional publishing paradigms, if the review process selects against non-intuitive hypotheses. However, a major concern is that these non-intuitive "splashy" results are not correct and are not replicable (Open Science Collaboration, 2015). Social science may be better off to have a set of valid findings that might be more ordinary, but that the research community has more confidence in sharing with society at large. Further,

---

[6] See: https://web.archive.org/web/20171115110444/http://www.psychologicalscience.org/publications/psychological_science/ps-submissions.

there is a set of research questions for which any answer—positive, negative, or null—is important and interesting. Perhaps these questions should be the ones the scholarly community tackles first. Nonetheless, most likely a subset of journals will experiment with results-blind review rather than journals moving en masse to the practice. These experiments will help us better understand potential tradeoffs between creativity and validity.

Conclusion

If social science is to thrive and succeed as an intellectual enterprise, we must be confident that published social science reflects an accurate and representative description of the research that has been conducted. Publication bias has compromised this objective. There are several forms that publication bias can take; whereas most readers are likely familiar with selection based on statistical significance, we have highlighted the underappreciated concern of selection based on inference. There is substantial evidence that both forms of publication bias have undermined literatures. Researchers and consumers of social science making inferences about the literature on a given research question should be aware of the potential for publication bias in the literature and be aware of or test for evidence that such publication bias has occurred. Moving forward, researchers should consider adopting practices that reduce publication bias in their own research, and the research community should consider adopting policies to prevent publication bias and mitigate this threat to scientific integrity. Many of the solutions we have discussed here–results-blind review, study registries, pre-analysis plans, registered reports–are not panaceas but would likely ameliorate problems with how scholarship is conducted. If the scholarly community does not address issues related to various forms of publication bias, then not only will science lose legitimacy, but society as a whole will also be harmed.

References

Banks, G. C., Rogelberg, S. G., Woznyj, H. M., Landis, R. S., & Rupp, D. E. (2016). Evidence on questionable research practices: The good, the bad, and the ugly. *Journal of Business and Psychology, 31*(3), 323–338.

Begg, C. B., & Berlin, J. A. (1988). Publication bias: A problem in interpreting medical data. *Journal of the Royal Statistical Society. Series A (Statistics in Society), 151*(3), 419–463.

Benjamin, D. J., Berger, J. O., Johannesson, M., Nosek, B. A., Wagenmakers, E-J., Berk, R., Bollen, K. A., Brembs, B., Brown, L., Camerer, C., Cesarini, D., Chambers, C. D., Clyde, M., Cook, T. D., De Boeck, P., Dienes, Z., Dreber, A., Easwaran, K, Efferson, C., ... Johnson V. E. (2018). Redefine statistical significance. *Nature Human Behaviour, 2*(1), 6–10.

Brodeur, A., Lé, M., Sangnier, M., & Zylberberg, Y. (2016). Star Wars: The empirics strike back. *American Economic Journal: Applied Economics, 8*(1), 1–32.

Casey, K., Glennerster, R., & Miguel, E. (2012). Reshaping institutions: Evidence on aid impacts using a preanalysis plan. *Quarterly Journal of Economics, 127*(4), 1755–1812.

Dickersin, K. (1990). The existence of publication bias and risk factors for its occurrence. *Journal of the American Medical Association, 263*(10), 1385–1389.

Findley, M. G., Jensen, N. M., Malesky, E. J., & Pepinsky, T. B. (2016). Can results-free review reduce publication bias? The results and implications of a pilot study. *Comparative Political Studies, 49*(13), 1667–1703.

Francis, G. (2014). The frequency of excess success for articles in *Psychological Science*. *Psychonomic Bulletin & Review, 21*(5), 1180–1187.

Franco, A., Malhotra, N., & Simonovits, G. (2014). Publication bias in the social sciences: Unlocking the file drawer. *Science, 345*(6203), 1502–1505.

Franco, A., Malhotra, N., & Simonovits, G. (2015). Underreporting in political science survey experiments: Comparing questionnaires to published results. *Political Analysis, 23*(2), 306–312.

Franco, A., Malhotra, N., & Simonovits, G. (2016). Underreporting in psychology experiments: Evidence from a study registry. *Social Psychological and Personality Science, 7*(1), 8–12.

Galiani, S., Gertler, P., & Romero, M. (2017). *Incentives for Replication in Economics*. No. w23576. National Bureau of Economic Research.

Gerber, A. S., Green, D. P., & Nickerson, D. (2001). Testing for publication bias in political science. *Political Analysis, 9*(4), 385–392.

Gerber, A., & Malhotra, N. (2008a). Do statistical reporting standards affect what is published? Publication bias in two leading political science journals. *Quarterly Journal of Political Science, 3*(3), 313–326.

Gerber, A. S., & Malhotra, N. (2008b). Publication bias in empirical sociological research: Do arbitrary significance levels distort published results? *Sociological Methods & Research, 37*(1), 3–30.

Gerber, A. S., Malhotra, N., Dowling, C. M., & Doherty, D. (2010). Publication bias in two political behavior literatures. *American Politics Research, 38*(4), 591–613.

Gill, J. (1999). The insignificance of null hypothesis significance testing. *Political Research Quarterly, 52*(3), 647–674.

Gross, N., & Simmons, S. (2014). The social and political views of American college and university professors. In N. Gross & S. Simmons (Eds.), *Professors and Their Politics* (pp. 19–50). Johns Hopkins University Press.

Honeycutt, N., & Freberg, L. (2017). The liberal and conservative experience across academic disciplines: An extension of Inbar and Lammers. *Social Psychological and Personality Science, 8*(2), 115–123.

Humphreys, M., Sierra, R. S., & van der Windt, P. (2013). Fishing, commitment, and communication: A proposal for comprehensive nonbinding research registration. *Political Analysis*, *21*(1), 1-20.

Inbar, Y., & Lammers, J. (2012). Political diversity in social and personality psychology. *Perspectives on Psychological Science*, *7*(5), 496-503.

Ioannidis, J. P. A., & Trikalinos, T. A. (2007). An exploratory test for an excess of significant findings. *Clinical Trials*, *4*(3), 245-253.

John, L. K., Loewenstein, G., & Prelec, D. (2012). Measuring the prevalence of questionable research practices with incentives for truth telling. *Psychological Science*, *23*(5), 524-532.

Kidwell, M. C., Lazarević, L. B., Baranski, E., Hardwicke, T. E., Piechowski, S., Falkenberg, L-S., Kennett, C., Slowik, A., Sonnleitner, C., Hess-Holden, C., Errington, T. M., Fiedler, S., & Nosek, B. A. (2016). Badges to acknowledge open practices: A simple, low-cost, effective method for increasing transparency. *PLoS Biology*, *14*(5), e1002456.

Kirkegaard, E. O. W. (2016, March 19, 9:53 p.m.). Twitter post. https://twitter.com/kirkegaardemil/status/711355039248416768

Light, R. J., & Pillemer, D. B. (1984). *Summing Up: The Science of Reviewing Research*. Harvard University Press.

Lovaglia, M., & Rogalin, C. (2006). Replication data for: The age-gender interaction effect on status expectations: Investigation and career implications. https://osf.io/q458t/

Lovaglia, M. J., Soboroff, S. D., Kelley, C. P., Rogalin, C. L., & Lucas, J. W. (2017). The status value of age and gender: Modeling combined effects of diffuse status characteristics. In S. R. Thye & E. J. Lawler (Eds.), *Advances in Group Processes* (pp. 81-101). Emerald Publishing Limited.

National Commission for the Protection of Human Subjects of Biomedical and Behavioral Research. (1978). *The Belmont Report: Ethical Principles and Guidelines for the Protection of Human Subjects of Research*.

Nguyen, H. D., & Ryan, A. M. (2008). Does stereotype threat affect test performance of minorities and women? A meta-analysis of experimental evidence. *Journal of Applied Psychology*, *93*(6), 1314-1334.

Open Science Collaboration. (2015). Estimating the reproducibility of psychological science. *Science*, *349*(6251), aac4716.

Roth, B., Becker, N., Romeyke, S., Schäfer, S., Domnick, F., & Spinath, F. M. (2015). Intelligence and school grades: A meta-analysis. *Intelligence*, *53*(Nov-Dec), 118-137.

Ryan, A. M., & Nguyen, H. D. (2017). Publication bias and stereotype threat research: A reply to Zigerell. *Journal of Applied Psychology*, *102*(8), 1169-1177.

Silberzahn, R., Uhlmann, E. L., Martin, D. P., Anselmi, P., Aust, F., Awtrey, E., Bahník, Š., Bai, F., Bannard, C., Bonnier, E., Carlsson, R., Cheung, F., Christensen, G., Clay, R., Craig, M. A., Dalla Rosa, A., Dam, L., Evans, M. H., Flores Cervantes, I., ... Nosek, B. A. (2018). Many analysts, one data set: Making transparent how variations in analytic choices affect results. *Advances in Methods and Practices in Psychological Science*, *1*(3), 337-356.

Simmons, J. P., Nelson, L. D., & Simonsohn, U. (2011). False-positive psychology: Undisclosed flexibility in data collection and analysis allows presenting anything as significant. *Psychological Science*, *22*(11), 1359-1366.

Simonsohn, U. (2012). It does not follow: Evaluating the one-off publication bias critiques by Francis (2012a, 2012b, 2012c, 2012d, 2012e, In Press). *Perspectives on Psychological Science*, *7*(6), 597-599.

Simonsohn, U. (2017, March 21). The funnel plot is invalid because of this crazy assumption: r(n,d)=0. http://datacolada.org/58

Skitka, L. J. (2012). Multifaceted problems: Liberal bias and the need for scientific rigor in self-critical research. *Perspectives on Psychological Science, 7*(5), 508–511.

Spencer, S. J., Steele, C. M., & Quinn, D. M. (1999). Stereotype threat and women's math performance. *Journal of Experimental Social Psychology, 35*(1), 4–28.

Steele, C. M., & Aronson, J. (1995). Stereotype threat and the intellectual test performance of African Americans. *Journal of Personality and Social Psychology, 69*(5), 797–811.

Zigerell, L. J. (2017). Potential publication bias in the stereotype threat literature: Comment on Nguyen and Ryan (2008). *Journal of Applied Psychology, 102*(8), 1159–1168.

14
Let's Peer Review Peer Review

Simine Vazire

In this chapter I will discuss how peer review is related to replicability and rigor in science. I will not cover the history and philosophy of peer review, nor the empirical studies that have been done on peer review. For thorough discussions of those topics I refer readers to Tennant et al. (2017). Rather, this chapter will present ideas and opinions based on my experience as someone who has played several roles in both the peer-review process and in the debates surrounding the replicability issues in psychology (i.e., the "credibility revolution"). My views are heavily influenced by my experiences in the field of social and personality psychology, and may not apply to other fields with very different norms. I do not have empirical evidence to back up most of these opinions, and I have refrained from adding "in my opinion" to the end of every sentence, but this chapter should be read as a very subjective, editorialized piece.

For context, here is a brief excerpt from Tennant et al.'s (2017) description of the history of peer review:

> Peer review in forms that we would now recognize emerged in the early 19th century. [. . .] Peer evaluations evolved to become more about judgments of scientific integrity, but the intention of any such process was never for the purposes of gate-keeping (Csiszar, 2016). [. . .] The current system of formal peer review, and use of the term itself, only emerged in the mid-20th century [. . .] *Nature,* now considered a top journal, did not initiate any sort of peer review process until at least 1967, only becoming part of the formalized process in 1973. (nature.com/nature/history/timeline_1960s.html)

The Reality of Peer Review Versus The Perception of Peer Review

Many people, including experienced scientists, act as if passing peer review at a prestigious journal is a very reliable marker of quality. Findings that pass this test are often treated as worthy of dissemination to the broader public and of building on in future research. Authors whose papers repeatedly pass this test are treated as accomplished scientists deserving of jobs, awards, promotion, and so forth.

This veneration of papers that have survived peer review at prestigious journals would be warranted if acceptance at such journals was a highly valid signal of research quality. However, peer review is quite fallible (Tennant et al., 2017), and therefore many papers that are rejected could easily have been accepted, and virtually all papers that are accepted at selective journals could easily have been rejected. Moreover, given the sheer volume of manuscripts submitted to prestigious scientific journals, there is no way to give each paper—even each promising paper (excluding the obviously flawed submissions)—the detailed scrutiny it would need to warrant the value we place on the seal of peer review. A set of three, four, or even 10 scientists volunteering a few hours to scrutinize a paper will not always catch errors, even glaring ones. There are many examples of embarrassing errors that should really have been caught before appearing in print in prestigious journals. In other words, peer review is a filter, but it is a very coarse one, and papers that pass through this filter are probably not much different from the much larger pool of papers that just barely fail to do so.

Thus, the first problem I see with peer review is not so much a problem with peer review itself, but with the reputation that peer review has. There is no reason to think that peer review can catch all or even most of the flaws in research, yet many people turn off their critical-thinking faculties when consuming research that has been published in a prestigious journal. While I would not do away with peer review, I do sometimes worry that the veneer of credibility that it lends to scientific findings may do a lot of harm, and not enough good. However, we can honestly acknowledge and try to fix the problems with peer review, including considering radical reforms such as moving to post-publication–only peer review, and open review (i.e., publishing the content of all peer reviews). In any case, we must peer review peer review.

Many scientists are uncomfortable with drawing attention to flaws in science, worried that it will undermine the public's trust in science. But a major pillar of the public's trust in science is the idea that we call out our own mistakes, that we are self-correcting. Thus, I think that allowing peer review to continue to enjoy its undeserved (and, probably, unachievable) reputation may, in the long run, do more harm to the public's trust in science if they eventually realize that peer review is actually a quite coarse filter. Instead, we should raise the standards for peer review, and acknowledge that flawed papers routinely get published in prestigious journals. Neither of these changes are popular, because both involve more harsh criticism (of not-yet-published and published papers, respectively).

Tone and Civility in Peer Review: A Call for More Effective Negativity

I share the concern that science is driving out many bright and capable junior scholars, particularly those from underrepresented groups. However, my perception is that harsh criticism is not the main culprit here. In my opinion, the main drivers of people leaving science are likely to include abusive mentors; impossible expectations that are incompatible with work/life balance and detrimental to mental health; sexual harassment; a lack of respect for cultural, political, and so forth, differences; and incentives that are not aligned with knowledge accumulation. My hypothesis is that when students decide to go into science, they understand and expect that their peers will point out when they are wrong, and won't always sugar coat their criticism. But they likely also expect that their work will be evaluated on its own merit, that stronger methods and more accurate interpretations will be valued over flashy but weak studies, and that they will be treated with respect, at least comporting to the standards of employment law.

All this is to say that when I call for more criticism during and after peer review, I am not dismissing concerns about creating an unwelcoming environment for junior scholars. I am saying that junior scholars can handle scientific criticism, and that our efforts at creating a more inclusive environment would be better spent elsewhere. Some of these bigger problems (harassment, abuse) sometimes occur within the context of peer review, and when they do they should not be tolerated. The extent to which this happens within the peer-review process seems to differ across fields (I've only ever seen one decision letter or review that crossed this line, out of the hundreds of decisions I've seen).

Isn't peer review already almost entirely negative? Yes, I suspect so—most reviews and decision letters focus on what is wrong or could be improved, which is as it should be (with some attention given to the strengths, as well). However, the focus of the criticism, at least in my field, is often misplaced. Reviewers and editors often point out that a manuscript's findings are not novel enough, do not fundamentally change the way we think about the topic. In other words, the criticisms are often that a paper is too boring, rather than placing more emphasis on whether the methods are solid and the findings are true and interpreted correctly. The degree to which the research question is interesting should of course play a role in evaluating a manuscript, but in many sciences today, there is too much emphasis on this, and not enough on rigor. If we have gotten to the point where we've weeded out most of the papers that are not rigorous, then we can and should use interestingness to select among the remaining submissions. But if we don't apply the rigor filter and select mainly on interestingness, that is a recipe for false positives (because most true claims are not as interesting as false claims).

Moreover, reviewers and editors sometimes do worse than ignoring rigor; they sometimes undermine it. For example, it is not uncommon for reviewers or editors to ask authors to reframe their predictions to anticipate the observed effect, even if the authors clearly state that they did not predict those results (i.e., "hypothesizing after the results are known," or HARKING; Kerr, 1998). Or, they may ask authors to reanalyze their data to see if they can bring a nonsignificant result in line with the others (i.e., p-hacking; Simmons et al., 2011). These are technically negative or critical comments, but they do not point out errors or improve the accuracy of the paper. All criticism is not created equal.

More generally, peer review too often takes the tone of "if I were an author on this paper, here's what I would have done" rather than evaluating the paper that was actually submitted and focusing on the fundamental strengths and flaws. Reviewers and editors should give priority to more objective dimensions of evaluation, and should resist the temptation to impose their subjective tastes and preferences on authors.

The more objective dimensions of evaluation are the dimensions we train undergraduate students in: those related to the basic validities (in psychology: construct, internal, external, and statistical). Many of the errors that peer review misses that lead to embarrassing post-publication critiques fall into one of these categories. The main focus of the replicability-related criticism has been on statistical validity (e.g., violations of the rules of null hypothesis significance testing), but the other three are long overdue for greater attention (e.g., Henrich et al., 2010). These are more important than whether the aesthetics of a paper are pleasing to the reviewers and editor. If a journal publishes boring papers on a regular basis, not much harm is done. But if a journal consistently publishes papers that lack one of these kinds of validity, those errors either persist in the scientific record or a great deal of energy needs to be expended to correct them (more on that later in the chapter). The most important task of peer review is to evaluate threats to validity and assess their magnitude, and interestingness should be secondary to this concern.

Peer review should have a negativity bias—and it does. But the focus of that negativity needs to change. In some ways, shifting the focus of peer review to emphasize validity and rigor more, and subjective dimensions like interestingness less, may actually lead to less overall negativity—it's easier for authors to anticipate what reviewers and editors will consider high versus low in validity than it is for authors to anticipate what reviewers and editors will find interesting. Thus, if peer review focuses mainly on validity, authors may start routinely meeting reviewers' and editors' expectations, leading to more positive reviews overall.

Status Bias

There is one category of papers that I suspect are not scrutinized nearly as harshly as others: papers authored by eminent scientists. There are a fair number of papers on status bias, and the evidence for this in reviews of manuscripts, conference submissions, and grants (e.g., Bravo et al., 2018; Le Goues et al., 2018; Tomkins et al., 2017) is convincing to me. Moreover, my own experiences have convinced me that status bias is a serious threat to the integrity of science, for two reasons. First, status bias leads to more false papers in the literature, which threatens the validity of science. Second, status bias violates the norm of universalism—the idea that scientific claims should be judged on their own merits and not based on who made them and what their status is (Merton, 1942/1973). One of the distinguishing features of science is that, in science, you can speak truth to power and if you're right, people will listen. That's the idea, anyway. If we compromise on that, we are at risk of losing what makes science different from pseudoscience, religion, politics, and so forth.

Status bias is hard to detect because it can be subtle and unintentional. The main reason I believe it exists is that I was engaging in it without realizing it. When I became an editor, I was not conscious of having any preference for papers with eminent authors. I rejected plenty of papers by famous authors (and once had an editor in chief ask me to reconsider, explicitly because the authors were famous people at a prestigious institution). I was pretty proud of my willingness to upset people if that was the price of making what I thought was the correct and fair editorial decision.

After having edited for a while, however, I decided to try something different (described in Vazire, 2016). I decided to first read each submission without knowing who the authors were or what institution they were at, and to decide whether to send the paper out for review or "desk reject" it before unblinding myself. Part of my reason for doing this was that I was finding it awkward to go to conferences, meet new people and sometimes hang out with them, and then receive their manuscripts a few days later. I thought it would be a lot more pleasant for me to make that initial decision without knowing who the authors were. It turns out it was actually very unpleasant, but in a good way.

Making a decision about whether to reject a manuscript without review, or send it out for review, without knowing who the authors are can be nerve-wracking. Even though I didn't think I was using information about the authors' identities to make decisions, making the decision without that information felt completely different. After I've written the desk rejection letter, but before I send it, I look at who the authors are (to make sure I don't have a conflict of interest), and sometimes I change some of the content (but never the ultimate decision) in the letter to acknowledge some of the authors' past work. The feeling of anxiety I have when I finally see the authors' names is how I know that I am influenced by status. If I've written a pretty harsh decision letter (with some hopefully helpful suggestions), my gut clenches a little if a famous person's name turns out to be on the paper. When I've decided not to reject a paper and I think it's an exceptionally good paper, I find myself being pleasantly surprised when it's by people I've never heard of at an institution I didn't know about. I'm not proud of these reactions. The fact that I have these reactions is part of the reason I'm convinced that status bias is a big problem.

When I talk to other editors, they frequently claim that they don't let the authors' identities influence their decisions. The editor in chief of *Nature*, in response to my question about why they don't keep authors' identities blind to reviewers, told me that he's not worried because they instruct reviewers not to let the authors' identities influence them. If that was all it took to eliminate bias, the world would be a much different place. When I hear these claims, my answer is always the same: Try blinding yourself and see if it feels different. I've yet to have anyone tell me that they tried it and didn't notice a difference (though to be honest, this is because I've yet to have someone take me up on the suggestion to try it).

There is no easy solution to the problem of status bias. Blinding editors and reviewers to authors' identities helps, and while complicated, such a system could in principle be developed (e.g., by using ORCID and having researchers upload a list of people with whom they have conflicts of interest to their ORCID profile). Indeed, the *American Political Science Review* has found a way to keep handling editors blind to authors' identities, so it is possible. I am in favor of blinding, and the best argument I've heard against it is that it doesn't always work (reviewers can sometimes guess who the authors are). That's certainly a reason to keep searching for a better solution, but it's not a reason not to have blind review in the meantime. The effectiveness of blinding will decrease as preprints become more common, so we should hurry up and think of other ways to curb status bias. Given how strong I think this bias is in virtually every human, it's going to be a big challenge.

Impact Bias

Sometimes, status bias is conscious and intentional. This is a result of journals inviting submissions—or being especially welcoming of submissions—from eminent authors in order to boost their profile.

For many journal editors and publication boards, one major aim of a journal is to publish impactful work. Impact is traditionally measured with the Journal Impact Factor (IF). The 2-year IF tells you, roughly, how many times papers published in a 2-year span (e.g., 2016–2017) were cited in the following year (2018), on average (the exact formula is not public). Journals and editors are frequently evaluated on this metric. This is not completely inappropriate given that many important decisions are influenced by IFs (e.g., whom to hire, promote, or recognize with an award, which papers to read and trust), so a journal that has a low IF may drop in popularity and may even be at risk of folding, for example if authors stop submitting there, or if their subscriptions drop too much. Unfortunately, it makes sense that journals care about their IFs, and try to keep IFs up, given the world we live in.

It makes sense, but it presents a big problem. Officially (according to guidelines published by the Committee on Publication Ethics), editors should not be motivated by finances or popularity—if their decisions are sound and fair, they should be prepared to let the chips fall where they may. The financial well-being of the journal should be looked after by a separate body that does not influence the editors of the journal. However, in reality, journal editors know that they will be evaluated, at least by some, according to the IF of the journal, and more generally according to how much positive attention the journal gets.

If impact and attention were strongly correlated with the quality of the studies published, this would not be a problem. But of course there are other factors that influence these outcomes, for example the eminence of the authors and the catchiness of the results. It seems inevitable that papers by eminent authors, and papers reporting especially eye-catching results, will get more attention. If those papers have serious flaws, perhaps that attention will backfire, but if they are mediocre or better, this will likely be a net plus for the journal's IF and reputation. Thus, unless an editor is preternaturally immune to popularity and praise, they will experience some temptation to have a lower threshold for publishing papers by eminent authors, and papers making sensational claims.

This bias for actively favoring papers that are likely to have greater impact, at the expense of quality, is often explicit. Some journals solicit (or "commission") submissions from particular authors, and those that do typically target famous authors, in part because publishing papers by those authors will raise the profile of the journal. Moreover, it is not uncommon for rejection letters to mention no justification for the rejection decision other than that the paper is not groundbreaking enough, not transformative enough, and so forth to meet the high standards of the journal. Perhaps this is just a convenient template for form decision letters, but if some rejections are actually based exclusively on this criterion (without regard for the rigor of the research), we are straying away from scientific publishing and moving into the world of entertainment. It can be very hard to tell whether a paper was rejected merely because the editor felt that it would hurt the journal's IF versus whether the editor genuinely believed that the topic is not interesting or worthy of study, but I suspect more than a few decisions are made on the basis of the former reason alone.

How Can We Make Peer Review Better?

There are plenty of essays on what criteria editors and reviewers should use to improve the quality of peer review (e.g., Vazire, 2017) though ironically, many of my favorite sources on this are not peer reviewed (e.g., Simmons, 2016). Instead of going into the specifics of what reviewers and editors should be doing as individuals, I will take a step back and ask: How can we change the system so that journals and editors prioritize scientific quality over all else?

Currently, the incentives that influence people who run journals (editors, publishers, professional societies, and publication committees) reward journals that maximize their reputation, which typically amounts to publishing high-impact papers by eminent authors on hot topics. There is little pressure on journals to aim to get it right above all else—it's unlikely journals will take the steps necessary to publish more true papers if that means taking a hit to the journal's IF or reputation/prestige. Thus, the key to incentivizing journals to get the science right is to make a journal's reputation heavily dependent on getting it right. This will likely require decoupling a journal's reputation from its IF, because citations are unlikely to ever become a strong signal of quality. In addition, it will require imposing costs and benefits for publishing papers with low versus high scientific validity.

As things stand now, if a journal is publishing many papers with false claims, there is little chance that this will be found out. Why do I believe this? Although it is easy to think of individual cases in which errors were detected in individual papers, testing whether a *journal* systematically publishes deeply flawed papers is a much more daunting task. This would require subjecting a large sample of a journal's published papers to intensive scrutiny (e.g., attempting to reproduce and/or replicate the studies, checking the validity of the measures and manipulations, conducting generalizability tests if generalizability claims were made). There is no group dedicated to this task, very little money available to support it, and virtually no glory to be had from conducting it, regardless of the outcome. The Reproducibility Project: Psychology (RP:P; Open Science Collaboration, 2015) is one of the few examples of such a coordinated effort to audit a few journals, and even that project targeted only three journals, and only 1 year's worth of issues. Moreover, there are many reasons (some good and some not so good) to be skeptical of the results of this project, and I am not aware of the three targeted journals openly acknowledging that the results motivated them to make changes to their peer-review practices. This raises the question: What would it take for journals to feel accountable for the validity of their published papers?

Perhaps one answer is more replication projects. Perhaps the RP:P wasn't enough, and if more journals were subjected to similar audits, this could shift the incentives. Moreover, the mere anticipation of frequent replication projects aimed at assessing the reproducibility of an entire journal could also have spillover effects on other journals not targeted. Certainly, if there was a credible threat of having something like the RP:P conducted on a randomly selected journal in a given subdiscipline, all of the journals in that group would likely start thinking a bit more seriously about reproducibility. The main drawback to this approach is that the effort required to do even one such project per year is exorbitant, and it is not clear that even a substantial increase in direct replications would have much impact if other aspects of the incentive structure do not change (Smaldino & McElreath, 2016).

What are some cheaper ways of holding journals accountable? One approach that is growing in popularity is open post-publication peer review. This can come in many forms, and typically entails posting criticisms (or praise) of specific papers online. This type of criticism can be very effective for correcting individual papers, but I have rarely seen it systematically applied to journals (cf., Lakens, 2018; Schimmack, 2017). While it is probably fair to hold authors more accountable for errors in individual papers, a pattern of publishing many papers with major errors should also reflect on the journal and its editors. Yet I rarely see journals or editors called out.

I suspect there are several reasons for this. One is that it is hard to tell whether there is a pattern without systematically looking for one. We are susceptible to memory biases, and our subjective impression that a journal has a good or a bad track record may not be very trustworthy. This brings us back to the problem of the resources and time necessary to conduct a thorough audit of a large enough sample of a journal's published articles. New tools are emerging to do this, but they often test a relatively narrow aspect of validity (e.g., GRIM [Brown & Heathers, 2017] and statcheck [Epskamp & Nuijten, 2016]) and are sometimes quite time intensive anyway (e.g., p-curve; Simonsohn et al., 2014).

Another reason I suspect journals and editors are rarely called out, even when a published paper is found to have serious errors that should have been caught during peer review, is that editors are treated with an excessive amount of respect. One thing I had not anticipated when I became an editor (though it seems naive in hindsight) is how rarely I would be criticized. It is not easy for scientists to call out journals, because they often rely on getting published in those journals for their own career advancement. Moreover, there are strong norms to assume editors are benevolent, fair, and hyper-competent. Even if all of that were true (it's not), it's unhealthy for science if scientists don't feel comfortable calling out suboptimal practices among journals and editors.

Again, criticism is distinct from harassment or abuse, and I'm not advocating for unscientific attacks on editors, of course. But it should be acceptable and common for scientists (and non-scientists, when they are capable) to publicly point out errors, and patterns of errors, in journals, and to put some of the blame on the journals/editors. In the years I've been editor, this has happened to me only three times, and all three times I learned something and adjusted my approach to editing. Not only is this kind of feedback immediately useful, but it also conveys to journals and editors that the scientific community values journals that are careful and minimize the number of unforced errors they publish. This can have an influence on the longer-term trajectory of the journal—with enough such pressure, it is more likely that the publication board of the journal will select future editors who prioritize getting it right, and the journal may implement policies that minimize such errors.

Conclusion

I have highlighted a number of threats to the integrity of peer review. These are not necessarily the biggest threats, but threats that I feel have not gotten the attention they deserve, and ones that I underestimated before I had seen peer review from both sides. A common theme among many of these problems is that editors and reviewers sometimes place too much emphasis on values that are not at the core of scientific rigor. Scientific journals serve many functions, but they are ultimately the place where we keep our primary scientific records, and they are treated by scientists and the rest of society as superior to other, unvetted records. If we are going to put peer-reviewed articles on a pedestal, we had better make sure that we do what we can to ensure the scientific validity of the findings published there. Alternatively, I am increasingly in favor of separating publication from peer review, and conducting all peer review after publication, in an open forum where everyone can see the content of the reviews (but not necessarily the identity of the reviewers).

We should also cultivate a culture of organized skepticism (another of Merton's scientific norms) about peer review and journals/editors. This means protecting the people who have the courage to raise concerns about journal and editor practices, and making sure their criticism is recognized as an important part of what makes science self-correcting.

Author Note

This chapter title is similar to a section of Tennant et al.'s (2017) paper. I came up with the title before reading their paper. It's also a relatively unoriginal title, so I suspect it has been used in many other places as well.

References

Bravo, G., Farjam, M., Moreno, F. G., Birukou, A., & Squazzoni, F. (2018). Hidden connections: Network effects on editorial decisions in four computer science journals. *Journal of Infometrics, 12*, 101–112.

Brown, N. J. L, & Heathers, J. A. J. (2017). The GRIM test: A simple technique detects numerous anomalies in the reporting of results in psychology. *Social Psychological and Personality Science, 8*, 363–369.

Epskamp, S. & Nuijten, M. B. (2016). statcheck: Extract statistics from articles and recompute p values. http://CRAN.R-project.org/package=statcheck. (R package version 1.2.2)

Henrich, J., Heine, S. J., & Norenzayan, A. (2010). The weirdest people in the world? *Behavioral and Brain Science, 33*, 61–83.

Kerr, N. L. (1998). HARKing: Hypothesizing after the results are known. *Personality and Social Psychology Review, 2*, 196–217.

Lakens, D. (2018, March). *The Journal of Personality and Social Psychology*: The good, the bad, and the ugly. http://daniellakens.blogspot.com/2018/03/the-journal-of-personality-and-social.html

Le Goues, C., Brun, Y., Apel, S., Berger, E., Khurshid, S., & Smaragdakis, Y. (2018). Effectiveness of anonymization in double-blind review. *Communications of the ACM, 61*, 30–33.

Merton, R. K. (1942/1973). *The Sociology of Science: Theoretical and Empirical Investigations*. University of Chicago Press.
Open Science Collaboration. (2015). Estimating the reproducibility of psychological science. *Science, 349*(6251):aac4716.
Schimmack, U. (2017, March). 2016 replicability rankings of 103 psychology journals. https://replicationindex.wordpress.com/2017/03/01/3950/
Simmons, J. P. (2016, September). What I want our field to prioritize. http://datacolada.org/53/
Simmons, J. P., Nelson, L. D., & Simonsohn, U. (2011). False-positive psychology: Undisclosed flexibility in data collection and analysis allows presenting anything as significant. *Psychological Science, 22*, 1359–1366.
Simonsohn, U., Nelson, L. D., & Simmons, J. P. (2014). P-curve: A key to the file drawer. *Journal of Experimental Psychology: General, 143*, 534–547.
Smaldino, P. E., & McElreath, R. (2016). The natural selection of bad science. *Royal Society Open Science, 3*, 160384.
Tennant, J. P., Dugan, J. M., Graziotin, D., Jacques, D. C., Waldner, F., Mietchen, D., Elkhatib, Y., Collister, L. B., Pikas, C. K., Crick, T., Masuzzo, P., Caravaggi, A., Berg, D. R., Niemeyer, K. E., Ross-Hellauer, T., Mannheimer, S., Rigling, L., Katz, D. S., Greshake Tzovaras, B., . . . Colomb, J. (2017). A multi-disciplinary perspective on emergent and future innovations in peer review. *F1000Research, 6*, 1151. doi: 10.12688/f1000research.12037.1
Tomkins, A., Zhang, M. & Heavlin, W. D. (2017). Reviewer bias in single- versus double-blind peer review. *Proceedings of the National Academy of Science USA, 114*(48), 12708–12713.
Vazire, S. (2016, June). Don't you know who I am? http://sometimesimwrong.typepad.com/wrong/2016/06/dont-you-know-who-i-am.html
Vazire, S. (2017, June). What is rigor? http://sometimesimwrong.typepad.com/wrong/2017/06/whatisrigor.html

15
Impact and Influence of the Institutional Review Board

Protecting the Rights of Human Subjects in Scientific Experiments

Alison Dundes Renteln

Scientific integrity is of vital importance for the pursuit of knowledge. Without a serious commitment to validity in method and interpretation, public acceptance of research findings will be undermined. In the 21st century, highly publicized incidents of academic fraud have called into question the credibility of the research enterprise in general.[1] The startling example of fabrication of data by a prominent Dutch psychologist forced academics around the world to face the reality that scientific integrity could not be taken for granted and, indeed, that existing mechanisms for validating research were ineffective.[2] Numerous scandals led President Barack Obama to issue a memorandum calling for the U.S. Office of Science and Technology Policy to ensure "the highest level integrity in all aspects of the executive branch's involvement with scientific and technological processes."[3]

The need for greater attention to best practices in research, whether biomedical or behavioral studies, compels us to ask what approaches institutions should take to achieve compliance with domestic and international standards. As research is becoming more transnational in scope, the special challenges posed by these collaborations across borders deserves much more

---

[1] In behavioral sciences, an egregious case of cheating involved a doctoral student in political science, Michael J. LaCour, who falsified data about attitudes toward same-sex marriage (Carey & Belluck, 2015). The senior author asked that the journal *Science* retract the study (Carey, 2015).

[2] Prominent mentors failed to supervise their protégés, and they have sometimes committed academic fraud, occasionally with tragic results. See, e.g., Johnson (2014).

[3] White House (2009, March 9). Memorandum for the Heads of Executive Departments and Agencies on Scientific Integrity. The directive mandated each agency to protect science from political influence and take steps to guarantee broad principles of scientific integrity. The Union of Concerned Scientists called for steps to protect scientific integrity originally in 2004 and renewed the call in 2017.

attention (Carome, 2014). To address widely recognized problems in the research process, more and more world conferences on scientific integrity are being convened (Steneck et al., 2018).[4] There is an urgent need to find legitimate ways to protect scientific integrity and human subjects via policies that can be enforced (Annas, 2009).

In the chapter I consider the role of institutional review boards (IRBs), mainly in the United States.[5] I discuss their purpose, historical background, and criticisms to ascertain whether they are adequate to the task of safeguarding scientific integrity. As a vast literature on this subject exists, I highlight the most commonly mentioned concerns about IRBs. One of the main challenges is harmonizing research ethics standards in different countries. Finally, I will present a case study that illustrates this global problem in comparative public policy.

IRBs: Historical Background and Function

The historical record reflects a longstanding lack of concern for the welfare of individuals who have been forced to be subjects in medical and scientific experiments.[6] The infamous Nazi experiments on Jewish people in concentration camps shocked the conscience of the world (Barondess, 1996; Grodin & Annas, 1996). These included the notorious hypothermia studies, Mengele's studies of 1,500 twins, and other horrendous research carried out in the name of science.[7] In response to these atrocities, after World War II, the Nuremberg Code was drafted. It reflected a global consensus that researchers must obtain informed consent from human subjects in scientific experiments. It states that "the voluntary consent of the human subject is absolutely essential. This means that the person involved should have the legal capacity to give consent." Further, the notion was that such protection should

---

[4] The World Conferences on Research Integrity drafted the Singapore Statement in 2010 and the Montreal Statement in 2013.

[5] Relatively little scholarship exists on the success of IRBs in safeguarding the rights of human subjects. But see Chapters 2 and 5 in Schrag (2019).

[6] It is beyond the scope of this essay to provide a survey of all the unethical experiments undertaken. For selected historical examples, see, e.g., Anon. (1964).

[7] In the hypothermia experiments, Jewish concentration camp prisoners were exposed to extreme temperatures to find out if they could be revived after being frozen. This was designed to help the German forces dealing with cold. The twin experiments were gruesome and entailed the killing and dissection of young persons. For the most part the experiments did not yield results of any scientific value. Even if they had, though, some contend the data should not be used out of respect for the individuals who died during the experiments.

be guaranteed as a fundamental principle; this was subsequently enshrined in the United Nations International Covenant on Civil and Political Rights (ICCPR) in Article 7.[8]

Despite this development, many other research projects, after the horrendous Nazi experiments, also failed to consider the ethical implications of using people as guinea pigs.[9] Studies that violated human rights and created the impetus for the creation of research boards include the Tuskegee and Guatemala syphilis experiments (Edgar, 2000; Jones, 1981; Reverby, 2018), the Willowbrook experiments on children, radiation experiments on indigenous peoples and prisoners (Anon., 1998; Johnston, 2007), and others.

Not only has biomedical research been called into question, but behavioral studies have been closely scrutinized as well. The conventional wisdom in the United States has been that Stanley Milgram's shock experiments at Yale University,[10] and the trauma students experienced because of them,[11] whether they were subjects or confederates, exerted pressure on the U.S. government to impose new, more stringent requirements on those receiving federal funding.[12]

An in-depth study of the historical development of IRBs attributes their creation to the expansion of biomedical research after World War II (Schrag, 2010, p. 24). The public health law massively increased the budgets of the National Institutes of Health (NIH) and the Public Health Corporation. The 1953 opening of the NIH clinical center was the impetus behind the first

---

[8] International Covenant on Civil and Political Rights, Article 7: "No one shall be subjected to torture or to cruel, inhuman or degrading treatment or punishment. In particular, no one shall be subjected without his free consent to medical or scientific experimentation."

[9] Pasteur tried out his rabies vaccine on a child who was violently ill, even though this would now be considered as a violation of research ethics. For an interesting account, see Guerrini (2003), pp. 94–102.

[10] For an interpretation of the significance of Milgram's (1964) study, see Brown (1986), Chapter 1. For a reconsideration of Milgram's legacy that challenges the harsh critiques by Baumrind and others, see Nicholson (2011). Nicholson comments that Milgram never acknowledged "the full extent of the harm he had inflicted" from data he collected himself from participants (p. 11).

[11] Although not all agree they experienced "trauma," Milgram himself recognized the impact of the experiments. According to Nicholson (2011, p. 5), Milgram "took steps to minimize the physical and psychological impact of the extreme stress his experiment engendered" and in his publications emphasized that all participates were debriefed or "dehoaxed," as he put it. Most likely, some students were more affected by the experiences than others.

[12] Although debate continues about the precise effects Milgram's work had on participants, it appears Milgram downplayed the deleterious potential of his research in his published work, but in unpublished material he acknowledged his recognition of the ethical questions his studies raised. "In his published work, Milgram hid issues of power, sadism, and self-aggrandizement behind the Holocaust and the pose of disinterested science. However, Milgram's unpublished doubts concerning the ethics and meaning of research suggest that darker personal motivations were an important factor in the study" (Nicholson, 2011, p. 18).

U.S. federal policy for the protection of human subjects (Wichman, 2012, p. 53).

Research boards, made up of at least five scholars in various disciplines, are authorized to review a protocol for a study to determine if the research design meets federal guidelines. As regulations stipulate that the board consider the impact of research on the larger society, one member must come from the community to represent the interests of society at large (Allison et al., 2008). In the United States, research must follow the Federal Policy for the Protection of Human Subjects, or the Common Rule.[13] IRBs are mandated to employ a utilitarian approach, a cost/benefit analysis to ensure that the potential risks of involvement in the research project do not outweigh the benefits.[14] Ordinarily a majority of those present must approve the study. Some projects are deemed "exempt"—that is, not subject to regulation—if they involve minimal risk (Petrosino & Mello, 2014, p. 278).

The principles that IRBs employ in evaluating protocols for studies include well-established norms from global bioethics such as beneficence, respect for persons, and justice.[15] The U.S. federal law is based on the landmark Belmont Study, which provided a comprehensive investigation of research ethics (Wichman, 1998).

Inasmuch as IRBs were initially constructed to evaluate biomedical research, policies were not originally formulated with the particular concerns of social scientists in mind.[16] The rules themselves have been modified over the years, so their scope of application has varied. In 2017 the federal government's Department of Health and Human Services Office for Human Research Protections announced that it would propose a significant change in the application of the rules. The new policy would exempt studies involving "benign behavioral interventions" (Murphy, 2017). Some construed this proposed change as giving social scientists license to determine whether their studies would be harmful to human subjects. The changes came into effect in 2018.

Particularly troubling in the reasoning of IRBs is the presumption that a utilitarian calculus is necessarily the appropriate mode of analysis. In general, they weigh risks and balances to judge whether to authorize researchers to

---

[13] The so-called Common Rule was revised in 2017. It exempted certain types of research and added a few requirements. See Shrag (2019).
[14] For a brief description of the reasoning process, see Freeza (2018).
[15] For the classic work on these, see Beauchamp and Childress (2009).
[16] For historical background on how government funding reflected ideological influences, see Solovey (2013).

proceed. IRBs are advised to approve protocols as long as they do not entail more than minimal risk.[17] Even assuming that it is the appropriate way to judge research, it is hardly clear how best to weigh benefits and risks in a particular study to ascertain the likely magnitude of the actual harm likely to be involved.

Using the utilitarian calculus may not function well if risks are unknown and researchers have an incentive to downplay them (Manson & O'Neill, 2007). Moreover, the risks associated with participation in research may truly be unknown. When research threatens to violate fundamental human rights, even if risks do not appear to be looming on the horizon, some studies should not be permitted. To be clear, even if individuals appear to be informed and voluntarily give consent, some types of research simply should be prohibited as a matter of principle. According to this rights-based approach, some research should be rejected, even if it may have benefits for the community.[18]

How should one assess benefits to the community and the human subject? It is unclear whether the frame of reference should be within national borders, or the world as a whole. Indeed, one of the major challenges of the 21st century is the growing trend toward conducting cross-national research. This phenomenon of "outsourcing" data collection raises serious questions about whether it is feasible to enforce the same standards used in North America and Europe to studies carried out in other countries. Not only is there a dire need to harmonize differing national policies, but there also exist explicit rules in international instruments that must be followed.[19] For instance, the International Ethical Guidelines for Biomedical Research Involving Human Subjects state that "The investigator must obtain the voluntary, informed consent of the prospective subject [or legally authorized representative] . . . Waiver of informed consent is to be regarded as uncommon and exceptional, and must in all cases be approved by an ethical

---

[17] Reference to weighing risks and benefits is the main approach. When exemptions are granted based on a conclusion that a protocol involves minimal risk, that implies use of this utilitarian calculus.

[18] It is beyond the scope of this paper to consider the contentious debate about whether data collected via unethical research, when of potential scientific value, should be used.

[19] After the Nuremberg Code, the Declaration of Helsinki was adopted, which incorporated principles to protect human subjects. Subsequently, in 1982, Council for International Organizations of Medical Sciences (ICIOMs), in collaboration with the World Health Organization, promulgated another instrument geared to "developing" countries; some, e.g., and Lomax (1997), consider this "paternalistic." It was revised in 2017.

review committee." Nascent research boards abroad may not have the same experience, nor do they necessarily interpret the international standards similarly.[20]

Criticisms

IRBs have been criticized on a number of grounds. In what follows, I highlight some of the most common concerns about their enforcement of policies.

Overzealousness and "Overreach"

Research on IRBs has shown dissatisfaction with aspects of the review process deemed overly cumbersome (Ceci et al., 1985, p. 996). Considerable resistance to IRBs stems from the perception that board members are "overzealous" in their enforcement of research standards; they seem more like a police force than a research board (Rosnow et al., 1993, p. 821). Much of the literature reflects a sense that these boards engage in censorship, thwarting serious efforts to undertake important studies (Bledsoe et al., 2007; Hamburger, 2004). By contrast, others contend that IRBs have proven to be too weak to enforce research standards, partly because they do not monitor the process of conducting research (Elliott, 2015).

Scope of Authority

That no consensus exists on the scope of authority of IRBs remains a significant problem. Generally, IRBs are not supposed to reject research on the basis of the content because their mandate is to protect human subjects from risk that outweighs the benefit.[21] While the review of biomedical and behavioral studies falls under the purview of IRBs, whether IRBs should also scrutinize research in the humanities and some branches of the social sciences has proven more controversial.

---

[20] For a compilation of national boards and regulations across the globe, see Office of Human Subjects Research Protection (2019).
[21] Some think that the time wasted in a worthless study should count for something and be a factor considered in the IRB approval process.

In the late 20th century, some questioned whether oral histories, journalism, and ethnographic work should be subject to review.[22] With respect to participant observation in anthropology and sociology, for instance, it may not be feasible to obtain informed consent, as it is with other methodologies (Lederman, 2009). While some argue that these types of social science should not be covered by IRB regulations, others on IRBs maintain that this research should receive scrutiny because of genuine concern about the privacy rights of subjects.[23] Although some types of research were made exempt from IRBs[24] (though researchers must still apply to request exemptions), the issue persists, as with, for instance, how to obtain informed consent in studies involving big data. The new U.S. rule mandated that a single IRB oversee multisite research. This has significant implications for conducting transnational research.

Defining and Assessing Risk

Another serious criticism is the inevitable existence of multiple interpretations of rules governing research (Henry et al., 2016; White, 2007). Partly this is a consequence of vagueness in the standards that IRBs are expected to apply to the evaluation of research protocols. Inasmuch as IRBs are expected to interpret what line of research involves "minimal risk," this leads to differing interpretations. While this is unavoidable to some extent, it gives the impression that IRBs may be arbitrary and capricious because institutions vary as to what they permit (Stark, 2014).

Bias

IRBs also face the challenge that their assessment reflects bias. Since their inception, IRBS have been accused of political bias (Ceci et al., 1973). They have

---

[22] For a discussion of the debate about whether these types of inquiry constitute "research," see Meeker (2012). In 2017 the government revised its policy to exclude oral histories from IRB scrutiny beginning in 2018 (Flaherty, 2017).

[23] In 2003 the federal Office for Human Research Protections issued a letter to the American Historical Association and the Oral History Association saying that oral history interviews need not be regulated by IRBs. Some historians hoped this would influence IRBs across the United States. For more, see Brainard (2003).

[24] Nichols et al. (2017).

also been charged with the more specific criticism of gender bias on the basis of their treatment of protocols involving reproductive health issues (Barnes & Munsch, 2015). The tendency of IRB regulations to reinforce hegemony is part of the critique. Consequently, feminist scholars have expressed concern with IRB regulations for imposing strict hierarchical power relations between IRB committees and researchers, and between researchers and human subjects (Barnes & Munsch, 2015, pp. 597–598). IRBs are accused of "perpetuating historically masculine epistemologies" and "inequality" (Barnes & Munsch, 2015, p. 598). Research demonstrates that IRBs in the United States have treated male and female researchers differently, particularly in evaluating gender-related projects such as infertility studies and gender identity surveys.[25]

An ethnographic study of IRB review noted that board members judged the quality of research protocols based on the character of researchers. This is problematic because it "accentuate[s] *ad hominem* biases in the review process" (Stark, 2014, pp. 181–182). A failure of IRB assessment is also the possibility that IRB members lack sufficient breadth in their knowledge of various types of methodologies.

Handling Deception in Research

Another problematic feature of IRB decision-making is how best to address research that involves deception. Some psychological studies require that human subjects not know the real reason for the research project. This premise means it is not possible for them to give truly informed consent. To handle this matter, IRBs often have asked researchers to "debrief" subjects after the conclusion of the study. When, however, the project is longitudinal, this renders such a compromise approach impractical. If the study depends on subjects not being aware of the true purpose of the research, debriefing while the study is ongoing would undermine the project. Debriefing can only occur at the conclusion of what may be multiple-year data collection. This means the potential damage caused by deception can be intensified because of its duration.

---

[25] In their provocative analysis, Barnes and Munsh note the dearth of scholarship on the efficacy of IRB protection. They rely on data available from IRB committees (p. 601).

Vulnerable Populations and Informed Consent

In reality, the primary concern of IRBs is to protect human subjects, particularly those belonging to vulnerable communities. This includes children, especially if institutionalized; pregnant women; active-duty military personnel; prisoners; individuals with intellectual and developmental disabilities; individuals at an educational or economic disadvantage; and indigenous peoples.[26] Given the controversies raging over research of this kind, views differ as to whether it should be entirely prohibited, allowed unconditionally, or partially permitted (Beauchamp & Childress, 2009, p. 90). As mentioned earlier, there is cause for alarm when individuals are not informed about the nature of the research or are coerced into participation in studies because of the long history of abuse in human experimentation. As one scholar puts it succinctly: "Throughout history, it has been marginalized people in society, including racial minorities, prisoners, and slaves, who have been most experimented on. These experiments attracted little criticism within 'educated' society of prevailing attitudes" (MacNeill, 2009, p. 4710; Moreno, 2001, pp. 29–36, 226–228).

Many of the researchers in the infamous studies showed utter disregard for the requirement that they obtain informed consent from participants in their experiments. For instance, the U.S. government funded research in Tuskegee, Alabama, and abroad in Guatemala (McNeil, 2010; Reverby, 2018) that followed individuals infected with syphilis who were left untreated for years, even when an effective cure was known to exist. To study the long-term effects of the disease, scientists at the Tuskegee Institute misled African American men in Macon County, Alabama, about the purpose of the research. The men did not know that they were receiving only aspirin, even after penicillin was readily available. After this came to light, because a journalist published an article about it, the Tuskegee experiments became known as one of the most notorious violations of the rights of individuals as human subjects in the U.S. history. It was the longest-running such experiment, lasting over three decades from the 1930s to 1972. Critics acknowledge that the data had medical value and helped develop "more reliable tests for syphilis (Duke, 2013, p. 116; Washington, 2006, pp. 117–118). President Bill Clinton offered an apology May 17, 1997, 25 years after the study was

---

[26] The Havasupai tribe in Arizona sued Arizona State University for taking hundreds of blood samples without obtaining informed consent. The lawsuit alleged failure of the university's IRB and cost the university almost $2 million (Harmon, 2010). See also Couzin-Frankel (2010).

publicly acknowledged (McNeil, 2010; Reverby, 2018, p. 38). Speaking before the eight men who were still alive, Clinton said that the shameful study "diminished the state of men by abandoning the most basic ethical principles." Paltry reparations were paid to those still alive, but only survivors of the experiments and not their relatives.[27]

It is noteworthy that many of the most egregious violations of the human rights of participants in research experiments have involved persons of color, often indigent ones. Indeed, Tuskegee has become a metaphor for historic injustices against African Americans (Reverby, 2018).[28] The furor over the extraordinarily cruel violation of human rights also created the impetus for new laws to protect human subjects (McNeil, 2010).

What transpired in the Tuskegee experiments is entirely unacceptable because it violates the basic principle that human subjects should give informed consent. The deception used was entirely incompatible with the principle of autonomy—that is, that individuals should decide whether to participate in research.

Children with Intellectual Disabilities

Children pose a different problem. The presumption is usually that those held in institutions are unable to give informed consent because the institutional setting induces them to agree to participate in research, even if it is actually not in their self-interest to do so. Much ink has been spilled on the matter of informed consent in these particularly coercive contexts. Furthermore, as the Nuremberg Code stipulates that voluntary consent must be given by those with legal capacity, it is unclear whether children should ever participate in experiments.

In some instances parents may give proxy consent to have their children participate in non-therapeutic research (McCormick, 1974). Whether the bioethics standards permit or require this is open to debate (Bartholome, 1976; Ramsey, 1976). Often children have been part of biomedical and behavioral science experiments while living in institutions.

---

[27] Debate about reparations continues as the heirs have requested that they receive what is left in the settlement fund; see Associated Press (2017).
[28] Reverby (2018).

One of the most infamous examples of parents consenting to the participation of their children in studies with no benefit to them is the sinister Willowbrook School case. Over a few decades in the mid-20th century, several thousand children institutionalized there were deliberately given hepatitis to study its effects. These studies were conducted after two prominent scholars, NYU Chair of Pediatrics Dr. Saul Krugman and Dr. Robert Ward, who joined the staff at Willowbrook in 1955. Krugman published papers based on the research and later won accolades based on the data gathered, including the Lasker Prize.[29]

While these scientists conducted experiments that are blatantly unethical by standards past and present, the parents were also complicit. They ostensibly agreed to have children be part of studies in order to have them housed there. Willowbrook actually came to be known as a "dumping ground" for these children.[30] Insofar as parents may not always have the best interests of their children at heart, proxy consent should be viewed with skepticism.

In the 1980s, after a national television program exposed the brutal abuses and dilapidated conditions in Willowbrook, plaintiffs filed a class action. After protracted litigation, they prevailed in *New York State Association for Retarded Children v. Carey* (1975); the school was closed and they received substantial compensation. This research had virtually no scientific benefit and offered no therapeutic benefit to the children. The lawsuit mobilized advocates to sponsor legislation to protect children with disabilities.

In another disturbing case, MIT researchers conducted research on the absorption of calcium in children with disabilities at the Fernald School in Waltham, Massachusetts. They gave the youngsters milk containing radiation. The parents were not informed that their children would be ingesting radiation, as the consent form only requested permission to have them participate in nutritional studies.

The failure to adhere to informed consent requirements is also evident abroad in the treatment of children in clinical trials conducted by U.S. pharmaceutical companies in Africa. In 2000 the *Washington Post* published a sensational story about a 1996 medical experiment in Kano, Nigeria (Annas, 2009). Two hundred children in Nigeria were used in experiments to test Trovan, an antibiotic drug for bacterial meningitis, and also ceftriaxone.

---

[29] Krugman (1986) continued to insist that his research was ethical.
[30] Goode et al. (2013) mention that the Willowbrook facility had become so notorious as a dumping ground for unwanted children that "children were even left in public places with signs on them saying 'Take Me to Willowbrook.'"

Their families consented to the treatment but were not told that a successful therapy existed. Several children died during the clinical trials—five from Trovan and six from taking a substantially reduced dose of ceftriaxone (compared to what the U.S. Food and Drug Administration recommended). Other children suffered "brain damage, paralysis or slurred speech (Smith, 2010). When the egregious nature of the research came to light, it sparked controversy and revived discussion about the ethics of outsourcing research. Why had Pfizer chosen to conduct the clinical trials in Nigeria if not to circumvent global bioethics standards?[31]

Families of the affected children sued Pfizer, the world's largest pharmaceutical company, in U.S. federal courts under the Alien Tort Claims Act. Although the district court dismissed the case for lack of subject matter jurisdiction, the U.S. Court of Appeals for the Second Circuit ruled in *Abdullahi v. Pfizer* (2009) that a foreign citizen may bring an action for a tort committed outside the United States involving a violation of that customary law norm that medical experiments may not be performed without obtaining informed consent. Reaffirming this global norm was an important victory.

The state of Kano and the federal government of Nigeria also brought suit against Pfizer. Although the entire litigation continued for 15 years, the parties eventually agreed to a settlement of $75 million. In late 2014 Pfizer paid compensation to the victims of the 1996 Trovan clinical trial in accordance with the 2009 settlement agreement. Payments were $175,000 to each family (Smith, 2011) and a fund of $35 million was created to compensate those affected. Pfizer also agreed to finance community health projects.

Those in Detention and Prisons

Of special concern here is the treatment of those who are detained by the state because they are out of sight and frequently subject to the most dehumanizing conditions. I turn now to the question of how IRBs address studies in which those in jail or prison are sought as subjects for research

---

[31] Why is it attractive for researchers to engage in "scientific tourism"? Drug companies conduct clinical trials abroad because it is more economical for them to do so (profit motive). They can circumvent the policies that exist in the country where they are based. There will be fewer drug interactions because people in "developing" countries cannot afford other medications. They do not have the same worries that they will be under IRB scrutiny. By carrying out clinical trials in other countries, they can avoid dealing with regulatory agencies. It is easier to recruit subjects because fewer incentives need to be provided.

(Gostin et al., 2007). This discussion shows how dangerous this research can be for the incarcerated.

Those in total institutions are among those most likely to be abused.[32] Not only are they out of the public eye, but they seldom have the means to challenge policies applied to them. In short, they lack access to justice because of resources and because the state prevents advocates from meeting with them. Prisoners have been brutalized in numerous ways; indeed, human rights advocates usually measure the humanity of a country by the treatment of inmates in its penitentiaries.[33] Furthermore, mass incarceration of individuals has increased dramatically, putting more and more individuals at risk for coercion, including pressure to participate in experiments (Alexander, 2010; Simon, 2014).

While domestic and international standards clearly guarantee prisoners' rights, the question is how they apply to their status as human subjects in scientific research. The Eighth Amendment to the U.S. Constitution protects prisoners from cruel and unusual punishment, yet it is unclear whether participation in experiments should necessarily be deemed a constitutionally proscribed form of punishment. What if prisoners wish to participate as part of rehabilitation and giving back to society?[34] Some maintain, based on U.S. constitutional law, that it would be unreasonable to have an absolute prohibition on research in prison, especially if the study offered a potential therapeutic benefit to the incarcerated. The American Bar Association Rules on Standards for Treatment of Prisoners, adopted in 2010, allow for the possibility that prisoners may be part of experiments.[35]

The formulation in international law is broader in scope as it prohibits cruel, inhuman, or degrading treatment or punishment, including experimentation. As mentioned earlier, Article 7 of the ICCPR specifically provides: "No one shall be subjected without his free consent to medical or

---

[32] For classics, see Goffman (1968) and Foucault (1979).

[33] See reports of the United Nations Special Rapporteurs on Torture or Cruel, Inhuman or Degrading Treatment of Punishment (http://www.ohchr.org/EN/Issues/Torture/SRTorture/Pages/SRTortureIndex.aspx).

[34] This issue emerged in the context of a debate over a proposed study about the effects of sodium in the diets of prisoners. Although Ruth Macklin notes that "Prisons are an inherently coercive environment"... that doesn't mean informed consent is impossible. She says some prisoners want to give back to society. (Kolata, 2018).

[35] The American Bar Association adopted Standard Rules; see Standard 23-7.11, "Prisoners as subjects of behavioral or biomedical research." Researchers claim prisoners do not object or feel exploited (Christopher et al., 2017). Of course, they are in prison (only one correctional facility) when answering questions for these studies as well.

scientific experimentation."[36] Some contend this clearly prohibits involuntary human experimentation (Rodley, 2009, p. 413). When prisoners are asked to "consent" to behavioral modification techniques, there is a tremendous potential for abuse "even where prisoners do consent. Where they do not, they are illegal under international law" (Rodley, 2009, p. 414).

The notion that inmates can "consent" is rather dubious. Experts convened by the International Association of Penal Law concluded that "the objective conditions of detention precluded the possibility" that a detained or imprisoned person could ever give "free consent" (Rodley, 2009, p. 414). Thus, medical experimentation on prisoners will almost always be construed as a violation of international human rights law.

Unfortunately, prisoners in the United States have often been used in many different types of experiments.[37] For instance, they were subjects in the notorious human radiation experiments for a decade, from 1963 to 1973 (Moreno, 2001, pp. 144–151). When the military expressed reservations about operating nuclear-powered airplanes because of their potential threat to male fertility, research was conducted to determine the effect of radiation on testicles. One hundred thirty-one prisoners in Oregon and Washington agreed to be part of experiments to evaluate the effects of radiation, funded by the Atomic Energy Commission. When this came to light, it forced review of the general proposition that prisoners could make "voluntary" decisions. The National Commission for the Protection of Human Subjects of Biomedical and Behavioral Research considered the matter in 1976,[38] and ultimately the commission recommended banning virtually all research on prisoners (Anon., 1998, p. 263). IRBs have approved very few of the studies undertaken in prisons (Gostin et al., 2007).

As a consequence of this policy of prohibition, scholars who wish to have prisoners as human subjects have been compelled to turn to other countries and engage in what might be called "scientific tourism."[39] This raises the question as to whether IRBs have or should have extraterritorial jurisdiction. Sometimes research committees may exist in places researchers wish

---

[36] In 1992 the Human Rights Committee issued a general comment interpreting Article 7. In paragraph 7 it emphasized the need to protect those under any form of detention or imprisonment.

[37] The NIH supported virus research on federal prisoners during the 1069s at the NIH clinical center in Bethesda, Maryland. More than 1,000 prisoners from 16 penitentiaries had been at the center to be part of the experiments (Stark, 2010). See also Hornblum (1998).

[38] For detailed discussion, see *The Human Radiation Experiments*, Chapter 9 "Prisoners: A Captive Research Population," pp. 263–283.

[39] The ban is not absolute because research that could benefit inmates (i.e., that is therapeutic) might be permitted.

to conduct their studies; in this situation, IRBs may be expected to defer to the judgment of research committees elsewhere. In other places, however, such committees may not yet have been established, in which case IRBs in the United States may have to impose their standards. This is increasingly likely with the 2018 shift to a single IRB scrutiny of multiple-site research. For universities lacking the capacity to manage large-scale research projects involving more than several sites, this is likely to lead to the use of independent for-profit IRBs (Craun, 2019).[40] It seems, generally speaking, that there is a lack of a global approach to solving this problem of bioethics. This poses a serious problem because of the increasing trend toward international research collaboration (Appelt et al., 2015).

Cross-Cultural Considerations

If international standards and U.S. federal policy stipulate that informed consent is necessary for research on human subjects, this means researchers and IRBs must demonstrate that studies conducted abroad are consistent with domestic and international requirements.[41] With the new requirement of a single IRB responsible for multiple-site research projects, this will necessitate more careful attention to compliance by those in charge of projects in other countries.

Admittedly, it may be difficult to ascertain whether human subjects across the globe acquiesce. Philosophers debate whether informed consent can be regarded as meaningful in "developing" countries (Aguila et al., 2015; Macklin, 2004). Some worry that language barriers preclude the possibility of obtaining it; in rural settings, an analog to this term may not exist or may be hard to identify. If the individuals are not literate, some fear it may be exceedingly difficult to ensure they have understood the protocol and potential risks of participation.

A researcher apparently encountered this type of cross-cultural barrier when conducting a study of a potential cure for breast cancer in Vietnam (Love & Fost, 1997), evidently because patients were not accustomed to

---

[40] USC has a memorandum of understanding the Western IRB.

[41] A vast literature exists on the subject of ethical issues associated with clinical trials in "developing" countries. Some questions whether it is ethical to use placebo-controlled studies in developing countries, as in Lurie and Wolfe (1997). It is beyond the scope of this essay to survey all the commentary, but see, e.g., Angell (1997) and Kass et al. (2003).

making decisions about their own health. In the literature the claim was that Vietnamese experts who were consulted stated that "application of American standards of informed consent would not be acceptable to Vietnamese physicians, political leaders in Vietnam, or the vast majority of Vietnamese patients" (Love & Frost, 1997, p. 424). The claim was that the paternalistic tradition was not to have patients participate in making health care decision. When the researcher asked the research committee at his American medical school to waive the informed consent requirement, after months of negotiation, they declined to do so, although they did modify the consent form, making it much less detailed (Luna & Macklin, 2009, pp. 460–461). In spite of these efforts, the researchers were unsure whether the women in the study understood the risks associated with the clinical trial (Luna & Macklin, 2008, p. 451). Although the women had the capacity to give consent, because of the failure to translate the relevant concepts properly, they lacked the information to make a decision. It remains unclear how to balance the desire to protect international standards with cultural sensitivity (Macklin, 2004, pp. 131–162). Luna and Macklin acknowledge the challenge:

> Cultural differences are challenging for research in the international arena and conducted in multicultural settings because of the tension between the ethical requirements of informed consent and the need to remain culturally sensitive, both of which are stated in international guidelines. (2008, p. 461).

Case Study: Study of Detainees in China

Researchers were interested in studying the anatomical structure of the brains of detainees accused of violent crimes who were awaiting trial and decided to conduct their research in China. The motivation for the study was to investigate whether there is a biological basis for or predisposition to homicide (Schug et al., 2011; Yang et al., 2010). Adrian Raine, a psychologist formerly at the University of Southern California (USC) and subsequently at the University of Pennsylvania, took the lead in this line of research.

Cross-national research of this sort must have raised a red flag for the IRB because of particular features of the Chinese legal system. First, the death penalty is imposed for over 100 different offenses, including white-collar crimes, and some contend that the presumption of innocence is not firmly established.[42] Second, if a defendant is convicted in China, execution occurs quickly, within a few weeks.[43] Third, inmates sometimes have their organs harvested before they gasp their last breath (Doffman, 2019). In view of the manner in which capital punishment is administered in China, it is reasonable for IRBs to be concerned about research that might influence the outcome of judicial decision-making. It is within the realm of possibility that brain scans of those accused of committing violent crimes, if they showed an "abnormality," could be used to win a conviction. The IRB could have legitimately been concerned about ensuring that the brain scans not be acquired by the prosecution and used to win a conviction.

In these circumstances, what is the proper role of the IRB in the United States? One possibility would be for the IRB to ask the researcher to conduct site visits to ensure that the scans are kept away from government officials. That might prove difficult inasmuch as U.S. researchers would not be given access to jails and prisons. Also, some might consider that excessive interference and suggest that the American researcher simply delegate monitoring to a Chinese colleague. If, however, the IRB permitted the researcher to entrust the colleague abroad with ensuring compliance with research ethics standards, this might conceivably put the university at risk for failure to enforce the law.

Even though the USC IRB withdrew its provisional approval of the study (Wagner, 2018), the researcher proceeded to complete the data collection and published the results with a statement that the USC IRB had approved it (Schug et al., 2011, p. 86). When it came to USC's attention that the scholar, by then at another university, had used the data and published it in a journal with a statement that the USC IRB had approved the protocol (when, in fact, it had not), university officials notified the editor of the journal (Craun, 2018). The editor responded that the journal would investigate the matter but responded only with an acknowledgment that the submitted materials had been received (Craun, 2019).

This case study reveals that recalcitrance on the part of some investigators may block efforts to ensure adherence to international human rights

---

[42] China is considered to be the country with the highest number of executions annually. Although this is treated as a state secret, it is estimated to be in the thousands, according to nongovernmental organizations such as Amnesty International and Reprieve. Discussion of the due-process aspects of the legal system can be found in Liang et al. (2016).

[43] The nongovernmental organization Dui Hua "determined that the average length of time a person sentenced to death waits until execution is two months" (https://duihua.org/resources/death-penalty-reform/).

standards and undermine compliance with bioethics rules designed to protect scientific integrity. If scholars and journals both ignore admonitions not to publish research not authorized by the IRB, it will be difficult to safeguard the validity of research processes. The defiant attitude on the part of researchers will likely undermine future efforts of IRBs to enforce standards.

Complicated issues will continue to arise when studies involve cross-national collaborations. This will necessitate more careful consideration of what is at stake in terms of human rights. Furthermore, given that the reputations of scholars and institutions are at stake, it seems advisable for IRBs not to sanction a "hands off" approach in this circumstance, despite the perception of research boards as "overzealous." Protection of the human rights of research subjects, particularly those who are members of vulnerable groups, may require that IRBs take a more proactive approach to cross-national research.

Recommendations

Research involving human subjects must continue to be evaluated carefully but in an expeditious manner. Those assessing protocols should have the appropriate expertise. If IRBs do not have members with this background, they should request expert opinions from ethicists. When dealing with multiple-site projects, the IRB should consult the appropriate research committee in the other countries. If such a research committee does not yet exist, then the researcher abroad should follow the requirements mandated by U.S. regulations and international law.

As human subjects research in other countries has become a matter of concern for the United Nations, initiatives are under way to develop effective means of ensuring compliance with global bioethics standards. A working group of the Council for International Organizations of Medical Sciences, set up by the World Health Organization (WHO) and UNESCO, began meeting in 2017 to formulate policies applicable to clinical trials in resource-limited settings. It would be ideal if this organization based on the WHO–UNESCO partnership resulted in the creation of a global research ethics board to handle disputes associated with transnational research projects. This body could establish panels of certified ethicists to review protocols that appear to jeopardize the rights of human subjects. It is conceivable that appeals could be made via an online system of dispute resolution comparable to that of the

World Intellectual Property Organization (WIPO) for appeals of domain name assignment by the Internet Corporation for the Assignment of Names and Numbers (ICANN). There appears to be a trend toward online dispute resolution (Katsh & Rabinovich-Einy, 2017).

World conferences on scientific integrity can also formulate new policies to pressure institutions to comply with rules and impose sanctions. By urging professional associations and learned societies can take the lead in promulgating stringent standards. Enforcement of the rules will necessitate the imposition of real sanctions. Researchers who fail to adhere to the requirement to provide informed consent could be fined, denied visas to travel to research sites, or prevented from joining prestigious professional organizations. Journals and presses that publish work that lacks proper certification could also be subject to sanctions.

With regard to prisoners specifically, the United Nations should also play a much more active role in monitoring penal institutions to guarantee the human rights of inmates by protecting them from human experimentation that constitutes an atrocity.[44] Unless there is an obvious therapeutic benefit from participation in an experiment, prisoner research should be almost entirely banned.

Ultimately, the only way to prevent scientific misconduct is to inculcate values that encourage the protection of international human rights standards. If we change the way people think about research so that the principles of respect for persons, non-maleficence, and justice are at the forefront, then it may be less necessary to insist upon obtaining informed consent. There would be less need to protect those in a weaker bargaining position.

So long as we must rely on obtaining informed consent, however, it will be crucial to modify the system to make it more effective. Neil Manson and Onora O'Neil, in *Rethinking Informed Consent in Bioethics* (2007), challenge the narrow view of the consent process as one merely conveying relevant information to human subjects.[45] In reframing the debate about the interpretation of what constitutes informed consent, they urge us to shift from conceiving of it as disclosure of information and rather as a decision-making process. They offer an imaginative way of strengthening the process of ensuring that individuals give informed consent that takes into

---

[44] Special rapporteurs attempt to gain access to penitentiaries, but states deny it. Members of the UN should be required to allow fact finding in prisons.

[45] For instance, it should be clear that individuals may refuse and renegotiate the consent (Luna, 2019, p. 626).

account different contexts; in some situations, they propose the use of a series of steps to ensure full understanding. Following this advice, the United Nations should mandate a global consent process that requires a series of conversations before individuals sign a written document in their own language. The consent form should be a short, clear document (Cressey, 2012).[46]

Interpreters, certified by the United Nations as fluent in the language of the prospective human subjects, should be present to answer any questions about the protocol. Although some, like Ruth Macklin (2004), assert that informed consent can be understood universally in substantive terms, that position ignores the reality that there may not be analogues in other belief systems and informed consent may be conceptualized differently in diverse cultural contexts (Grady, 2015; Sellos Simoes, 2010; Sprumont, 2015; Sullivan, 2017).[47] However, if this right to language is afforded protection, then this will increase the chances that human subjects will be informed and make an autonomous decision to participate or not.

The partnership between the WHO and UNESCO should lead to the creation of a research board that provides independent experts to evaluate experiments that may involve unusual techniques and members of vulnerable groups. Eventually this organization might consider setting up an online dispute settlement system modeled after the WIPO arbitration system to handle domain name appeals from ICANN.

When the system breaks down, organizations like Public Citizen and others should receive grants to provide annual reports documenting the behavior of universities and pharmaceutical companies known to have engaged in dubious practices.

---

[46] Bioethics commentators increasingly call for simplified consent forms: "Institutions in developed countries are expanding clinical trials in Africa and Asia and most focus on the signing of the consent form rather than on the exchange of information between researchers and potential participants. Information should be culturally adjusted, taking local factors into account. These might include degrees of illiteracy, native dialects of ethnic minorities, a lack of suitable vocabulary, a preference for communal decision-making, and stigmatization by local authorities if people do not sign" (Guerrier et al., 2012).

[47] Macklin (2004) does concede that informed consent may require contextual analysis for the "procedural" aspects of obtaining consent. This distinction between substantive and procedural aspects of informed consent is not persuasive.

Conclusion

Although IRBs have come under fire for their aggressive efforts to enforce research standards, they actually struggle to achieve their goals. The lack of clear guidelines, the challenges associated with cross-national research, and the smug attitude of investigators undermine sincere efforts by IRBs to achieve compliance with domestic and international standards.

Balancing the right to scientific inquiry with the rights of human subjects is challenging. The reality that IRBs are confronted with many obstacles does not mean they should cease efforts to promote scientific integrity. It does mean that commentators should offer thoughtful recommendations about how to review studies in a fair, timely manner. Greater support of IRBs combined with clearer rules will help institutions reach the right balance between academic freedom and human rights.

References

Abdullahi v. Pfizer, Inc., 2002 U.S. Dist. LEXIS 17436 at *1 (S.D.N.Y. September 17, 2002).
Abdullahi v. Pfizer, Inc., 2005 U.S. Dist. LEXIS 16126, at *23 (S.D.N.Y., August 9, 2003).
Abdullahi v. Pfizer, Inc., 2005 U.S. Dist. LEXIS 16126 (S.D.N.Y., August 9, 2005).
ACHRE. (1996). *Final Report of the Advisory Committee on Human Radiation Experiments*. Oxford University Press.
Addessi, K. S. (2017). How the Willowbrook Consent Decree Has Influenced Contemporary Advocacy of Individuals with Disabilities. Master's thesis, CUNY, New York.
Aguila, E., Cervera, M. D., Martinez, H., & Weidmer, B. A. (2015). Norms and regulations for human-subject research in Mexico and the United States. In E. Aguila et al., *Developing and Testing Informed-Consent Methods in a Study of the Elderly in Mexico*. RAND Corporation.
Alexander, M. (2010). *The New Jim Crow: Mass Incarceration in the Age of Colorblindness*. Harvard University Press.
Allison, R. D., Abbott, L. J., & Wichman, A. (2008, September–October). Nonscientist IRB members at the NIH. *IRB: Ethics and Human Research*, 30(5), 8–15.
Angell, M. (1997). The ethics of clinical research in the Third World. *New England Journal of Medicine*, 337(12), 847–849.
Annas, G. (2009). Globalized clinical trials and informed consent. *New England Journal of Medicine*, 360(20), 2050–2053.
Anon. (1964, January 21). Hospital accused on cancer study; live cells given to patients without their consent, director tells court. *New York Times*.
Apelt, S., van Beuzekom, B., Galindo-Rueda, F., & de Pinho, R. (2015). Which factors influence international mobility of research scientists? In A. Geuna (Ed.), *Global Mobility*

of Research Scientists: The Economics of Who Goes Where and Why (pp. 177–213). Academic Press/Elsevier.

Associated Press. (2017, July 16). Kin of syphilis study victims seek leftover settlement fund. *New York Times*, p. A16.

Barnes, L. W., & Munsch, C. L. (2015). The paradoxical privilege of men and masculinity in institutional review boards. *Feminist Studies, 41*(3), 594–622.

Barondess, J. A. (1996). Medicine against society: Lessons from the Third Reich. *Journal of the American Medical Association, 276*(20), 1647–1661.

Bartholome, W. B. (1976). Parents, children, and the moral benefits of research. *Hastings Center Report, 6*(6), 44–45.

Beauchamp, T. L., & Childress, J. F. (2009). *Principles of Biomedical Ethics* (6th ed.). Oxford University Press

Bhattacharjee, Y. (2013). The psychology of lying: Diederik Staple's audacious academic fraud. *New York Times Magazine*, pp.

Bledsoe, C. H., Sherin, B., Galinsky, A. G., Headley, N. M., Heimer, C. A., Kjeldgaard, E., Lindgren, J., Miller, J. D., Roloff, M. E., & Uttal, D. H. (2017). Regulating creativity: Research and survival in the IRB iron cage. *Northwestern University Law Review, 101*(2), 593–642.

Brainard, J. (2003, October 31). Federal agency says oral-history research is not covered by human-subject rules. *Chronicle of Higher Education*, p. A25.

Brown, R. (1986). *Social Psychology* (2nd ed.). Free Press.

Carey, B. (2015, May 29). Study on attitudes toward same-sex marriage is retracted by a scientific journal. *New York Times*, p. A16.

Carey, B., & Belluck, P. (2015, May 26). Maligned study on gay unions is shaking trust. *New York Times*, pp. A1, A11.

Carome, M. (2014, October). Unethical clinical trials still being conducted in developing countries. *Public Citizen*.

Ceci, S. J., Peters, D., & Plotkin, J. (1985). Human subjects review, personal values, and the regulation of social science research. *American Psychologist, 40*(9), 994–1002.

Christopher, P. P., Stein, M. D., Johnson, J. E., Rich, J. D., Friedmann, P. D., Clarke, J. G., & Lidz, C. W. (2016). Exploitation of prisoners in clinical research: Perceptions of study participations. *IRB, 38*(1), 7–12.

Couzin-Frankel, J. (2010, April 30). DNA returned to tribe, raising questions about consent. *Science, 328*(5978),558. doi:10.1126/science.328.5978.558. PMID: 20430983.

Craun, K. (2018, January 8). Personal communication from USC Director of the University Park Institutional Review Board.

Craun, K. (2019, July 29). Personal communication from the USC Director of the University Park Institutional Review Board.

Cressey, D. (2012, February 2). Informed consent on trial. *Nature, 482*, 16.

De Roubaix, M. (2008). Are there limits to respect for autonomy in bioethics. *Medicine & Law, 27*, 365.

Diekema, D. S. (2006). Conducting ethical research in pediatrics: A brief historical overview and review of pediatric regulations. *Journal of Pediatrics, 149*(1), S3–S11.

Doffman, Z. (2019, June 18). China killing prisoners to harvest organs for transplant, tribunal finds. *Forbes*.

Duke, N. (2013). Situated bodies in medicine and research: Altruism versus compelled sacrifice. In M. Goodwin (Ed.), *The Global Body Market: Altruism's Limits*. Cambridge University Press.

Edgar, H. (2000). Outside the community. In S. M. Reverby (Ed.), *Tuskegee's Truths: Rethinking the Tuskegee Syphilis Study* (pp. 489–494). University of North Carolina Press.

Elliott, C. (2015, May 26). Minnesota's medical mess. *New York Times*, p. A17.

Emanuel, E. J., Wendler, D., & Grady, C. (2000). What makes clinical research ethical? *Journal of the American Medical Association, 283*(20), 2701–2711.

Flaherty, C. (2017, January 20). Oral history no longer subject to IRB approval. *Inside Higher Ed*.

Foucault, M. (1978). *Discipline and Punish: The Birth of the Prison.* Vintage Books.

Frezza, E. E. (2018). Clinical research and institutional review board (IRB). In E. E. Frezza, *Medical Ethics: A Reference Guide for Guaranteeing Principled Care and Quality* (pp. 203–209). Productivity Press.

Goffman, E. (1968). *Asylums: Essays on the Social Situation of Mental Patients and Other Inmates.* Aldine Transaction.

Goode, D., Hill, D., Reiss, J., & Bronston, W. (2013). *A History and Sociology of the Willowbrook State School.* American Association on Intellectual and Developmental Disabilities.

Gostin, L., Vanchieri, C., & Pope, A., (Eds.) (2007). *Ethical Considerations in Research on Prisoners.* Institute of Medicine; National Academies Press.

Grady, C. (2015). Enduring and emerging challenges of informed consent. *New England Journal of Medicine, 372*(9), 855–862.

Grodin, M. A., & Annas, G. (1996). Legacies of Nuremberg: Medical ethics and human rights. *Journal of the American Medical Association, 276*(20), 1682–1683.

Guerrier, G., Sicard, D., & Brey, P. T. (2012, March 1). Informed consent: Cultural differences. *Nature, 483*, 36.

Guerrini, A. (2003). *Experimenting with Humans and Children: From Galen to Animal Rights.* Johns Hopkins University Press.

Gunderson, L. C. (Ed.) (2018). *Scientific Integrity and Ethics in the Geosciences.* American Geophysical Union and John Wiley & Sons, Inc.

Hamburger, P. (2004). The new censorship: Institutional review boards. *Supreme Court Review*, 271–354.

Harmon, A. (2010, April 21). Indian tribe wins suit to limit use of its DNA. *New York Times*.

Henry, S. G., Romano, P. S., & Yarborough, M. (2016). Building trust between institutional review boards and researchers. *Journal of General Internal Medicine, 31*(9), 987–989.

Hill, D. B. (2016). Sexual admissions: An intersectional analysis of certifications and residency at Willowbrook State School (1950–1985). *Sexuality and Disability, 34*(2), 103–129.

Hornblum, A. M. (1998). *Acres of Skin: Human Experiments at Holmesburg Prison.* Routledge.

Human Rights Committee. (1992, March 10). CCPR General Comment No. 20: Article 7 (Prohibition of Torture, or Other Cruel, Inhuman or Degrading Treatment or Punishment). https://www.refworld.org/docid/453883fb0.html

Johnson, C. Y. (2014, August 5). Coauthor of retracted stem cell papers commits suicide. *Boston Globe*.

Johnston, B. R. (Ed.) (2007). *Half-Lives & Half-Truths: Confronting the Radioactive Legacies of the Cold War.* School for Advanced Research.

Jones, J. H. (1981). *Bad Blood: The Tuskegee Syphilis Experiment.* Free Press.

Kass, N., Dawson, L., & Loyo-Berrios, N. I. (2003). Ethical oversight of research in developing countries. *Ethics and Human Rights, 25*(2), 1–10.

Katsh, E., & Rabinovich-Einy, O. (2017). *Digital Justice and the Internet of Disputes*. Oxford University Press.

Kolata, G. (2018, June 5). Looking to prison for a health study: Inmate volunteers may be the ideal subjects for a look at salt. *New York Times*, p. D3.

Krimsky, S. (2017). The ethical and legal foundations of scientific "conflict of interest." In T. Lemmons & D. Waring (Eds.), *Law and Ethics in Biomedical Research Regulation, Conflict of Interest and Liability* (pp. 63–81). University of Toronto Press.

Krugman, S. (1986) The Willowbrook hepatitis studies revisited: Ethical aspects. *Reviews of Infectious Diseases, 8*(1), 157–162.

Lederman, R. (2009, September). Comparing ethics codes and conventions. *Anthropology News*, 11–12.

Liang, B., Lu, H., & Hood, R. (2016). *The Death Penalty in China: Policy, Practice, and Reform*. Columbia University Press.

London, L. (2002). Ethical oversight of public health research: Can rules and IRBs make a difference in developing countries. *American Journal of Public Health, 92*(7), 1079–1084.

Love, R. R., & Fost, N. C. (1997). Ethical and regulatory challenges in a randomized control trial of adjuvant treatment for breast cancer in Vietnam. *Journal of Investigative Medicine, 45*, 423–431.

Luna, F. (2019). Research in developing countries. In B. Steinbock (Ed.), *Oxford Handbook on Bioethics* (pp. 621–647). Oxford University Press.

Luna, F., & Macklin, R. (2009). Research involving human beings. In H. Kuhse & P. Singer (Eds.), *A Companion to Bioethics* (2nd ed., pp. 448–457). Wiley-Blackwell.

Lurie, P., & Wolfe, S. (1997). Unethical trials of interventions to reduce perinatal transmission of the human immunodeficiency virus in developing countries. *New England Journal of Medicine, 337*(12), 853–855.

Macklin, R. (2004). *Double Standards in Medical Research in Developing Countries*. Cambridge University Press.

MacNeil, P. U. (2009). Regulating experimentation in research and medical practice. In H. Kuhse & P. Singer (Eds.), *A Companion to Bioethics* (2nd ed., pp. 469–486). Wiley-Blackwell.

Manson, N. C., & O'Neill, O. (2007). *Rethinking Informed Consent in Bioethics*. Cambridge University Press.

McCormick, R. A. (1997). Proxy consent in the experimentation situation. *Perspectives in Biology and Medicine, 18*(1), 2–20.

McNeil, D. G., Jr. (2010, October 1). U.S. apologizes for syphilis tests in Guatemala. *New York Times*. https://www.nytimes.com/2010/10/02/health/research/02infect.html

Meeker, M. (2012). The Berkeley compromise: Oral history, human subjects and the meaning of "research." In C. B. Potter & R. C. Romando (Eds.), *Doing Recent History: On Privacy, Copyright, Video Games, Institutional Review Boards, Activist Scholarship, and History That Talks Back* (pp. 115–138). University of Athens Press.

Milgram, S. (1974). *Obedience to Authority*. Tavistock.

Moreno, J. D. (2001). *Undue Risk: Secret State Experiments on Humans*. Routledge.

Murphy, K. (2017, May 22). Some social scientists are tired of asking for permission. *New York Times*.

New York State Association for Retarded Children, Inc., et al. v. Hugh L. Carey, 393 F. Supp. 715 (1975).

Nicholson, I. (2011). Torture at Yale: Experimental subjects, laboratory torment and the "rehabilitation" of Milgram's "Obedience to Authority." *Theory and Psychology, 21*(6), 737–761.

Nicols, L., Brako, L., Rivera, S. M., Tahmassian, A., Jones, M. F., Pierce, H. H., & Bierer, B. E. (2017, August 18). What do revised U.S. rules mean for human rights? The updated Common Rule raises many questions. *Science, 357*(6352), 650–651.

Office of Human Subjects Research Protection, U.S. Department of Health and Human Services. (2019). *International Compilation of Human Subjects Research*. https://www.hhs.gov/ohrp/international/index.html

Onlineuniversities.com. (2012, February 27). The 10 Greatest Cases of Fraud in University Research. http://www.onlineuniversities.com/blog/2012/02/the-10-greatest-cases-of-fraud-in-university-research/

Petrosino, A., & Mello, D. (2014). Institutional review boards. In *Encyclopedia of Criminal Justice Ethics* (pp. 476–480). SAGE.

Ramsey, P. (1976). The enforcement of morals: Nontherapeutic research on children. *Hastings Center Report, 6*(4), 21–30.

Reverby, S. M. (2018). "So what?" Historical contingency, activism, and reflections on the studies in Tuskegee and Guatemala. In *Bioethics in Action* (pp. 32–54). Cambridge University Press.

Reverby, S. M. (Ed.) (2000). *Tuskegee's Truths: Rethinking the Tuskegee Syphilis Study*. University of North Carolina Press.

Rodley, N. (2009). *The Treatment of Prisoners Under International Law* (3rd ed.). Oxford University Press.

Rothman, D., & Rothman, S. (2017). *The Willowbrook Wars*. Routledge. (Originally published in 1984 by Harper and Rowe.)

Schrag, Z. M. (2019). Vexed Again: Social Scientists and the Revision of the Common Rule, 2011–2018 *Journal of Law, Medicine & Ethics, 47*, 254–263.

Schrag, Z. M. (2010). *Ethical Imperialism: Institutional Review Boards and the Social Sciences, 1965–2009*. Johns Hopkins University Press.

Schug, R. A., Yang, Y., Raine, A., Han, C., Liu, J., & Li, L. (2011). Resting EEG deficits in accused murderers with schizophrenia. *Psychiatry Research: Neuroimaging, 194*, 85–94.

Shweder, R. A. (2006). Protecting human subjects and preserving academic freedom: Prospects at the University of Chicago. *American Ethnologist, 33*(4), 507–518.

Simoes, L. C. S. (2010). Informed consent: The medical and legal challenge of our time. *Revista Brasileira de Ortopedia, 45*(2), 191–195.

Simon, J. (2014). *Mass Incarceration on Trial*. New Press.

Smith, D. (2011, August 12). Pfizer pays out to Nigerian families of meningitis drug trial victims. *The Guardian*.

Solovey, M. (2013). *Shaky Foundations: The Politics-Patronage-Social Science Nexus in Cold War America*. Rutgers University Press.

Sprumont, D. (2015). Informed consent: Do not be afraid. *Journal of the Formosan Medical Association, 116*, 322–323.

Stark, L. (2010, October 8). Closing the ethics gap in medical research. *Los Angeles Times*, p. A19.

Stark, L. (2014). IRBs and the problem of "local precedents." In I. G. Cohen & H. Fernandez Lynch (Eds.), *Human Subjects Research Regulation: Perspectives on the Future* (pp. 173–186). MIT Press.

Steneck, N. H., Maryer, T., Anderon, M. S., & Kleiner, S. (2018). The origin, objectives, and evolution of the World Conferences on Research Integrity. In L. C. Gunderson (Ed.), *Scientific Integrity and Ethics in the Geosciences*. American Geophysical Union and John Wiley & Sons.

Stern, J. E., & Lomax, K. (1997). Human experimentation. In D. Elliott & J. E. Stern (Eds.), *Research Ethics: A Reader* (pp. 286–295). University Press of New England.

Subramanian, S. (2017, February 26). Worse than Tuskegee. *Slate*. http://www.slate.com/articles/health_and_science/cover_story/2017/02/guatemala_syphilis_experiments_worse_than_tuskegee.html

Sullivan, L. S. (2017). Dynamic axes of informed consent in Japan. *Social Science & Medicine, 174*, 159–168.

Union of Concerned Scientists. (2004). *Scientific Integrity in Policymaking: An Investigation into the Bush Administration's Misuse of Science*. https://www.ucsusa.org/our-work/center-science-and-democracy/promoting-scientific-integrity/reports-scientific-integrity.html#.WxqoPqknZMA

Union of Concerned Scientists. (2017). *Preserving Scientific Integrity in Federal Policymaking*. https://www.ucsusa.org/center-science-and-democracy/promoting-scientific-integrity/preserving-scientific-integrity#.WxqocaknZMA

Wagner, M. (2018, January 8). Personal communication from former Chair of the University Park Institutional Review Board.

Washington, H. (2006). *Medical Apartheid: The Dark History of Medical Experimentation on Black Americans from Colonial Times to the Present*. Harlem Moon, Broadway Books.

White House. (2009, March 9). Memorandum for the Heads of Executive Departments and Agencies on Scientific Integrity. https://obamawhitehouse.archives.gov/the-press-office/memorandum-heads-executive-departments-and-agencies-3-9-09

White, R. F. (2007). Institutional review board mission creep: The Common Rule, social science, and the nanny state. *Independent Review, 11*(4), 547–564.

Wichman, A. (1998). Protecting vulnerable research subjects: Practical realities of institutional review board review and approval. *Journal of Health Care Law and Policy, 1*(1), 88–104.

Wichman, A. (2012). Institutional review boards. In J. I. Gallin & F. P. Ognibene (Eds.), *Principles and Practice of Clinical Research* (3rd ed., pp. 53–65). Academic Press; Elsevier.

Yang, Y., Raine, A., Han, C., Schug, R. A., Toga, A. W., & Narr, K. L. (2010). Reduced hippocampal and paraphippocampal volumes in murderers with schizophrenia. *Psychiatry Research: Neoroimaging, 182*, 9–13.

16
Viral Science and the Tragedy of the Scientific Commons

Tanya Menon and Christopher Winship

Introduction

On Thursday, April 12, 2018, two African American men were arrested in a Philadelphia Starbucks for trespassing after staff had called police. The two men, who had not yet bought anything, had asked to use the restroom as they waited for a third person to join them. A customer recorded this arrest on video and it immediately went viral. For Starbucks, this was a public relations disaster. The company responded with an announcement that all Starbucks stores would close for a day in May so that its entire staff could participate in implicit bias training. In the wake of this incident, many diversity and public relations experts congratulated Starbucks for its response (McGregor, 2018). Although implicit bias training, Starbucks' chosen method to address this incident, is a well-established method within the diversity training sector in which companies spend approximately $8 billion annually, a few articles emerged in the wake of the Starbucks declaration questioning whether implicit bias training actually works (Feintzeig & Jargon, 2018; Lipman, 2018; Mak, 2018).

Our goal here is not to critique implicit bias research or the training programs that it has produced. We believe that implicit bias, like "dark matter" in physics, may well turn out to be enormously important even if it is not well understood at present. Nor, when looking at social and hard scientists, is our goal to assess the boundary between scientist and science—for example, whether scientific peer review is an adequate regulatory process for determining whether a researcher's ideas, data, and analysis should be considered "scientific knowledge." Rather, our focus is on the relationship between science and the public and the fate of any given scientific research in the hands of the public.

Tanya Menon and Christopher Winship, *Viral Science and the Tragedy of the Scientific Commons* In: *Research Integrity*. Edited by: Lee J. Jussim, Jon A. Krosnick, and Sean T. Stevens, Oxford University Press. © Oxford University Press 2022. DOI: 10.1093/oso/9780190938550.003.0016

By *public*, we refer to the various external audiences who consume research outside academia, including curious individuals, the media, governmental agents, public policy leaders, and corporate actors seeking best practices. Our issue is with the largely *unregulated* boundary between science and the public—that is, the fate of research ideas, whether representing accepted science or not, as they are transmitted, translated, and transformed once they enter public consciousness. Given the lack of a formal gatekeeper (such as peer review), this pathway is regularly crossed by intellectual pundits, "policy entrepreneurs" (Rein & Winship, 1997), and management gurus, whose ideas and interpretations are not always based on research broadly accepted by the academic community.

Our concern is that when scientific research is presented so that it is conducive to rapid transmission, it is likely to be transmitted via emotionally evocative (Heath et al., 2001), persuasive storytelling (i.e., orally, anecdotally in popular nonfiction, and in viral news stories). This process can give research the characteristics of folklore, possessing a truth status that is disconnected from actual empirical reality. As it is processed and presented to a mass audience, the research is often simplified and nuance is lost as findings are imbued with "strong causality" (Rein & Winship, 1999): that is, far more powerful causal links are asserted than are warranted by the empirical evidence, such that what is claimed becomes little more than superstition (Vyse, 2013). From conception through implementation, implicit bias research and associated implicit bias training programs simply represent a single illustrative example of these processes. Through a study of implicit bias research and the ways in which research on implicit bias is transmitted to the public, we address a much larger concern, namely how scientific research is generally transformed into viral content as it is used and misused by the public broadly, and in public policy, legal, and corporate settings.

A Brief History of Implicit Bias Research

In 1995, Anthony Greenwald and Mahzarin Banaji published a now-classic paper indicating that people's attitudes are found not just in their conscious realm of awareness, but at an implicit level in cognitive associations that are inaccessible to individual or group introspection (Greenwald & Banaji, 1995). Grounded in psychology's rediscovery of the unconscious, the paper initiated an influential research program that touched on important questions in social psychology including intergroup bias, prejudice, and racism. They argued that the unconscious mind was not dominated by Freudian urges for sex and aggression. Instead, a decision maker traveled along the *System 1* pathway whereby automatic, involuntary, fast, first impressions dominate the more careful, well-reasoned *System 2* processing (Kahneman, 2011; Tversky & Kahneman, 1974). In spite of a person's best intentions, Tversky and Kahneman showed, these involuntary mental processes could hijack decision-making and release inner racist prejudices.

In an attempt to address these "inner racist prejudices," Greenwald et al. (1998) unveiled the Implicit Association Test (IAT) as a scientific measure of implicit bias. It is a timed reaction test where one is given instructions to associate the terms "good" or "bad" or other valanced stimuli with pictures of two categories of people. Which type of person is associated with each adjective is then reversed. For example, subjects in a laboratory might be shown faces of White and Black individuals. In the first condition, they might be asked to push a button on a computer representing "good" every time they saw a White face, and a different button representing "bad" every time they saw a Black face. The test is timed over a series of comparisons. The difference in the time it takes individuals to do the association task when Whites are paired with "good" and Blacks with "bad" versus the reverse is then considered a measure of a person's implicit racial bias. Initial research revealed that 70% of people show preference for White to Black faces. The test has been employed using a variety of groups. Readers can take the test and find a summary of the research at https://implicit.harvard.edu/implicit/ . Unsurprisingly, this research has inspired hundreds of papers (see Fazio & Olson, 2002, for an early review).

Many questions have been raised about the IAT. What does this association actually indicate? Are implicit associations a bona fide pipeline to people's true selves (Fazio et al., 1995)? Could it be that implicit biases don't tap an individual's unconscious biases, but instead simply capture associations in the environment (Payne et al., 2017)? Are measures of implicit bias actually predictive of discriminatory behavior (Blanton et al., 2009)? Social scientists have also focused on the instability of implicit associations over time: People may show a particular preference on one day but a different preference the following week (Gawronski et al., 2017). Still other researchers have wondered whether these results were context specific: Could the findings in a laboratory, where the IAT asks people to make split-second responses to hypothetical faces, reliably be generalizable to relationships and interaction in real-world contexts (Chakravarti et al. 2014)? Concerns have even been raised by the pioneering researchers themselves on implicit bias, including Russell Fazio, who has described the IAT as "noisy," and has said, "It has a potential to be a remarkably powerful tool. But as traditionally implemented, it really has problems" (Azar, 2008).

None of these questions suggest that the research is wrong; indeed, the basic findings of the IAT have been replicated repeatedly. Instead, the concern is that while academics were in the midst of critically assessing these findings—what they meant, when they mattered, and how they were tested— these scientific ideas crossed the boundary from academia into public spaces, including courtrooms and corporations. While scientific research might have once resided in narrow academic conversations, it now travels with ease and speed to diverse corners of society. Within a few years, the research on implicit attitudes and bias had become a centerpiece of corporate trainings, where people took the test, received their quantitatively "precise" implicit bias scores, and discussed their results, often in the context of recognizing how their own biases might influence their management decisions such as hiring and promotion.

The rush to apply the research in these potentially exciting ways risks significant overreach by generalizing the research into contexts, tasks, and situations far beyond the claims made by the original empirical researchers (Blanton et al., 2009; Mitchell & Tetlock, 2017). In addition to external validity concerns, the research has moved from the lab to corporations without trainings and interventions being directly assessed for their effectiveness in actually reducing biases (see Lai et al., 2014; Lai et al., 2016, for more recent assessments). Despite significant investments of time and money in diversity training and testing, the question remains whether they offer real, stable correctives for bias (Bezrukova et al., 2016), or if they make them worse (Kalev et al., 2006). If the latter, these training seminars are not simply a waste of corporate time and money: they affect careers and corporate practices and, when incorporated into law enforcement training, they have life-and-death implications (James, 2018). For example, as companies like Walmart have faced litigation on workplace discrimination, the larger social psychological body of research on discrimination has been used (and criticized) in the courtroom (U.S. Supreme Court, 2011). Implicit bias research was presented to support arguments that the unconscious offered a different, perhaps more valid, report of one's true self, despite denial of biased intent by defendants.

Science and the Public: What Is the Problem?

Many of the chapters in this volume address how science institutionally manages the transformation of research into scientific knowledge, focusing on the boundary between researchers and the scientific community that certifies research through peer review. Thus, a key question in these chapters is what institutional practices could science, particularly social science, improve or adopt to increase the fidelity of this internal process. By contrast, this chapter's focus is on the boundary between the scientist and the public.

Researchers and the public alike have often called for expanded public access to scientific research.[1] As expressed in the mission statement of the Boston Foundation's *Science for the Public*: "Modern democratic society depends on an informed public in a global community. Citizens today require an understanding of basic scientific concepts, new developments in science, and numerous science-related issues."[2] That is, when the public remains ignorant of basic science, this ignorance weakens the public's ability to make informed choices. In contrast, a basic understanding of scientific research might potentially inoculate people against false information and irrational beliefs. Furthermore, the public is hungry for scientific research, as evidenced by bestselling books that popularize scientific research and numerous scientifically themed TED talks that millions have viewed. As science is often funded with public money, it is appropriate and important that public investment is returned through useful knowledge.

Our concern is with potential and actual failures in the flow of scientific information to the public and what might be done so that the process is traversed with discretion, integrity, and appropriate epistemic humility. We note that these problems are particularly pronounced with social sciences because the technical and mathematical language of the hard sciences presents a natural barrier that often makes them relatively impenetrable to the public. Due to the more accessible language of the social sciences, communication can occur in a highly accelerated and unfiltered fashion. This has led to three distinct but related effects: (1) unclear norms about what to communicate, how to communicate, and what the scientist's role is in this process, and thus (2) a lack of fidelity in the translation/transfer of research,

---

[1] See: https://obamawhitehouse.archives.gov/blog/2013/02/22/expanding-public-access-results-federally-funded-research

[2] See: http://www.scienceforthepublic.org/about

resulting in, finally, (3) reputational effects for both individual scientists and the broader scientific community.

Viral Science: A Changing Relationship Between Science and the Public

As noted by Gregory Mitchell and Philip Tetlock (2017, p. 164), "it is difficult to find a psychological construct that is so popular, yet so misunderstood," as the IAT. This tension between popularity and misunderstanding is likewise captured in scholarship on the transmission of urban legends and viral news, which commands interest based on emotional content regardless of informational content or even truth value (Heath et al., 2001). We define *viral science* as the transmission of scientific research in a manner that prioritizes emotional, persuasive content that can rapidly circulate, as compared to content with pure informational value. We contend the unregulated nature and unclear norms of this transmission sometimes prioritize elements that facilitate rapid proliferation at the expense of accuracy.

Public Access: Hunger for "Research" or Meaning?

The potential benefit or harm of public access to social scientific research is influenced by different goals such as (from the scientist's point of view) a need for nuanced content and a faithful representation of the evidence as it is represented in academic journals; or, from the public's point of view, the presence of content that is personally meaningful, interesting, and apparently useful. Social science is particularly well equipped to inform people about their own lives and therefore enjoys a unique position in public interest. It offers people not just a sense of what "is" in the world but also a broader tool kit of meaning (Swidler, 1986), occasionally treading into the "ought" and the "should," to help people manage their environment. Arie Kruglanski describes human learners such as these as lay epistemologists (Kruglanski, 1980): They seek to know via a quasi-scientific method of generating hypotheses and validating them. However, rather than consistently abiding by the stringent requirements of the scientific method, their hypothesis testing can be interrupted by particular motivational forces. For instance, as people are placed under time pressure, they are more likely to engage in epistemic freezing—that is, accepting an idea while ignoring alternative hypotheses and inconsistent data (Kruglanski & Freund, 1983). Similarly, as evaluation apprehension decreases (Kruglanski & Freund, 1983)—that is, they are less accountable to an audience who might recognize their errors (Tetlock, 1985)—they again engage in epistemic freezing. In these situations, the need to simply appear to "know" in a stable manner—even if the content is inaccurate—is heightened.

The drive to seek stable answers, whether true or not, is particularly pronounced when people experience a loss of personal control in their environments (Whitson & Galinsky, 2008). In these situations, people search for epistemic structures that make the world seem predictable, and they heighten their beliefs in the existence of controlling external actors such as God and the government (Kay et al., 2009; Wang, Whitson, & Menon, 2012; Whitson & Galinsky, 2008; Whitson, Galinsky, & Kay, 2015). Thus, people who feel a lack of personal control are also more likely to succumb to superstitious beliefs such as horoscopes (Wang et al., 2012) and explain events via stable patterns, including conspiratorial beliefs (Whitson et al., 2019). While these knowledge structures place significant power in the hands of controlling external actors, they also offer people a consistent, coherent-seeming way to try to understand, predict, and order the world.

Science, like superstitions, religion, government, and conspiracy theories, offers a source of definitive answers. Indeed, science operates as a highly organized cultural meaning system—in other words, a "tool kit of symbols, stories, rituals, and worldviews" (Swidler, 1986, p. 273). While each of these sources of definitive answers has its own audience, its own truth-content, and its own reliability, Swidler (1986, p. 281) has found that in settled times, more people rely on the "undisputed authority of habit, normality, and common sense," while in unsettled times, a multitude of cultural meaning systems compete with science, normality, and common sense.

Wicked Problems

Beyond meaning-making, the public also expects scientists to provide solutions—that is, to put content into action in a purposeful fashion to address pressing problems. These solutions do not just live as ideas in the mind but also become rituals, practices, and lived culture (Geertz, 1973).

According to Swidler (1986, p. 273), "people may use their chosen tool kits in varying configurations to solve different kinds of problems."

However, although scientific research has transformed cultural practice in various domains, the questionable results of some of these "scientific" solutions and their underlying "scientific" methodologies (and, indeed, their funding) have led to concerns that the truth status of research is disconnected from empirical reality. As one example, pseudoscientific research (typically sponsored by the sugar industry) seemed to offer a clear-cut solution to the obesity epidemic with the low-fat diet (O'Connor, 2016). This dominant solution, which conveniently shifted attention away from sugar, transformed dietary patterns to low-fat, high-carbohydrate diets while also introducing a multitude of new product lines and marketing opportunities for manufactured foods. Only after decades of skyrocketing obesity rates have these recommendations been reconsidered.

Another example of scientific research that altered cultural practices is the so-called education flat line—that is to say, the realization that "countless public and private initiatives, site-based innovations, dramatic increases in per-pupil spending, wordy symposia and books, laws upon laws" have essentially attained "small gains from an unacceptably low base" (Gordon, 2006: p. 8). These research-based solutions transformed how teachers worked on a daily basis, and how children were educated and tested, with questionable results.

In the case of the IAT, this research did not simply offer people personal insight. It has also provided managers with a solution at hand as they attempt to navigate the pressing challenges of workplace diversity. By offering trainings based on validated, peer-reviewed research, managers could address, though not necessarily fix, a key issue affecting the culture of their organizations. With IAT, organizations could demonstrate positive action with compliance issues as well as provide positive evidence for the organization in the event of lawsuits. Additionally, the trainings offered moral credentialing: By offering the trainings, managers were able to feel good about their moral identities (Monin & Miller, 2001). And finally, instituting IAT answered the universal human need to *do something*.

All of these problems—the obesity epidemic, educational shortfalls, and managing diversity in the workplace—are examples of what researchers describe as "wicked problems" (Churchman, 1967; see discussion in Menon & Thompson, 2016, pp. 6–8). These are a particular class of problems that:

1. Lack an algorithm for structured problem solving (e.g., there is a formula for solving certain math problems, but not reducing the obesity epidemic without completely disrupting the entire American agricultural industry)
2. Lack demonstrable answers (e.g., a math problem has a clear numerical answer; eliminating bias does not)
3. Lack clear tests for the proposed solutions (e.g., it's possible to measure a computer's processing speed but more complicated to say if an intervention has actually "improved" people's racial beliefs/behaviors)
4. Arise from interdependencies with multiple problems (e.g., issues like obesity, education, and racism are tied to other complex socioeconomic and political issues).

People facing tough wicked problems are particularly prone to grasp for solutions that may be readily available but offer little real traction on the issues. In our noisy, overloaded world in which true signals are hard to capture, Cohen et al. (1972) describe the garbage can model, whereby people, problems, and solutions float like pieces of garbage in a garbage can, coming together somewhat haphazardly. Thus, sometimes there are problems looking for solutions and occasionally there are even solutions looking for problems. The fact that an idea rises to the top of the garbage can doesn't imply that it has risen in the hierarchy from data to wisdom or usefulness.

People grasping for solutions for wicked problems are trapped in action without traction because they do not have a clear mental model or valid causal map of how things work, the true causes of an issue, and likely effects (Menon & Thompson, 2016) of the proposed "solutions." For example, one cognitive psychology study showed that people implicitly operate from a mental model that thermostats function like gas pedals (Kempton, 1986). This meant that they cranked up the temperature on the thermostat hoping to heat their homes faster even though it would have been just as effective to simply set the temperature to the desired level. Their action was misdirected by an incorrect causal map of the process. Likewise, without a clear mental model of the problems, people are also vulnerable to solutions that solve substitute problems (Kahneman & Fredrick, 2002). That is, rather than solving the true hard problem (e.g., managing diversity in a productive manner), people locate an easier substitute problem (e.g., showing we care about diversity or checking the boxes on diversity for compliance purposes).

Idea Entrepreneurs

Solutions, however, do not simply become available in a haphazard process. Idea entrepreneurs play a significant role in bridging the boundary between academia and the public by marketing solutions and making them stick, regardless of their intrinsic value. We define an *idea entrepreneur* as an individual—either a scientist or someone else—who comes to be attached to and, indeed, personifies particular ideas and publicizes, sells, and profits from those ideas. These individuals operate as brokers (Burt, 1992) who can translate the abstruse ideas of academia to the public in an easily digestible manner. Unlike policy entrepreneurs who peddle public policy recommendations to political actors (e.g., poverty or education policy; Rein & Winship, 1997), idea entrepreneurs market ideas to the public more generally. Idea entrepreneurs differ also from public intellectuals whose op-ed pieces and mainstream media work present ideas for critical appraisal. Idea entrepreneurs see "science" as something that is commodified (i.e., has economic value and is owned, bought, sold, and traded), operating via their own rules and norms.

Challenges to Managing the Boundary Between Science and the Public

There are two potential barriers to a healthy and appropriate relationship between science and the public. First, there are the techniques that idea entrepreneurs use to convey research in a narrative structure that is simple, persuasive, and easily digestible—and, often, not (entirely) true to the original scientific findings. Second, as an idea is imbued with purpose and stretched beyond the original empirical evidence, the power and strength of effects may be overstated. Within these two major barriers, we examine three specific concerns: (1) the tendency to convey research in a manner that involves stronger-than-warranted causality (Rein & Winship, 1999); (2) elastic effects (stretching to contexts beyond the original zone of validity in empirical tests); and (3) the desire for definitive answers when the science does not yield a provable, definitive answer (Kruglanski, 1980). We then consider how these processes transform the scientist and the scientific method.

The Psychology of Believing—Persuading the Audience

Consistent with Swidler's (1986) notion of "unsettled times," scientists today are among many content producers in the marketplace of ideas, competing for attention alongside news, opinion, and YouTube. Just as 24-hour news has forced the news media to produce faster, more easily digestible content, scientists have also increased their speed, reach, and accessibility, perhaps at the expense of nuance and accuracy. As one example, the IAT has several notable features that easily feed into an environment that prioritizes rapid production and easily consumable sound bites. While we could choose many different research programs from various disciplines as instructive case studies, our point is simply that several features of IAT research and how it was "processed" for public consumption promoted its rapid spread into the mainstream spaces and consciousness before the test's viability in addressing implicit bias was proven.

In a paper on urban legends, Heath (1996) consider how ideas are selected for transmission, suggesting that the veracity of an idea is not the sole force and sometimes not even the main factor determining which ideas spread. Ideas are often selected on their emotional power, namely their ability to evoke emotions such as fear or anger or their ability to unify a tribe. In considering the power of implicit bias research, several elements heightened its power:

1. Storytelling: Storytelling has become a critical element of research transmission. This involves a folkloric, word-of-mouth process of spreading wisdom within the tribe and community, creating warmth, emotion, and coherent narratives. One of the most famous idea entrepreneurs, Malcolm Gladwell, has noted: "I am a story-teller, and I look to academic research . . . for ways of augmenting story-telling" (Chabris, 2014). In the same way, in IAT trainings, research often becomes attached to specific, highly charged news stories (e.g., police shootings, the 2018 racial incident at Starbucks) and personal experiences, often presented in collective settings.
2. Data become attached to the self. The IAT test is interactive and offers instant, individualized feedback. Information about the self is attention-grabbing and makes the data personally meaningful.

3. Negativity bias: The IAT tends to deliver a negative message that is more attention-grabbing than positive information (Kahneman & Tversky, 1979; Rozin & Royzman, 2001).
4. Counterintuitive effects: While people readily deny their own racism, particularly their own biases, the IAT test belies these claims, offering people the powerful emotion of surprise. Research suggests that distinct, surprising information is more easily recalled (Hunt & Worthen, 2006; see Heath, 1996, for an exception that suggests that people prefer to transmit less surprising news). Worse, a study of rumor cascades on Twitter (spread by 3 million people) indicated that wrong ideas might in fact travel faster, further, and deeper than truth (Vosoughi et al., 2018), an effect arising from the novelty and emotionally evocative nature of that information.
5. Extremity: The implication that most people are secret racists is dramatic. Research on urban legends indicates that more extreme versions of a story evoke more emotion and are more likely to be repeated (Heath et al., 2001; "emotional snowballing"). Arousal (both positively and negatively valanced) increases social transmission of information (Berger & Schwartz, 2011).

When selected based on their emotional power and potential for viral transmission, ideas (and parts of ideas) with more accurate informational content but fewer of these evocative elements may well be crowded out. However, inclusion of these folkloric elements need not diminish the scientific legitimacy of an idea or proposal. Associations with scientists, prestigious universities, peer-reviewed journals, and quantitative data that appear precise and meaningful can render ideas scientifically legitimate despite having emotional and folkloric elements or presentations.

Strong Causality
One mechanism that cognitively simplifies an idea so that it is conducive to rapid transmission is *strong causality*. According to Rein and Winship (1999), strong causality occurs when a research finding with a small to modest association between a variable and an outcome (and thus, at best, a weak causal relationship) is interpreted as a fully deterministic relationship. Essentially, this hardens causal links such that causes and effects are neatly and inexorably linked. This eliminates any consideration of heterogeneous causal

effects or consideration of boundary conditions in either time or space. This is not about p-hacking the data; rather, it is overselling the effect. The canonical example in this paper is the claim that discussions of implicit bias might address organizational and social inequality, particularly without addressing structural factors in a meaningful way.

The claims of deterministic causality essentially producing illusory relations (Hamilton & Gifford, 1976) and connecting unrelated causes with effects are a defining feature of superstitious reasoning. Superstitious beliefs involve causation that is not explicable based on "known laws of nature or . . . what is generally considered rational in society" (Kramer & Block, 2008, p. 784). Superstitions offer seemingly stable beliefs when people face sense-making difficulty. Since the age of Enlightenment and the advancement of science, scientists have held these irrational beliefs to account. The irony is that in a marketplace prioritizing rapid transmission, science in its public manifestation might be distorted sufficiently to assume the characteristics of superstition.

Elastic Effects
It is often claimed, we think correctly, that research has scientific value even when results are not generalizable, or, in more technical language, when it lacks external validity (Mook, 1983). A potential issue in all research, generalizability is particularly acute in laboratory studies and ethnographies that are confined to a single site and population. While affirming the scientific value of these empirical findings, the question is how to extract applicable lessons and appropriately apply them to other contexts (legal, policy, corporate). While strong causality strengthens causal links, elastic effects stretch the applicability of a finding by neglecting the social context and assuming that effects in one context readily translate to another. People regularly simplify social reality by committing fundamental attribution errors, elevating the causal power of individual actors and ignoring the nuances of social context (Ross, 1977).

Researchers fall prey to an analogous cognitive bias when they elevate the causal power of their own effects by failing to account for the social context and population to which they apply. While strong causality positions ideas to become purposeful and solution-ready fixes (sometimes marketed as life-changing hacks), elastic effects allow these solutions to apply broadly, in a misguided attempt to cure many complex problems. For instance, the U.S. Supreme Court's (2011) decision in *Walmart v. Dukes et al.* was arguably the most important class-action employment decision in decades. The case involved a contention that women at Walmart were discriminated against both in terms of wages and promotions. In finding for Walmart, the Court severely curtailed the future potential effectiveness of class-action gender- and race-based employment discrimination lawsuits (U.S. Supreme Court, 2011). The expert witness for the plaintiffs, the sociologist William Bielby, relied mainly on social psychological research, as he had in close to a hundred other cases. Specifically, in his report he claimed that implicit bias based on stereotyping was universally present in all organizations (Bielby, 2005), but the Supreme Court refused to accept the applicability of research on the universal presence of implicit bias to the specific Walmart case.

The research that Bielby used to support his claim was almost entirely based on experiments in psychology laboratories where at best individuals interacted with complete strangers and at worst only saw videos. In the 5–4 majority opinion Justice Scalia attacked Bielby's use of social science research multiple times, concluding that a key problem was the failure of social science to establish the external validity of the research he relied on. It is not that Bielby's claims were wrong, but rather that the research needed to support its applicability hadn't and to a great degree still hasn't been done (U.S. Supreme Court, 2011). For example, the IAT's zone of validity involves interactions in the "extreme short term, i.e., people's split-second, first impressions about (often hypothetical) people of other races" (Banaji & Greenwald and Banaji, 1995; Fazio et al., 1995), as compared to real, long-term, and interdependent relationships (Chakravarti et al., 2014, p. 1217). And, organizational contexts implicate other dynamics of discrimination such as hierarchical power. In these diverse contexts, discrimination might emerge in dramatically different ways. In spite of this, the IAT has been stretched to diverse empirical contexts, including police and corporate trainings (James, 2018; Nordell, 2017). As the world faces a host of deep questions with respect to race, gender, and identity, there has been a convenient but unproven match between the problem and this implicit bias training solution (Cohen et al., 1972).

Definitive Answers
President Harry Truman famously stated, "Give me a one-handed economist! . . . All my economists say 'on the one hand . . . on the other.'"[3] Presidents and the public alike would typically prefer science to provide

---
[3] See: https://www.economist.com/node/2208841

definitive answers. It is, however, constitutive of the scientific method to qualify any claim. Rather than effects that are with certainty true or false, scientific progress is simply "a cumulative process of uncertainty reduction" (Nosek et al., 2015, pp. 4716–4717). However, whereas confidence is persuasive (Moscovici et al., 1969), tentative claims, even when more truthful, are often less persuasive: They don't make for interesting headlines, they don't sell books, and they don't win court cases. As a result, the media, publishers, and lawyers in litigation look to scientists or experts who will take strong, one-sided opinions and operate as persuasive advocates rather than as individuals who see a phenomenon or a set of empirical findings as more complicated. As such, scientists face external pressures to overreach in their claims.

Moscovici demonstrated that persuasive confidence has a stronger influence than a reasoned, balanced presentation of alternatives. In a classic research study, Tetlock (2005) compared the predictions of international relations experts to measure levels of persuasive confidence versus accuracy of predictions. Tetlock asked the experts to make a variety of predictions about a future time period, and, after it passed, he assessed the accuracy of their predictions. In general, the quality of predictions was poor, but political scientists who advocated for a singular theory and made strong definitive predictions did particularly poorly. Those who were generalists—basically, two-handed political scientists—did better. In short, the scientists or experts who made the strongest claims were the ones most likely to be wrong.

The Psychology of Selling

It is not only the scientific idea that is transformed as it becomes broader, faster, and stronger, but also the researcher who transmits it. The concern is that the scientist who operates as an idea entrepreneur loses the ability to perform the scientific method and, particularly, tends to falsify hypotheses. Specifically, when ideas are commodified, the individual scientist who has come to be associated with them faces both financial conflicts of interest and identity challenges that can lead to a psychological entrenchment (Cialdini, 2006).

Financial Conflicts of Interest

Today, academics find themselves with new ways to commercialize their ideas (keynotes, popular books), and they are also evaluated on new criteria in universities as well. For instance, "media mentions" are a new component of academic vitas that has emerged in recent years, and many universities publish a regular list of such mentions. As idea entrepreneurs are financially and professionally invested in their ideas, falsifying them—the basic requirement of performing the scientific method—is directly counter to self-interest. Further, while people readily detect others' biases, researchers struggle to recognize their own biases and conflicts of interest (Pronin et al. 2004), so scientists acting as idea entrepreneurs may self-identify as scientists while failing to recognize that they've crossed the line into sales.

Commitment and Consistency
If the job of a scientist is to falsify hypotheses, it is psychologically difficult to do so when you are publicly committed to an idea (Cialdini, 2006). Indeed, aside from financial benefits, the simple act of standing in front of an audience produces internal commitment to that idea. The person's identity becomes meshed with the idea. For example, during the Korean War, the Chinese made American POWs read positive statements about communism in public to brainwash them. In an elegant formulation of the underlying principle used by the Chinese and idea entrepreneurs, people may not say what they believe, but they believe what they say (Cialdini, 2006). This unfortunately sets in motion psychological entrenchment and confirmation bias (Klayman & Ha, 1987) rather than a drive to disprove one's own hypotheses. In other words, idea entrepreneurs are susceptible to faith-based belief, as compared to dispassionate science.

Esteemed social psychology professor Daryl Bem, who published work on extrasensory perception (ESP) in a leading psychology journal, is an instructive example of a scientist taking on the role of persuader and faith-based believer. After a failed replication led him to attempt to "squeeze droplets of confirmation" from those data, an interviewer asked if he would ever "budge on his beliefs," and he described his beliefs as his "religion":

> If things continue to fail on that one, I'm always willing to update my beliefs. But it just seems unlikely. There's too much literature on all of these experiments... so I doubt you could get me to totally switch religions... I'm all for rigor, but I prefer other people do it. I see its importance—it's fun for some people—but I don't have the patience for it... If you looked at all my past experiments, they were always rhetorical devices. I gathered data to show how my point would be made. I used data as a point of persuasion,

and I never really worried about, "Will this replicate or will this not?" (Engber, 2017)

The ESP research directly led to Simmons et al.'s (2011) papers on how "psychologists could theoretically prove anything true" through methodologies that served their confirmation biases. But beyond the methodological points, the ESP example also raises deeper questions about the scientist's personally defined role identity. Specifically, Bem embraces the scientist-as-persuader identity, viewing what should be his hypothesis as his religion and data as simply a point for persuasion, an overt rejection of the scientific method.

Implicit Bias Research Today

Strong claims were initially made for the research findings on implicit research and particularly the validity of the IAT as a measure of implicit bias. Similarly, strong claims have also been made about the efficacy of implicit bias training. What is its status today?

While many evaluations of the IAT have been carried out by critics (e.g., Blanton et al., 2009; Oswald et al., 2015), the recent meta-analysis (based on 295 studies) carried out by the originators of the IAT, Greenwald and Banaji, and their collaborators (Kurdi et al., 2018) is unlikely to be influenced by negative priors. Their key finding is the low average effect size of 0.14 for the IAT.[4] Forscher et al. (2019) have carried out a meta-analysis of 494 studies of efforts to change implicit bias (also see Lai et al., 2014; Lai et al., 2016). Most effects were weak (<0.30). Most importantly, they demonstrated that changes in implicit bias do not lead to changes in behavior. Although Forscher et al.'s and Lai et al.'s research does not directly evaluate the effectiveness of corporate implicit bias training programs on behavior, their work raises serious questions about their likely effect. We not that the originators of the IAT and their associates should be commended for publishing these results, given its potential implications.

---

[4] The general rule of thumb is that an effect size of 0.2 is considered small, 0.5 is medium, and 0.8 is large (Cohen, 1992).

The Tragedy of the Scientific Commons

The dynamics we have described present a unique commons dilemma: The individual idea entrepreneur, whose legitimacy rests on the authority of science to support his or her claims, has an incentive to operate in ways that potentially undermine that authority. Ideas are *not* the scarce resource in this commons dilemma. Indeed, we are in a state of overload and noisy overcommunication where there is an oversupply of ideas. But as particular idea entrepreneurs over-communicate, over-claim, and over-extend across this boundary, it is the trust, legitimacy, and authority of science that becomes the collective resource that individual researchers have motivation to overuse, even exploit.

The growing mistrust of science—and authority in general—is a broader social phenomenon that goes beyond idea entrepreneurs and their actions, though it is often generated by idea entrepreneurs and their actions. Gillian Tett notes, "In our everyday lives, we are moving from a system based around vertical axes of trust, where we trust people who seem to have more authority than we do, to one predicated on horizontal axes of trust: we take advice from our peer group."[5] Specifically, whereas people are more skeptical of vertical players—from government to academic experts—they are increasingly comfortable learning horizontally, within tribes of those with like-minded belief.

One strategy idea entrepreneurs have often adopted as they've crossed the academia/public divide is to join the tribe: operating as a horizontal player, sharing chatty stories by the campfire, and dispensing personal advice. In the process, however, these tribal scientists have often shaped the viewpoint that all scientists are merely part of a very particular tribe—politically left-wing, and antagonistic to conservatives (Cofnas, 2015; Gross, 2013; Jussim et al., 2016; Martin, 2000; Redding, 2001) in the case of social scientists researching implied bias, for example, and politically right-wing and anti-liberal and anti-centrist, in the case of television scientists who deny the climate crisis, as another. This tribalism means that scientific ideas are owned—not only by science in general or even by specific individuals—but by particular political tribes. As a further example, we note that implicit bias and "checking one's privilege" are embraced by "woke" liberals, and the heretics who question this orthodoxy risk being labeled "racists."

---

[5] https://www.ft.com/content/24035fc2-3e45-11e6-9f2c-36b487ebd80a

The reputational danger for the scientific commons in this dynamic is that science becomes just one of many content producers competing for eyeballs in a "post-truth society" where the veracity of an idea may be irrelevant to the attention it receives, its dissemination, and its acceptance (Keyes, 2004). What is more relevant than truth is that an idea is interesting, extreme, and emotional and aligns with preexisting beliefs. In Frankfurt's even starker terms (1988), viral science involves producing content in a bullshit culture—that is to say, where speech is designed to persuade without regard for truth (also see Wakeham, 2017). When scientists own, sell, and operate as partisan advocates for ideas, science becomes a part of this dynamic, rather than remaining above it.

Moving Forward

At this point the reader may well be totally discouraged about the prospects for a healthy relationship between science and the public. What might fix this wicked problem? Certainly, the prospect of the public becoming a sufficiently effective agent of accountability seems doubtful. In viral science, it is public demand that motivates scientists and the media to transform research into fast, convenient, easily digestible fragments that resemble folklore. The public does not hold science accountable for the pseudoscience they are fed because their hunger for what is meaningful, interesting, and apparently useful crowds out what is true. This incentive structure sets in motion the dilemma of the scientific commons and ends with diminishing public trust over the long run in scientific authority. The question, then, is whether there is any hope that science, perhaps in partnership with the media, might have the ability to establish effective norms of accountability. History provides some possible guidance.

The Hutchins Commission?

During World War II, the publisher Henry Luce and Robert Hutchins (president of the University of Chicago) formed the Hutchins Commission (Commission on the Freedom of the Press) to clarify the role of media in democracy. At the time—similar to ours in the early 21st century—journalists were under scrutiny, facing suspicions about their sensationalistic tactics designed to entertain rather than educate and inform. The Commission noted that the power of the media had become concentrated in fewer and fewer hands with the more powerful technologies of radio and mass-published newspapers gaining power over local news and other media, and that those with this control had not served the public in a socially responsible manner. As such, Luce and Hutchins asserted, society needed to take control for its own protection. While the Commission noted Charles Beard's point that at its inception, freedom of the press had "little or nothing to do with truth telling" (1947, p. 131), the loss of public trust had become a dilemma without a perfect solution. The Commission sought methods to raise media standards and social responsibility. While suspicious of government regulation, it hoped to see self-regulation emerge from the media itself (Blanchard, 1977). The Commission's strategies included encouraging more communication outlets (to counteract the concentration of ownership) and more public and direct criticism (to correct biased, false information). In addition and most relevant here, the Commission produced a conversation about journalistic ethics, particularly adhering to truth and accuracy, which now forms the basis for critical components of the curriculum in journalism schools. These standards are now formalized in the Society of Professional Journalists Code of Ethics, the first section of which is titled "Seek Truth and Report It" (https://www.spj.org/ethicscode.asp).

A New Hutchins Commission?

We suggest that now may well be the time for a new commission, involving academic professional associations in the social and physical sciences and the media. Academic associations have a clear vested interest in maintaining the authority of science. Most, if not all, academic associations have a code of ethics, so establishing guidelines for what the appropriate norms for the interactions between scientists and the media should be would easily fall under their jurisdiction.[6]

---

[6] Although we believe that it is important to encourage academic disagreement, we also recognize it can be painful for the community: what one side might see as healthy debate that is a natural part of self-correction in science, another might see as bullying and indeed, methodological terrorism (https://www.businessinsider.com.au/susan-fiske-methodological-terrorism-qa-2016-9). The public learns little when academic controversy devolves into mud-slinging. Clarifying the norms of engagement, perhaps via professional code of conduct, could well be beneficial.

New expectations of scientists are needed. Rather than operating as simply content producers, scientists should first and foremost transfer the rules of the scientific method, with clear tests and demonstrable outcome measures, to the public and the media. For instance, a year after the Starbucks incident and all the publicity surrounding implicit bias training as a solution, we have not seen any measures of accountability: that is, has this training actually improved the situation? We note one unfortunate incident at a Starbucks after the company-wide training where a Filipino American customer and former veteran had his name changed from "John" to "Chang" on his coffee order by an employee. This occurred a week after that store held its implicit bias training (Murdock, 2018). At present, even in universities, where scientists should appreciate and demand empirical evaluation, diversity training, including IAT-based programs, has proliferated with few demands to demonstrate proof of their effectiveness.

In addition to demanding proof of effectiveness, replication should be another expectation. As the social sciences navigate their relationship with journalists, it is important that there be an openness to new findings and skepticism until they have been extensively replicated. In the hard sciences, no finding is considered established until it has been replicated multiple times.[7]

The media also has a vested interest in maintaining its authority. Here the question would be the need to extend journalism's current norms. Recently, Jack Beatty, a highly regarded and honored journalist, suggested, in the context of fact-checking President Trump, that the news media, especially major TV outlets, should not provide access to people if there is a reasonable possibility that their statements are inaccurate or untrue (WBUR, On Point, January 11, 2019). This is a most interesting suggestion. Obviously, if the president of the United States makes a statement and the news media reports on it, there is no factual issue as to what the president said; there is, however, the question of whether what was claimed is in fact accurate or true. Beatty's suggestion seems to be that members of the media have not only the obligation to accurately report what someone says, but the responsibility to ensure the accuracy and truthfulness of the statement's content.

Perhaps a similar principle should apply to the media's reporting on scientific findings. In the context of science, the Beatty proposal could be

---

[7] One positive example of accountability in the social sciences is the Reproducibility Project, a collaboration of 270 researchers coordinated by Brian Nosek. This team replicated approximately 40% of 100 studies in top psychological journals (Baker 2015), an outcome reported widely in the media.

understood as requiring that the media only report science that has gone through peer review and been replicated or, at the least, indicate the degree of acceptance of the reported findings within the scientific community. As we noted earlier, many researchers have raised questions about the applicability of lab-based implicit bias research and in particular the IAT in workplace settings. Although some of this was reported in the media, it was done in separate stories, not in the original articles, so it has been difficult for laypeople to know that there has been serious academic disagreement.

How might a new commission come about? It would certainly take strong leadership from both academia and journalism. It could be a worthy project for the National Academy of Sciences, although it would also require foundation support. Perhaps there are other, better alternatives. In suggesting a new Hutchins-type commission, we advance only one possible way of moving forward.

Conclusion

We contend that scientific content, conveyed in a viral form by idea entrepreneurs, can undermine the public authority of science. The public in its hunger for meaning is more likely to be persuaded by the emotive content of a message, its consistency with their existing beliefs, and the degree to which it provides solutions to existing problems than with the actual veracity of the report. Academics are sometimes motivated by both money and fame to promote their research. In doing so they are likely to be become overly committed to their research findings in contradistinction, as required by the scientific method, to searching for disconfirming evidence. In doing so, there is the danger that in making their research as attractive to the public as possible, they will overstate the strength of their findings (strong causality), the breadth of their applicability (elastic effects), and the reliability of their results. This confluence of scholarly and public incentives creates the potential for a "tragedy of the commons" where individual scientists are motivated to exploit the public authority of science at the potential long-term cost of greatly diminishing science's overall perceived integrity and reliability.

We argue that scientists should transfer scientific content to the public accurately and with epistemic humility. However, they should openly and publicly embrace the scientific method's cycle of claim—refutation—claim. Although we have discussed a number of cases in this chapter, our principal focus to examine the effect of public expectations and idea entrepreneurship on the role of science in the world is on the use of implicit bias research by corporations and other institutions in bias-reduction training. We do not question the research itself, but rather the ease with which it has been unquestionably applied outside the research laboratory. We end by proposing a new Hutchins Commission of academics and journalists, the goal of which would be to produce appropriate and effective norms for scholars and the media for transferring scientific research to the public.

Acknowledgments

We would like to thank Jonathan Imber, Lee Jussim, and Greg Mitchell for comments on an earlier draft. Genevieve Butler and Rahel O'More provided excellent editorial assistance. Of course, any issues with the paper are the authors' responsibility.

Authors' Note

The chapter authors are listed in alphabetical order.

References

Azar, B. (2008). IAT: Fad or fabulous? *APA Monitor, 39*, 7. http://www.apa.org/monitor/2008/07-08/psychometric.aspx

Baker, M. (2015). Over half of psychology studies fail reproducibility test. *Nature News, 27*.

Berger, J., & Schwartz, E. M. (2011). What drives immediate and ongoing word of mouth?. *Journal of Marketing Research, 48*(5), 869–880.

Bezrukova, K., Spell, C. S., Perry, J. L., & Jehn, K. A. (2016). A meta-analytical integration of over 40 years of research on diversity training evaluation. *Psychological Bulletin, 142*(11), 1227–1274.

Bielby, W. T. (2005). Applying social research on stereotyping and cognitive bias to employment discrimination litigation: The case of allegations of systematic gender bias at Wal-Mart stores. In *Handbook of Employment Discrimination Research* (pp. 395–408). Springer, New York, NY.

Blanchard, M. A. (1977). The Hutchins Commission, the press and the responsibility concept. *Journalism Monographs*, 49.

Blanton, H., Jaccard, J., Klick, J., Mellers, B., Mitchell, G., & Tetlock, P. (2009). Strong claims and weak evidence: Reassessing the predictive validity of the race IAT. *Journal of Applied Psychology, 94*(3), 567–582.

Burt, R. S. (1992). *Structural holes*. Cambridge, MA: Harvard University Press.
Chabris, C. (2013). The trouble with Malcolm Gladwell. *Slate*. http://www.slate.com/articles/health_and_science/science/2013/10/malcolm_gladwell_critique_david_and_goliath_misrepresents_the_science.html
Chakravarti, A., Menon, T., & Winship, C. (2014). Contact and group structure: A natural experiment of interracial college roommate groups. *Organizational Science*, 25(4), 1216–1233.
Churchman, C. W. (1967). Wicked problems. *Management Science*, 14(4), B141–B146.
Cialdini, R. B. (2006). *Influence: The Psychology of Persuasion* (rev. ed.). Harper Business.
Cofnas, N. (2015). Science Is Not Always 'Self-Correcting': Fact–Value Conflation and the Study of Intelligence. *Foundations of Science*, 21, 477.
Cohen, J. (1992) A power primer. *Psychological Bulletin*, 112(1), 155.
Cohen, M. D., March, J. G., & Olsen, J. P. (1972). A garbage can model of organizational choice. *Administrative Science Quarterly*, 17(1), 1–25.
Engber, D. (2017, May 17). Daryl Bem proved ESP is real. *Slate*. https://slate.com/health-and-science/2017/06/daryl-bem-proved-esp-is-real-showed-science-is-broken.html
Evans, J. A., & Foster, J. G. (2011). Metaknowledge. *Science*, 331, 721–725.
Fazio, R., Jackson, J., Dunton, B., & Williams, C. (1995). Variability in automatic activation as an unobtrusive measure of racial attitudes: A bona fide pipeline? *Journal of Personality and Social Psychology*, 69, 1013–1027.
Fazio, R., & Olson, M. (2002, August 6). Implicit measures in social cognition research: Their meaning and use. *Annual Review of Psychology*, 54, 297–327.
Feintzeig, R., & Jargon, J. (2018, May 26). In antibias training, Starbucks enlists hip-hop artist Common, chairman Howard Schultz. *Wall Street Journal*. https://www.wsj.com/articles/in-anti-bias-training-starbucks-enlists-hip-hop-artist-common-chairman-howard-schultz-1527332400?mod=e2f
Forscher, P., Lai, C., Axt, J., Ebersole, C. R., Herman, M., Devine, P. & Nosek, B. (2019). A meta-analysis of change in implicit bias.
Foundation for Child and Development and the Brookings Institution. (2006, March 28). The Education Flatline: Causes and Solutions. https://www.brookings.edu/wp-content/uploads/2016/06/0328education_haskins.pdf
Frankfurt, H. 1988. *On Bullshit. The Importance of What We Care About: Philosophical Essays*. Cambridge University Press.
Gawronski, B., Morrison, M., Phills, C. E., & Galdi, S. (2017). Temporal stability of implicit and explicit measures: A longitudinal analysis. *Personality and Social Psychology Bulletin*, 43(3), 300–312.
Geertz, C. (1973). *The Interpretation of Cultures*. Basic Books.
Gordon, D. (2006). A Short History of School Reform. Paper presented at The Foundation for Child Development and the Brookings Institution, pp. 8–17. https://www.brookings.edu/wp-content/uploads/2016/06/0328education_haskins.pdf
Greenwald, A. G., & Banaji, M. R. (1995). Implicit social cognition: Attitudes, self-esteem, and stereotypes. *Psychological Review*, 102, 4–27.
Greenwald, A. G., Banaji, M. R., Rudman, L., Farnham, S., Nosek, B. A., & Mellott, D. (2002). A unified theory of implicit attitudes, stereotypes, self-esteem, and self-concept. *Psychological Review*, 109, 3–25.
Greenwald, A. G., McGhee, D. E., & Schwartz, J. K. L. (1998). Measuring individual differences in implicit cognition: The Implicit Association Test. *Journal of Personality and Social Psychology*, 74, 1464–1480.

Gross, N. (2013). *Why Are Professors Liberal and Why Do Conservatives Care?* Harvard University Press.

Hamilton, D. L., & Gifford, R. K. (1976). Illusory correlation in interpersonal perception: A cognitive basis of stereotypic judgments. *Journal of Experimental Social Psychology, 12*, 392–407.

Heath, C. (1996). Do people prefer to pass along good news or bad news? Valence and relevance of news as a predictor of transmission propensity. *Organizational Behavior and Human Decision Processes, 68*, 79–94.

Heath, C., Bell, C., & Sternberg, E. (2001). Emotional selection in memes: The case of urban legends. *Journal of Personality and Social Psychology, 81*, 1028–1041.

Hunt, R. R., & Worthen, J. B. (2006). *Distinctiveness and Memory*. Oxford University Press.

James, T. (2018, December 23). Can cops unlearn their unconscious biases? *The Atlantic*. https://www.theatlantic.com/politics/archive/2017/12/implicit-bias-training-salt-lake/548996/.

Jussim, L., Crawford, J. T., Stevens, S. T., Anglin, S. A., & Duarte, J. L. (2016). Can high moral purposes undermine scientific integrity? In J. Forgas, L. Jussim, & P. van Lange (Eds.), *The Social Psychology of Morality* (pp. 173–195). Taylor and Francis.

Kahneman, D. (2011). *Thinking, Fast and Slow*. Farrar, Straus & Giroux.

Kahneman, D., & Fredrick, S. (2002). The Psychology of Intuitive Judgment, Thomas Gilovich, Dale Griffin, Daniel Kahneman, Heuristics and Biases.

Kahneman, D., & Tversky, A. (1979). Prospect theory: An analysis of decision under risk. *Econometrica, 47*(2), 263.

Kalev, A., Dobbin, F., & Kelly, E. (2006). Best practices or best guesses? Assessing the efficacy of corporate affirmative action and diversity policies. *American Sociological Review, 71*(4), 589–617.

Kay, A. C., Whitson, J. A., Gaucher, D., & Galinsky, A. D. (2009). Compensatory control achieving order through the mind, our institutions, and the heavens. *Current Directions in Psychological Science, 18*(5), 264–268.

Keyes, R. (2004) *The Post-Truth Era: Dishonesty and Deception in Contemporary Life*. St. Martin's Press.

Klayman, J., & Ha, Y. (1987). Confirmation, disconfirmation, and information in hypothesis testing. *Psychological Review, 94*(2), 211–228.

Kramer, T. & Block, L. (2008), Conscious and non-conscious components of superstitious beliefs in judgment and decision-making. *Journal of Consumer Research, 36*, 783–793.

Kruglanski, A. W. (1980). Lay epistemology process and contents. *Psychological Review, 87*, 70–87.

Kruglanski, A. W., & Freund, T. (1983). The freezing and unfreezing of lay-inferences: Effects on impressional primacy, ethnic stereotyping, and numerical anchoring. *Journal of Experimental Social Psychology, 19*, 448–468.

Kurdi, B., Seitchik, A. E., Axt, J., Carroll, T., Karapetyan, A., Kaushik, N., Tomezsko, D., Greenwald, A. G., & Banaji, M. R. (2018, March 2). Predicting intergroup discrimination using the Implicit Association Test: Meta-analysis and recommendations for future research. http://doi.org/10.17605/OSF.IO/SVNTJ

Lai, C. K., Marini, M., Lehr, S. A., Cerruti, C., Shin, J. L., Joy-Gaba, J. A., Ho, A. K., Teachman, B. A., Wojcik, S. P., Koleva, S. P., Frazier, R. S., Heiphetz, L., Chen, E., Turner, R. N., Haidt, J., Kesebir, S., Hawkins, C. B., Schaefer, H. S., Rubichi, S., ... Nosek, B. A. (2014). Reducing implicit racial preferences: I. A comparative investigation of 17 interventions. *Journal of Experimental Psychology: General, 143*, 1765–1785.

Lai, C. K., Skinner, A. L., Cooley, E., Murrar, S., Brauer, M., Devos, T., Calanchini, J., Xiao, Y. J., Pedram, C., Marshburn, C. K., Simon, S., Blanchar, J. C., Joy-Gaba, J. A., Conway, J., Redford, L., Klein, R. A., Roussos, G., Schellhaas, F. M. H., Burns, M., ... Nosek, B. A. (2016). Reducing implicit racial preferences: II. Intervention effectiveness across time. *Journal of Experimental Psychology: General, 145*, 1001–1016.

Lipman, J. (2018, January 25). How diversity training infuriates men and fails women. *Time*. http://time.com/5118035/diversity-training-infuriates-men-fails-women/

Mak, A. (2018, April 20). What can Starbucks accomplish? *Slate*. https://slate.com/technology/2018/04/does-implicit-bias-training-work-starbucks-racial-bias-plan-will-probably-fail.html

Martin, B. (2000). Directions for liberation science. *Philosophy and Social Action, 26*, 9–21.

McGregor, J. (2018, April 19). Anatomy of a PR response: How Starbucks is handling its Philadelphia crisis. *Washington Post*. https://www.washingtonpost.com/news/on-leadership/wp/2018/04/19/anatomy-of-a-pr-response-how-starbucks-is-handling-its-philadelphia-crisis/

Menon, T., & Thompson, L. (2016). *Stop Spending, Start Managing: Five Ways to Transform Wasteful Habits*. Cambridge, MA. Harvard Business Review Press.

Mitchell, G., & Tetlock, P. (2017). Popularity as a poor proxy for utility: The case of implicit prejudice. In S. O. Lilienfeld & I. D. Waldman (Eds.), *Psychological Science Under Scrutiny: Recent Challenges and Proposed Solutions*. Virginia Public Law and Legal Theory Research Paper No. 2017-32. https://ssrn.com/abstract=2973929

Monin, B., & Miller, D. T. (2001). Moral credentials and the expression of prejudice. *Journal of Personality and Social Psychology, 81*(1), 33.

Mook, D. G. (1983). In defense of external invalidity. *American Psychologist, 38*, 379–387.

Moscovici, S., Lage, E., & Naffrechoux, M. (1969). Influence of a consistent minority on the responses of a majority in a color perception task. *Sociometry, 32*, 365–380.

Murdock, J. (2018, December 3). Starbucks barista changed Filipino-American Air Force veteran's name from John to Chang. https://www.newsweek.com/starbucks-barista-changed-filipino-american-customers-name-john-chang-1240548

Nordell, J. (2017, May 7). Is this how discrimination ends? *The Atlantic*. https://www.theatlantic.com/science/archive/2017/05/unconscious-bias-training/525405/

Nosek, B. A., Greenwald, A. G., & Banaji, M. R. (2005). Understanding and using the Implicit Association Test: II. Method variables and construct validity. *Personality and Social Psychology Bulletin, 31*(2), 166–180.

O'Connor, A. (2016, September 9). How the sugar industry shifted blame to fat. *New York Times*. https://www.nytimes.com/2016/09/13/well/eat/how-the-sugar-industry-shifted-blame-to-fat.html

Oswald, F., Mitchell, G., Blanton, H., Jaccard, J., & Tetlock, P. E. (2015). Revisiting the predictive validity of the Implicit Association Test. *Journal of Personality and Social Psychology, 105*, 171–192.

Payne, B. K., Burkley, M. A., & Stokes, M. B. (2008). Why do implicit and explicit attitude tests diverge? The role of structural fit. *Journal of Personality and Social Psychology, 94*, 16–31.

Project Implicit. https://implicit.harvard.edu/implicit/

Pronin, E., Gilovich, T., & Ross, L. (2004). Objectivity in the eye of the beholder: Divergent perceptions of bias in self versus others. *Psychological Review, 111*(3), 781.

Redding, R. E. (2001). Sociopolitical diversity in psychology: The case for pluralism. *American Psychologist, 56*(3), 205.

Rein, M., & Winship, C. (1997). Policy entrepreneurs and the academic establishment: The bell curve controversy. In E. White (Ed.), *Intelligence, Political Inequality and Public Policy* (pp. 18–47). Praeger.

Rein, M., & Winship, C. (1999). The dangers of strong causal reasoning: Root causes, social science, and poverty policy. *Society*, 38–46.

Ross, L. (1977). The intuitive psychologist and his shortcomings: Distortions in the attribution process. In *Advances in experimental social psychology* (Vol. 10, pp. 173–220). Academic Press.

Rozin, P., & Royzman, E. B. (2001). Negativity bias, negativity dominance, and contagion. *Personality and Social Psychology Review*, 5, 296–320.

Simmons, J., Nelson, L., & Simonsohn, U. (2011). False-positive psychology: Undisclosed flexibility in data collection and analysis allow presenting anything as significant. *Psychological Science*, 22, 1359–1366.

Swidler, A. (1986). Culture in action: Symbols and strategies. *American Sociological Review*, 51(2), 273–286.

Tetlock, P. E. (1985). Accountability: The neglected social context of judgment and choice. In B. Staw & L. Cummings (Eds.), *Research in Organizational Behavior* (Vol. 7, pp. 297–332). JAI Press.

Tetlock, P. E. (1994). Political psychology or politicized psychology: Is the road to scientific hell paved with good moral intentions? *Political Psychology*, 15, 509–530

Tetlock, P. E. (2005). *Expert Political Judgment: How Good Is It? How Can We Know?* Princeton University Press.

Tetlock, P. E. (2012). Rational and irrational prejudices: How problematic is the ideological lopsidedness of social-personality psychology? *Perspectives in Psychological Science*, 7, 519–521.

Tversky, A., & Kahneman, D. (1974). Judgment under uncertainty: Heuristics and biases. *Science*, 185, 1124–1131.

U.S. Supreme Court. (2011). *Wal-Mart Stores, Inc. v. Dukes et al.*, Certiorari to the United States Court of Appeals for the Ninth Circuit, No 10-277. https://www.supremecourt.gov/opinions/10pdf/10-277.pdf

Vosoughi, S., Roy, D., & Aral, S. (2018). The spread of true and false news online. *Science*, 359(6380), 1146–1151.

Vyse, S. A. (2013). *Believing in magic: The psychology of superstition-updated edition*. Oxford University Press.

Wakeham, J. (2017). Bullshit as a problem of social epistemology. *Sociological Theory*, 35(1), 15–38.

Wang, C. S., Whitson, J. A., & Menon, T. (2012). Culture, control, and illusory pattern perception. *Social Psychological and Personality Science*, 3(5), 630–638. https://www.wbur.org/radio/programs/onpoint/archive/2019/01/11

Whitson, J. A., & Galinsky, A. D. (2008). Lacking control increases illusory pattern perception. *Science*, 322(5898), 115–117.

Whitson, J., Kim, J., Wang, J., Menon, T., & Webster B. (2019). Regulatory focus and conspiratorial perceptions: The importance of personal control. *Personality and Social Psychology Bulletin*, 45(1), 3–15.

Index

For the benefit of digital users, indexed terms that span two pages (e.g., 52–53) may, on occasion, appear on only one of those pages.

Tables and figures are indicated by *t* and *f* following the page number.

Abdullahi v. Pfizer, 381
academic associations, 415
academic culture. *See* scientific culture
academic misconduct. *See* misconduct
accommodational hypothesizing. *See* HARKing
accountability, establishing norms of, 414–17
accumulation of evidence, focusing on, 31–32
accuracy
  causes of problematic behaviors, 18–20
  overview of issues in scientific practice, 5
  proposed solutions, 26–30
accuracy goals, and motivated reasoning, 229–30
accuracy in social psychology textbooks
  Asch conformity experiments, 129–30
  Berkowitz and LePage weapons effect, 138–39
  Darley and Latané bystander intervention, 139–42, 140*t*, 141*t*
  Festinger and Carlsmith forced compliance dissonance, 133–35
  Jones and Harris correspondent inferences, 137–38
  Milgram obedience research, 135–37
  overview, 129
  Rosenthal and Jacobson teacher expectations, 142–43, 143*t*
  Sherif intergroup competition, 131–33
admissions at Berkeley, 232
adversarial collaborations, 59–60, 246–48

African Americans
  racial stereotype threats and test performance of, 237–38
  syphilis experiments on, 378–79
aggregation bias, 332–34
aggression, weapons effect on, 127–29, 138–39, 145–46, 146*t*
Akert, R. M., 124–30, 126*t*, 132–33, 134–35, 136–38, 139, 140–41, 142–44
Albers, C. J., 232–33
aleatoric probability, 176–77
alpha (α) level, 74–75, 309
alternative hypotheses
  in frequentist testing, 183
  pitting against each other, 248–49
American Bar Association Rules on Standards for Treatment of Prisoners, 382
American Economic Association (AEA) Randomized Controlled Trial Registry, 50–52, 52*f*, 54
American Political Science Review (journal), 363
American Statistical Association, 188, 243
ampliative inference, 180
analytical methods, improved, 45–50. *See also specific analytical methods*; statistical inference
Anderson, M. L., 49
Angrist, J. D., 43
Annual Review of Psychology (journal), 234–35
antidepressants, scientific myths about, 227–28
Arizona State University, 378n.26

424   INDEX

Aronson, E., 124–30, 126t, 132–33, 134–35, 136–38, 139, 140–41, 142–44
Aronson, J., 237–38
Asch, S. E., 127–30, 145–46, 146t
assumptions, statistical
  generalizing Type IV error, 325–27
  role in type III errors, 317–18
  and type III error definitions, 323–24
as-you-go scientific communication, 276n.5
Augusteijn, H. E. M., 167
author bias, 39–40, 42. *See also* publication bias
authority of institutional review boards, 375–76
authors
  gift authorship, 271–72
  impact bias related to, 364–65
  questionable research practices initiated by, 270–72, 273
  status bias related to, 361–63

Babbage, C., 109
Bacon, F., 248
bacteria, as primary cause of ulcers, 226–27
badges, for transparency, 22–23
bad results, publishing good research with, 276–77
Banaji, M. R., 239, 397–98, 412
Banerjee, P., 249
Banks, G. C., 346
Barber, T. X., 295n.1
Bargh, J. A., 240
Barnes, L. W., 377n.25
Bayes, T., 179
Bayes factor, 190, 191, 192–93, 193f
Bayesian probability. *See* epistemic probability
Bayesian statistical approaches, 298
  embracing methodological rigor, 280–81
  estimation, 193–97, 195f
  general discussion, 198–99
  limiting questionable interpretive practices, 243–44
  mathematical likelihood, 191
  and origins of frequentist inference, 181
  overview, 176
  "scientific" property of probability, 178–79
  software, 197–98, 198f
  statistical inference, 180
  testing overview, 190–91
  testing with likelihood ratios, 192–93, 193f
  type III or IV errors in, 334
  updating, 188–89
Bayes' theorem, 178–80, 181, 189
Beatty, J., 416–17
Becker, B. J., 162
behavioral priming, 76–77
behavioral research. *See* research integrity; *specific aspects of research integrity*
Beilock, S. L., 78
believing, psychology of, 406–10
Belmont Study, 373
Bem, D., 82–83, 411–12
Bem Sex-Role Inventory (BSRI), 328–30
benign behavioral interventions, exemptions for, 373
benign neglect approach to replicability crisis, 84–86
Benjamini, Y., 50
Berge, L. I. O., 57, 58
Berkeley, University of California at, 232
Berkowitz, L., 127–29, 138–39, 145–46, 146t
Bertrand, M., 46–47
Best Practices in Science Conference, 3
between-groups analysis of variance, 325–26
bias-corrected meta-analyses
  fail-safe N and trim and fill, 162–63
  general discussion, 167
  meta-regression, 166–67
  overview, 162
  selection models, 163–65
bias(es). *See also* gender bias; implicit bias research; publication bias; questionable interpretive practices
  aggregation, 332–34
  causes of problematic behaviors, 16–18
  citation, 233–35, 233t, 234t
  confirmation, 250, 295–96, 296t
  disconfirmation, 295–96, 296t
  empirical research questions about, 10
  gray-literature, 101

INDEX   425

impact, 363–65
of institutional review boards, 376–77
investigator, types of, 295–96, 296t
negativity, 407
overturn, 344–45
overview of possible solutions, 6
reporting, and creation of scientific myths, 228
researcher, stimulus sampling connections to, 206
risk of, assessing in systematic reviews, 159–60, 161
selection, 154, 156
small-study, 101–2
social desirability, 235–36
status, 361–63
stimulus sampling connections to, 206
Bickel, P. J., 232
Bielby, W., 408–9
binomial test, Bayesian, 197–98, 198f
biomedicine. *See also* institutional review boards
creation of scientific myths in, 226–27
statistical inference in, 198–99
Bishop, D. V. M., 301–2
bistable perception, 192–93, 194–97
blinded data analysis, 244, 309
blind peer-review process, 270–73, 362–63
blind spots, 231–35, 233t, 234t
Bonferroni correction, 49
Boston Foundation *Science for the Public*, 400
Boston Medical and Surgical Journal, 275, 276–77
Boyle, R., 109
Brodeur, A., 39–40, 44, 45–46, 342–43
BSRI (Bem Sex-Role Inventory), 328–30
bullshit culture, 414
Buss, D. M., 328–29, 330–31, 332
bystander intervention
accuracy of presentation in textbooks, 139–42, 140t, 141t
as core social psychology experiment, 127–29
retention of information by students, 145–46, 146t

caliper test, 40, 301
canonization, 225–26, 242–43, 251, 251t

capitalization on chance, 295–96, 296t
Card, D., 47, 48
caring about research question, relation to problematic behavior, 16–17
Carlin, J., 298, 321–22, 323–24
Carlsmith, J. M., 127–29, 133–35, 145–46, 146t, 212–13
Carpenter, K. M., 321–22, 323–24
Carter, E. C., 83, 155, 163, 165, 167
Caruso, E. M., 78
Casey, K., 50, 54–56, 55t, 61
causal components of theory, type III error and, 321–22
causal map, lack of valid, 404
Ceci, S. J., 233–34, 233t, 235–36
cell means, focusing on, 324–25
Center for Advanced Study in the Behavioral Sciences (CASBS) Scientific Integrity Group, 3
Center for Drug Evaluation and Research (CDER), 52–53
Center for Open Science, 51–52
chance, as kind of probability, 176–77
Chartrand, T. L., 240
cherry-picking
erroneous interpretations under, 54–56, 55t
in narrative reviews, 159
as questionable interpretive practice, 231–35, 233t, 234t
children with intellectual disabilities, research involving, 379–81
China, study of detainees in, 385–87
chrysalis effect, 5, 263
CI (confidence interval), in frequentist estimation, 186–88
Cialdini, R. B., 124–30, 126t, 132–33, 134–35, 136–38, 139, 140–41, 142–44
citation biases, 233–35, 233t, 234t
citation coercion, 272, 273
citation counts, as cause of problematic behaviors, 13–14
citation errors, empirical research questions about, 11–12
civility, in peer review, 359–61
Class 1 designation, 86–87, 88
Class 2 designation, 86–87, 88
Class 3 designation, 86–87, 88

classic findings in social psychology
  Asch conformity experiments, 129–30
  Berkowitz and LePage weapons effect, 138–39
  Darley and Latané bystander intervention, 139–42, 140t, 141t
  Festinger and Carlsmith forced compliance dissonance, 133–35
  general discussion, 146–48
  identification of, 123–29, 125t, 126t
  Jones and Harris correspondent inferences, 137–38
  Milgram obedience research, 135–37
  overview, 122–23
  retention of information by students, 144–46, 145t, 146t
  Rosenthal and Jacobson teacher expectations, 142–43, 143t
  Sherif intergroup competition, 131–33
classic studies, references to in textbooks, 6
clear mental model, lack of, 404
clinical trial registry, 50–52, 52f, 54
clinical trials involving children, 380–81
Clinton, W., 378–79
Cochrane reviews, 161–62
coding issues, in meta-analysis, 156
coding materials, openly sharing, 22
Coffman, L. C., 58
cognitive dissonance experiment
  accuracy of presentation in textbooks, 133–35
  as core social psychology experiment, 127–29
  retention of information by students, 145–46, 146t
cognitive neuroscience, 85–86
cognitive psychology, credibility crisis in, 84–86. See also credibility crisis in psychological literature
Cohen, M. D., 404
collaborations limiting questionable interpretive practices, 246–48
collective, in frequentist notion of probability, 177
comment sections, for journals, 27–28
Commission on the Freedom of the Press (Hutchins Commission), 414–15

commitment to ideas, 411–12
Common Rule (Federal Policy for the Protection of Human Subjects), 373n.13
communication of research to public. See public, relationship between science and
competing-point hypothesis, in Bayesian testing, 192–93, 193f
Competitive Reaction Time Task (CRTT), 157–58
complete transparency, 15–16
complexity, role in problematic behaviors, 19–20
conceptual boundaries, stimulus definitions with respect to, 214
confidence interval (CI), in frequentist estimation, 186–88
confirmation bias, 250, 295–96, 296t
confirmatory data analysis, 318–19
conflicts of interest, financial, 410–11
conformity experiments
  accuracy of presentation in textbooks, 129–30
  as core social psychology experiment, 127–29
  retention of information by students, 145–46, 146t
conjugate families of distributions, 194–97, 195f
conservative labeling proposal, 86–88
conservative political ideology, 345–46
conspiracist ideation, 241
constrained greed p-hacking, 304–5, 314, 315f
construct validity
  need for attention to in peer review, 360–61
  related to stimulus sampling, 211–12
  type III errors related to, 328–30
context, stimulus definitions with respect to, 215
continuing education, reducing questionable research practices through, 277–78
controversial studies, p-hacking in, 306–7, 307f, 308

core experiments in social psychology
    Asch conformity experiments, 129–30
    Berkowitz and LePage weapons effect, 138–39
    Darley and Latané bystander intervention, 139–42, 140t, 141t
    Festinger and Carlsmith forced compliance dissonance, 133–35
    general discussion, 146–48
    identification of, 123–29, 125t, 126t
    Jones and Harris correspondent inferences, 137–38
    Milgram obedience research, 135–37
    retention of information by students, 144–46, 145t, 146t
    Rosenthal and Jacobson teacher expectations, 142–43, 143t
    Sherif intergroup competition, 131–33
correcting for multiple tests, 48–50
correlations, confusing with means, 241
correspondent inferences experiment
    accuracy of presentation in textbooks, 137–38
    as core social psychology experiment, 127–29
    retention of information by students, 145–46, 146t
Council for International Organizations of Medical Sciences, 387–88
counterintuitive effects/papers, 128
    and incentives, 13–14, 32
    and research transmission, 407
    and results-blind review, 352–53
courageous collaborations, 246–48
Crawford, J. T, 246–47, 248
credibility crisis in psychological literature, 260–61, 263. *See also* crisis narrative about science; questionable research practices; research integrity
    arguments about overstated nature of, 74–80
    benign neglect approach to, 84–86
    emergence of, 71–72
    honest conservative labeling proposal, 86–88
    meta-analyses to correct for, 81–84
    overview, 70–71
    recent evidence of widespread published error, 72–74
    suggestions for dealing with, 81–88
crisis narrative about science, 260–61, 263. *See also* research integrity; *specific problematic behaviors*
    false research findings, 102–4
    general discussion, 112–15
    increase in prevalence and impact, evidence on, 109–12
    non-replicability of research, 104–9
    number of scientists engaging in misconduct, 94–95
    overview, 93–94
    prevalence of misconduct and questionable practices, 95–102
criterial control systems, 297
critical appraisal, in systematic reviews, 159–60, 161
criticism
    open post-publication peer review, 366–67
    in peer review, call for more effective, 359–61
    relation to problematic behavior, 17–18
    selective calls for rigor, 235–36
cross-cultural considerations for institutional review boards, 384–87
cross-cultural differences in mate preferences, 330–31
cross-national research, 374–75, 380–81, 383–89
cross-sectional comparison, nonexperimental, 34
CRTT (Competitive Reaction Time Task), 157–58
culture. *See also* scientific culture
    considerations for institutional review boards, 384–85
    and mate preference, 330–31
    scientific research transforming, 402–4
Cumming, G., 298
CVs, creating new type of, 32–33

Darley, J. M., 127–29, 139–42, 140t, 141t, 145–46, 146t, 297
data, open, 22, 350

data analysis. *See also* epistemic errors; *specific analytical methods*; statistical inference; statistical methods
  detective work metaphor for, 318–21
  improved methods of, 45–50
data blinding, 309
data collection, research questions about, 10
data dredging, 295–96, 296t
data fabrication, data falsification, and plagiarism (FFP). *See also* credibility crisis in psychological literature; questionable research practices
  increase in prevalence and impact, evidence on, 109–12
  number of scientists engaging in, 94–95
  prevalence, 97–98, 263–64
data misinterpretation/misrepresentation. *See* questionable interpretive practices
data-related questionable research practices
  unreported changes to methods, 267
  unreported changes to results, 268–70
  unreported changes to theory and hypotheses, 264–67
data sharing, increasing transparency through, 279
debriefing, 377
deception in research, handling, 377
decision errors. *See* epistemic errors
decline effect, 12, 18–19, 104–9
deductive inference, 180
definitive answers, preference of public for, 405, 409–10
demographic diversity, as component of intellectual diversity, 245
Dennett, D. C., 298
descriptive norms regarding questionable research practices, 276–77
Design of Experiments, The (Fisher), 87–88
detainees, research involving, 381–84, 385–87, 388
detective work metaphor for data analysis, 318–21
De Vries, Y. A., 227–28
Dienes, Z., 280–81

Dijksterhuis, A., 78
directional goals, and motivated reasoning, 229–30
disconfirmation bias, 295–96, 296t
dissemination of social psychology research findings
  Asch conformity experiments, 129–30
  Berkowitz and LePage weapons effect, 138–39
  Darley and Latané bystander intervention, 139–42, 140t, 141t
  Festinger and Carlsmith forced compliance dissonance, 133–35
  general discussion, 146–48
  identification of core experiments, 123–29, 125t, 126t
  Jones and Harris correspondent inferences, 137–38
  Milgram obedience research, 135–37
  overview, 122–23
  retention of information by students, 144–46, 145t, 146t
  Rosenthal and Jacobson teacher expectations, 142–43, 143t
  Sherif intergroup competition, 131–33
distributions, conjugate families of, 194–97, 195f
diversity, embracing intellectual, 244–46
dosage of stimuli, 214–15
double-blind review process, 270–73
Doucouliagos, H., 48, 166
dropping of hypotheses, 265
duplications, problematic, 97–98
Durante, K. M., 332–34
Dutch grant funding investigation, 232–33

Easterbrook, P. J., 41
economic research. *See* research integrity; *specific aspects of research integrity*
editor-initiated questionable research practices, 270, 272–73. *See also* peer review
education, reducing questionable research practices through, 277–78
education flat line, 403
effectiveness, accountability related to, 416

effective prior sample size, 196
effect sizes. *See also* meta-analyses; statistical inference; statistical methods
  and publication bias, 339–41, 340f
  relation to sample size, 268–69, 342
Egger, M., 166
ego depletion, 83, 153–54
elastic effects, 405, 408–9
Election Research Preacceptance Competition, 56–57
Ellemers, N., 234–35, 240
Elson, M., 157–58
embargoing of project details, 54
eminent authors
  impact bias related to, 364–65
  status bias related to, 361–63
emotional power, role in spread of ideas, 406–7
empirical research. *See also specific aspects of research integrity*
  general discussion, 34–35
  investigating research questions, 33–34
  need for, 7–8
  questions about causes of problematic behaviors, 13–20
  questions about proposed solutions, 20–33
  questions about questionable practices, 8–12
  questions and conference sessions, 3
epistemic errors. *See also* type I errors; type II errors
  detective work metaphor for data analysis, 318–21
  improving science by use of type III and IV errors, 334–35
  overview, 316–17
  specific examples of type III errors, 327–31
  specific examples of type IV errors, 327, 332–34
  type III error definitions, 317–18, 321–24
  type IV error definition, 324–25
epistemic freezing, 401–2

epistemic probability, 176–77, 178–79, 180. *See also* Bayesian statistical approaches
errors. *See also* credibility crisis in psychological literature; epistemic errors; questionable interpretive practices; *specific error types*
  empirical research questions about, 11
  proposed solutions, 26–31
  in psychological literature, 71
errors of the third kind. *See* type III error
estimation
  Bayesian, 193–97, 195f
  frequentist, 186–88
ethnic diversity, as component of intellectual diversity, 245
Etz, A., 193f
evaluation errors. *See* type IV errors
evidence
  focusing on accumulation of, 31–32
  issue with p-values as measures of, 185–86
evidence map (systematic maps), 160
evolutionary psychology literature, type III and IV errors in, 327–34
execution, procedural errors related to, 320–21. *See also* epistemic errors
experimentally demonstrable effect, 87–88
experiments. *See also* core experiments in social psychology; institutional review boards; stimulus sampling; subject sampling
  improved analytical methods, 45–46
  investigating research questions with, 8
expert, motivation to appear like, 18
explicit policies for accessing data and transparency, 24
exploration section, in journals, 25
exploratory data analysis, 318–21
external validity
  elastic effects, 408–9
  need for attention to in peer review, 360–61
  of stimuli, 203–4
extreme bounds analysis, 46

extremity, and research transmission, 407
Eysenck, H. J., 154, 156–57

fabrication, falsification, and plagiarism (FFP). *See also* credibility crisis in psychological literature; questionable research practices
　increase in prevalence and impact, evidence on, 109–12
　number of scientists engaging in, 94–95
　prevalence, 97–98, 263–64
fail-safe N, 162
failure, as central part of science, 265
faith-based belief, 411–12
false discovery rate (FDR), controlling, 50
false interpretations, 228–29. *See also* questionable interpretive practices
false negatives. *See* type II errors
false positives. *See* type I errors
false research findings, prevalence of, 102–4
falsification. *See also* credibility crisis in psychological literature; questionable research practices
　explicit statements regarding, 250
　increase in prevalence and impact, evidence on, 109–12
　number of scientists engaging in, 94–95
　overview, 3–4
　prevalence in literature, 97–98
family-wise error rate (FWER), controlling, 49–50
famous authors
　impact bias related to, 364–65
　status bias related to, 361–63
Fanelli, D., 263–64
FAT (funnel asymmetry test), 47–48
Fazio, Russell, 398–99
federal minimum wage, 59–60
Federal Policy for the Protection of Human Subjects (Common Rule), 373n.13
Fein, S., 124–30, 126t, 132–33, 134–35, 136–38, 139, 140–41, 142–44
femininity, and desired number of sexual partners, 328–30
Fernald School experiments, 380
Festinger, L., 127–29, 133–35, 145–46, 146t, 212–13

Feynman, R. P., 278
FFP. *See* credibility crisis in psychological literature; fabrication, falsification, and plagiarism; questionable research practices
Fiedler, K., 75–76, 77, 266, 267, 299
field experiments
　investigating research questions with, 33
　observing multiple stimuli in natural settings, 219–20
file drawer problem. *See* publication bias
financial conflicts of interest, 410–11
financial incentives for transparency, 23
findings section, in journals, 25
Finkelstein, A., 56, 57
fire sale authorship, 271–72
Firestone, C., 249
Fisher, R., 87–88, 181–82, 183–84
fishing for significant effects, 27, 42–45, 295–96, 296t
Flake, J. K., 157
forced compliance dissonance paradigm. *See* cognitive dissonance experiment
Forscher, P., 412
Fox, N. W., 266–67
fractional publication output, 110, 111–12
Francis, G., 342–43
Franco, A., 38–39, 341, 343–44
Frankfurt, H., 414
fraud, 3–4, 72–73, 82–83. *See also* credibility crisis in psychological literature; questionable research practices
Freberg, L., 345–46
free step-down resampling method, 49
frequentist statistical approaches
　basics of testing, 183–84
　criticisms of estimation, 188
　criticisms of testing, 184–86
　estimation overview, 186–87
　general discussion, 198–99
　misconceptions and misuses, 175–76
　origins of, 181–82
　to probability, 177–78
　"scientific" property of probability, 178
　statistical inference, 180
fundamental alteration or qualification of hypotheses, 265–66

fundamental attribution error, 137
funnel asymmetry test (FAT), 47–48
funnel plots
    illustrating publication bias, 339–42, 340f, 348–49
    improved publication bias tests, 47
    trim and fill, 162–63
FWER (family-wise error rate), controlling, 49–50

Galbraith, R. F., 47
Galiani, S., 344–45
gamesmanship. *See* questionable research practices
Ganimian, A., 53
gap map (systematic maps), 160
garbage can model, 404
garden of forking paths. *See* questionable research practices
Gaspelin, N., 85–86
gatekeeper-initiated questionable research practices, 270, 272–73
Gelman, A., 43–44, 280–81, 298, 321–22, 323–24
gender
    differences in desired number of sexual partners, 328–30, 332
    diversity, as component of intellectual diversity, 245
    and mate preference, 330–31
gender bias
    and citation biases, 233–35, 233t, 234t
    by institutional review boards, 376–77
    and selective calls for rigor, 235–36
    and Simpson's paradox, 232–33
generalizability, elastic effects and, 408–9
generalizations based on stimulus sampling, 203–4, 208–10, 211–12, 216
genetic association studies, 103–4
Genovese, K., 139
Gerber, A., 40, 301, 342–43
gift authorship, 271–72
Gigerenzer, G., 280–81
Gladwell, M., 406
Glass, G. V., 151, 154, 156–57
Glennerster, R., 53
goal-oriented incentives for transparency, 23–24

GoBifo project, 54–56, 55t
Goode, D., 380n.30
good research with bad results, publishing, 276–77
gray literature, 83, 101
greedy p-hacking
    constrained, 304–5, 314, 315f
    general discussion, 308–10
    overview, 300f, 301–2
    predicted effects of, 304–5, 305f
    significance rates for, 314t
    susceptibility to across empirical literatures, 305–6
Greenhouse, J. B., 165
Greenwald, A. G., 239, 397–98, 412
Gross, N., 345
Guatemala syphilis experiments, 378–79

Haddaway, N. R., 160–61
Hagger, M. S., 83
HARKing (hypothesizing after the results are known). *See also* questionable research practices
    defined, 296t
    versus other forms of investigator bias, 295–96
    overview, 96
    in peer review, 360
    unreported changes to hypothesis, 264–65
Harris, C. R., 333
Harris, V. A., 127–29, 137–38, 145–46, 146t
Hartgerink, C. H. J., 276n.5, 301–2
Harvey, C. R., 50
Hauser, M., 3–4
Havasupai tribe, 378n.26
health insurance expansion, 56
Heath, C., 406
helping behavior experiment, 139–42, 140t, 141t
heterogeneity, causes of problematic behaviors, 18–19
Hevelius, J., 310
Hochberg, Y., 50
Hoekstra, R., 188
Hollenbeck, J. R., 264–65
Holm, S., 49

432 INDEX

honest conservative labeling
 proposal, 86–88
Honeycutt, N., 345–46
human radiation experiments involving
 prisoners, 383
human subjects research. *See* institutional
 review boards
Humphreys, M., 43–44
hunting for significant effects. *See* fishing
 for significant effects
Hutchins, R., 414–15
Hutchins Commission (Commission on
 the Freedom of the Press), 414–15
hypothermia studies, 371n.7
hypotheses
 alternative, pitting against each
  other, 248–49
 in Bayesian testing, 190–91,
  192–93, 193f
 changing, 5
 explicit statements regarding
  falsification of, 250
 questionable research practices related
  to, 264–67
 statistical, 180
 testing, 183, 184–85, 188
 unreported changes to, 264–67
hypothesizing after the results are known.
 See HARKing; questionable research
 practices

ICCPR (International Covenant
 on Civil and Political Rights),
 372n.8, 382–83
idea entrepreneurs
 overview, 405
 persuading audience, 406–10
 psychology of selling, 410–12
 tragedy of the scientific
  commons, 413–14
image duplications, problematic, 97–98
imagined political behavior, ovulation
 and, 332–34
impact bias, 363–65
Impact Factor (IF), 363–64
implementation errors. *See* type III errors
Implicit Association Test (IAT), 239,
 398–99, 401, 403, 406, 412

implicit bias research
 accountability related to, 416
 brief history of, 397–99
 elastic effects, 408–9
 power of, 406–7
 and relationship between science and
  public, 396, 397
 status of today, 412
improper rounding of p-values, 99
inaccuracy. *See also* accuracy in social
 psychology textbooks
 causes of problematic behaviors, 18–20
 proposed solutions, 26–30
 of stereotypes, as phantom fact, 240
incarcerated populations, research
 involving, 381–84, 385–87, 388
incentives
 causes of problematic behaviors, 13–16
 changing culture of, 32–33
 empirical research questions
  about, 9–10
 overview of issues in scientific
  practice, 4
 for selection for statistical
  significance, 344
 for transparency, 22–24
index tests, 48–49
inductive inference, 180
inference, selection on. *See also* statistical
 inference
 evidence for, 344–49, 348t
 general discussion, 353
 overview, 339–42, 340f
 procedures for reducing, 349–53
informed consent
 cross-cultural considerations, 384–87
 under Nuremberg Code, 371–72
 primary concerns of institutional
  review boards, 378–84
 recommendations for, 388–89
injunctive norms regarding questionable
 research practices, 277–78
in-principle acceptance, 58–59
in principle acceptance (IPA), 168
institutional review boards (IRBs)
 case study, 385–87
 criticisms of, 375–77
 cross-cultural considerations, 384–85

general discussion, 390
historical background and function, 371–75
overview, 370–71
recommendations, 387–89
vulnerable populations and informed consent, 378–84
instructors, dissemination of social psychology findings by. *See* dissemination of social psychology research findings
instruments, procedural errors related to, 320–21. *See also* epistemic errors
integrity, research. *See* credibility crisis in psychological literature; crisis narrative about science; research integrity; *specific problematic behaviors*
intellectual disabilities, research involving children with, 379–81
intellectual diversity, embracing, 244–46
intelligence tests, correlation between school grades and, 349
intent, in analysis of p-hacking, 298, 299
intentional behavior, 10. *See also* questionable research practices
interactions, and replicability crisis, 80
interaction terms, incorrectly interpreting, 324–25
intergroup competition experiment
  accuracy of presentation in textbooks, 131–33
  as core social psychology experiment, 127–29
  retention of information by students, 145–46, 146*t*
internal validity, need for attention to in peer review, 360–61
International Association of Penal Law, 383
International Covenant on Civil and Political Rights (ICCPR), 372n.8, 382–83
International Ethical Guidelines for Biomedical Research Involving Human Subjects, 374–75
international research, 374–75, 380–81, 383–89

interpretive practices. *See* questionable interpretive practices
interrupted intervention designs, 6
interventions, unintentional errors related to, 30–31
inverse probability, 180, 188–89. *See also* epistemic probability
investigator bias, 295–96, 296*t*, *See also specific bias types*
investment in research question, relation to problematic behavior, 16–17
Ioannidis, J., 20, 74, 102, 271–72, 303–4, 342–43
IPA (in principle acceptance), 168
IRBs. *See* institutional review boards
irreproducible research. *See* non-replicability of research
iterative strategies of p-hacking, 82
Iyengar, S., 165

Jacobson, L., 127–29, 142–43, 143*t*, 145–46, 146*t*
JASP software, 197–98, 198*f*
Jeffreys, H., 87
John, L. K., 267, 282, 299, 342–43
Jones, B. C., 79
Jones, E. E., 127–29, 137–38, 145–46, 146*t*
journals. *See also* peer review; publication bias
  allotting space for replication studies, 280
  errors in, 6
  online comment sections, 27–28
  registered reports, 168
  results-blind peer review, 58–59
  retraction policies, 109–10
  transparency policies, 15–16, 24–25
Jung, K., 46–47
Jussim, L., 232

Kahneman, D., 59–60, 76, 397–98
Kaiser, H. F., 321–22, 323
Kano, Nigeria, experiments on children in, 380–81
Kasser, T., 331
Kassin S., 124–30, 126*t*, 132–33, 134–35, 136–38, 139, 140–41, 142–44
Kenrick, D. T., 124–30, 126*t*, 132–33, 134–35, 136–38, 139, 140–41, 142–44

Kidwell, M. C., 350
Kimball, A. W., 317–18, 324
King, Gary, 309–10
Kirkegaard, E. O. W., 349
Kirsch, I., 41
Klein, R. A., 80
Kling, J. R., 48–49
knowledge, lack of
   causes of problematic behaviors, 18–20
   overview of issues in scientific practice, 4, 6
   proposed solutions, 26–30
knowledgeable expert, motivation to appear like, 18
Krawcyzk, M., 301–2
Krueger, A. B., 47, 48, 59–60
Kruglanski, A., 401–2
Krugman, S., 380
Kühberger, A., 269–70
Kuhn, T. S., 250

labeling, honest conservative, 86–88
laboratory experiments. *See* core experiments in social psychology; experiments; institutional review boards; stimulus sampling; subject sampling
LaCour, M. J., 370n.1
Lai, C. K., 412
Lakens, D., 169, 243–44, 281
LaLonde, R. J., 43
large-scale preregistered trials, 167–69
Latané, B., 127–29, 139–42, 140t, 141t, 145–46, 146t
lay epistemologists, 401–2
Leamer, E. E., 42–43, 46
LeBel, E. P., 73–74
Lee, S., 49
LePage, A., 127–29, 138–39, 145–46, 146t
"Let's Take the Con Out of Econometrics" (Leamer), 42–43
Levin, J. R., 324–25
Levine, D., 59–60
Lewandowsky, S., 241
liberal political ideology, selection on inference and, 345–46
likelihood function, in Bayesian testing, 191–93

List, J. A., 49
literature, psychological. *See* credibility crisis in psychological literature; dissemination of social psychology research findings
literature reviews. *See also* meta-analyses; peer review
   honest conservative labeling proposal for, 86–88
   meta-analyses and, 158–59
   versus systematic reviews, 159–62
Loeb, A., 245
Loersch, C., 76–77
Loken, E., 43–44
long-run frequency, 177–78
Lovaglia, M., 347–48, 348t
low-fat diet, 403
Luce, H., 414–15
Luck, S. J., 85–86
Luna, F., 384–85

Macklin, R., 382n.34, 384–85, 389
magnitude (type M) errors, 323–24
Mahalik, J. R., 329–30
Makel, M. C., 73–74
Malhotra, N., 40, 301, 342–43
Manson, N., 388–89
many cultures dataset, 330–31
Many Labs study, 80, 106–7
Marascuilo, L. A., 324–25
Markus, H. R., 124–30, 126t, 132–33, 134–35, 136–38, 139, 140–41, 142–44
Marshall, B., 226–27
Marsman, M., 73
Martinson, B. C., 267
masculinity, and desired number of sexual partners, 328–30
masked phenomena. *See* questionable interpretive practices
Massey, Walter, 278–79
mate preferences, cross-cultural differences in, 330–31
mathematical likelihood, 191
Matthew effect, 270–71
Mayo, D. G., 298
McCrary, J., 41–42, 308–9
McCullough, M. E., 83
McElreath, R., 281

McKenzie, D., 53
mean effect, 48–49
meaning, public hunger for, 401–2
measures, as pitfall of
    meta-analysis, 156–58
media
    accountability of, 414–15, 416–17
    interpretation errors on part of, 12
media psychology, stimulus sampling
    in, 210–13
mental model, lack of clear, 404
Merton, R. K., 244–45, 273
meta-analyses
    alternatives to and supplements
        for, 158–69
    bias-corrected, 162–67
    history of, 151
    and narrative reviews, 158–59
    overview, 6, 150
    pitfalls of, 152–58
    preregistration and registered
        reports, 167–69
    promise and strengths of, 151–52
    publication bias as threat to, 338
    recommendations for, 169
    and replicability crisis in psychological
        literature, 81–84
    and systematic reviews, 159–62
meta-regression, 166–67
methodological implementation errors.
    See type III errors
methodological rigor, embracing,
    280–81
methods
    pitfalls of meta-analysis, 156–58
    questionable research practices related
        to, 267
    reproducibility of, 105–6
Mickes, L., 333
Milgram, S., 127–29, 135–37, 145–46,
    146*t*, 372
minimum wage, 59–60
misconduct. *See also* questionable research
        practices; *specific misconduct*
    increase in prevalence and impact,
        evidence on, 109–12
    number of scientists engaging in,
        94–95

prevalence in literature, 95–102
as red herrings, 260–61
misinterpretation/misrepresentation of
    data. *See* questionable interpretive
    practices
misspecification errors. *See* type III errors
Mitchell, Gregory, 401
Mitura, K., 331
model uncertainty, improved analytical
    methods regarding, 46–48
moderated multiple regression
    tests, 268–69
moderation analysis, 324–25, 330–31
moderators
    overlooked, role in replicability
        crisis, 77–80
    selection and coding of
        meta-analytic, 156
Moher, D., 161–62
Moreno, S. G., 163
Moscovici, S., 410
Moss-Racusin, C. A., 233–34,
    233*t*, 235–36
Mosteller, F., 321–22, 323
motivated reasoning, and questionable
    interpretive practices, 229–30
motivation to engage in questionable
    research practices, 14–15, 275–78
Mullainathan, S., 46–47
multiple regression tests,
    moderated, 268–69
multiple-site research, 383–84
multiple stimuli in natural settings,
    designs observing, 219–20
multiple testing corrections, 48–50
multiverse analyses, 243–44
Munsch, C. L., 377n.25
Myers, D. G., 124–30, 126*t*, 132–33, 134–
    35, 136–38, 139, 140–41, 142–44
mythmaking, 226–28, 231, 236–39

name recognition, capitalizing on, 270–71
narrative reviews. *See also* meta-analyses;
    peer review
    honest conservative labeling proposal
        for, 86–88
    meta-analyses and, 158–59
    versus systematic reviews, 159–62

"NASA Faked the Moon Landing—
  Therefore (Climate) Science is a
  Hoax" (Lewandowsky et al.), 241
National Institutes of Health (NIH),
  372–73, 383n.37
natural settings, designs observing
  multiple stimuli in, 219–20
Nature (journal), 93–94
Nature: Physics (Loeb), 245
Nazi experiments on human
  subjects, 371–72
negativity, in peer review, 359–61
negativity bias, and research
  transmission, 407
Neuberg, S. L., 124–30, 126t, 132–33,
  134–35, 136–38, 139, 140–41, 142–44
Neumark, D., 59–60
neuroscience, cognitive, 85–86
new challenges narrative about
  science, 113
Newton, I., 338
*New York State Association for Retarded
  Children v. Carey*, 380
Neyman, J., 181, 182, 183, 187
Nguyen, H. D., 348–49
NHST. *See* null-hypothesis significance
  testing
Nicholson, I., 372n.10, 372n.11
Niederle, M., 58
Nigeria, experiments on children
  in, 380–81
noncumulative methods and measurement,
  in meta-analysis, 156–58
nonexperimental cross-sectional
  comparison, 34
noniterative strategies of p-hacking, 82
nonprospective studies, preregistration
  of, 59–61
nonpublication of statistical null findings.
  See publication bias
non-replicability of research. *See also*
  replicability crisis in psychological
  literature
  causes of problematic behaviors, 18–19
  empirical research questions about, 11
  increase in prevalence and impact,
    evidence on, 109–12
  overview, 2
  prevalence of, 104–9

proposed solutions, 30–33
stimulus sampling connections to, 205–6
nonsignificant findings, nonpublication
  of. *See* publication bias
nonstandard measurement, as pitfall of
  meta-analysis, 156–58
null findings, nonpublication of. *See*
  publication bias
null hypothesis, in frequentist testing,
  181–82, 183–84
null-hypothesis significance
  testing (NHST)
  alternatives to, 243–44, 280–81
  arguments for other normative
    approaches, 298
  canonization, 242–43
  changing ways of thinking about, 31
  as exemplar of criterial control
    systems, 297
  false positives as byproduct of, 102
  as incapable of disproving null, 250
  results-related questionable research
    practices, 269–70
  versus strong inference, 249
  Type I and II errors and, 317
  type III error and, 321–22
Nuremberg Code, 371–72, 379

Oakes, M. W., 184–85
Obama, B., 370
obedience to authority experiment
  accuracy of presentation in
    textbooks, 135–37
  as core social psychology
    experiment, 127–29
  retention of information by students,
    145–46, 146t
objective dimensions of evaluation, in peer
  review, 360–61
O'Boyle, E. H., 263, 266–67, 268–69, 308
observational studies
  investigating research questions
    with, 33–34
  preregistration of, 59–61
Olken, B. A., 57, 58
O'Neil, O., 388–89
one-parameter selection models, 163–65
online comment sections for
  journals, 27–28

open data practices, 22, 350
open nature of science, erosion of, 84–86
openness. *See* transparency
open post-publication peer review, 366–67
Open Science Collaboration, 73, 75
Open Science Framework (OSF), 51–52, 54
operationalization of theory components, errors of. *See* type III errors
ordinary least squares (OLS) multiple regression analysis, 326–27
Oregon Health Plan (OHP), 56
outliers influencing desired number of sexual partners, 332
overgeneralization, empirical research questions about, 10
overreach by institutional review boards, 375
overstatement of results, stimulus sampling connections to, 207
overturn bias, 344–45
overzealousness of institutional review boards, 375
ovulation, and imagined political behavior, 332–34

PAPs. *See* pre-analysis plans
parapsychology, 82–83
parents, consent to participation of children in studies, 379–80
Payne, B. K., 76–77
p-curves, 308n.5
　in attempts to correct for publication bias, 40–41, 82–83
　bias-corrected meta-analysis, 163–65
　detection of p-hacking, 98–99
　overview, 6
Pearson, E., 181, 182, 183
Pedersen, W. C., 332
"peek-a-boo" moderators, 79
peer review
　general discussion, 367–68
　history of, 357
　impact bias, 363–65
　improving, 365–67
　overview, 357
　post-publication, 28–29
　questionable research practices in, 270–73
　reality of versus perception of, 358–59

results-blind, 25, 58–59, 351, 352–53
selection on inference in, 344–46, 351–52
status bias, 361–63
tone and civility in, 359–61
peer-reviewed registrations of systematic reviews, 160
PEESE (Precision Effect Estimate with Standard Error), 83–84, 166–67
perceptions
　of research findings, 5–6
　of science, effect of transparency on, 26
perceptual studies, credibility crisis in, 85–86. *See also* credibility crisis in psychological literature
persuading audience, 406–10
PET (Precision Effect Test), 48, 83–84, 166–67
Pfizer clinical trials involving children, 380–81
p-hacking, 40–41
　and bias-corrected meta-analysis, 164–65
　causes of, 4
　defined, 296t
　discovery of practice, 72
　effects of raising statistical power, 313, 314t
　empirical research questions about, 8–10
　general discussion, 308–10
　increase in, evidence on, 111
　iterative versus noniterative strategies, 82
　overview, 295–98
　in peer review, 360
　pitfalls of meta-analysis, 155
　possible solutions overview, 6
　predicted effects of styles, 302–5, 303f, 304f, 305f, 306f
　prevalence in literature, 98–99
　as results-related questionable research practice, 268–70
　stimulus sampling connections to, 206–7
　styles of, 299–302, 300f
　susceptibility to across empirical literatures, 305–8, 307f
phantom facts, 231, 239–41
philosophy of science perspectives, 250

Pischke, J.-S., 43
plagiarism. *See* fabrication, falsification, and plagiarism
Platt, J. R., 248, 250
point estimate, in frequentist estimation, 186
point null hypothesis, in Bayesian testing, 192–93, 193*f*
political behavior, ovulation and imagined, 332–34
political diversity
  as component of intellectual diversity, 245–46
  relation to problematic behavior, 17–18
political ideology, selection on inference and, 345–46
Popper, K., 247–48, 250
posterior distribution, in Bayesian estimation, 194–97, 195*f*
posterior probability
  in Bayesian testing, 190–91
  in Bayesian updating, 189
post-publication peer review, 28–29, 366–67
post-truth society, 414
powering studies, 30
pp-value, 41
pre-analysis plans (PAPs)
  examples of, 54–57, 55*t*
  general discussion, 61–62
  observational studies, 59–61
  overview, 52–54
  reducing publication bias via, 350–51
  strengths, limitations, and other issues, 57–59
Precision Effect Estimate with Standard Error (PEESE), 83–84, 166–67
Precision Effect Test (PET), 48, 83–84, 166–67
preregistration
  collection and analysis of less biased data, 167–69
  increasing transparency through, 20, 21–23, 279
  reducing publication bias via, 350
  as reform to fix p-hacking, 309
pressures to publish, increase in, 110
priming, 76–77, 85

prior distribution, in Bayesian estimation, 194–97, 195*f*
prior elicitation, 194–95
prior probability
  in Bayesian testing, 190, 191
  in Bayesian updating, 189
prisoners, research involving, 381–84, 385–87, 388
probability
  Bayesian testing, 190–91, 192–93, 193*f*
  Bayesian updating, 188–89
  mathematical likelihood, 191
  origins of frequentist inference, 181
  "scientific" property of, 178–79
  types of, 176–78
problematic research behaviors. *See* misconduct; questionable research practices; research integrity; *specific problematic behaviors*
procedural errors of data analysis, 319–21. *See also* epistemic errors
Proceedings of the National Academy of Sciences USA (journal), 233–34, 233*t*
professional incentives. *See* incentives
prospective experimental studies, 45
protocols for systematic reviews, 160
PRRR project, 86
pseudoscientific research, 403
psychological research. *See* credibility crisis in psychological literature; research integrity; *specific areas of research integrity; specific misconduct*
Psychological Science (journal), 350, 351–52
psychology of selling, 410–12
public, relationship between science and
  brief history of implicit bias research, 397–99
  challenges to managing, 405–12
  failures in flow of scientific information, 400–1
  future of, 414–17
  general discussion, 417–18
  idea entrepreneurs, 405
  implicit bias research today, 412
  overview, 396–97
  persuading audience, 406–10
  psychology of selling, 410–12

public access to research, 401–2
tragedy of the scientific
  commons, 413–14
viral science, 401
wicked problems, 402–4
public access to research, 400, 401–2
publication
  changing ways of thinking about, 31–33
  incentives related to, 13–14
  increase in pressures to publish, 110
  questionable research practices
    in, 270–73
  of replication studies, 280
  uncoupling from rewards, 275–78
publication bias
  attempts to correct for, 81–84
  caliper test, 301
  and creation of scientific myths, 227–28
  defined, 296t
  evidence for selection for statistical
    significance, 342–44
  evidence for selection on inference,
    344–49, 348t
  evidence on problems with, 38–42
  general discussion, 353
  improved tests for, 47–48
  increase in, evidence on, 111
  overview, 338
  versus p-hacking, 295–96, 297
  pitfalls of meta-analysis, 152–54
  prevalence in literature, 99–102
  procedures for reducing, 349–53
  proposed solutions, 31–32
  stimulus sampling connections to, 207
  study registration as solution for,
    50–52, 52f
  types of, 338–42, 340f
published error. See credibility crisis in
  psychological literature
p-uniform model, 163–65
p-values. See also p-curves; p-hacking
  American Statistical Association
    statement about, 188
  criticisms of, 184–86
  difficulty of addressing issues with, 4
  empirical research questions about, 10
  in frequentist testing, 183–84
  improper rounding of, 99

limiting questionable interpretive
  practices, 243–44
multiple testing corrections, 48
origins of, 181–82
selection for statistical significance,
  338–39, 342–43
shifting use and focus of, 31
specification searching, 44
Pygmalion in the Classroom (Rosenthal &
  Jacobson), 142

quality assessment, in systematic reviews,
  159–60, 161
quantitative synthesis of research
  evidence. *See* meta-analyses
quasi-experimental research
  designs, 45–46
questionable interpretive practices (QIPs)
  blind spots and cherry-picking, 231–35,
    233t, 234t
  canonization, 225–26, 251, 251t
  creation of scientific myths, 226–28
  empirical research questions
    about, 11–12
  general discussion, 251–52
  mythmaking and "wow" effects,
    231, 236–39
  overview, 5–6, 224–26, 230
  phantom facts, 231, 239–41
  potential solutions to, 242–50
  researcher role in, 228–29
  selective calls for rigor, 231, 235–36
  specific practices, 242, 246–50
  strategic approaches, 242–46
  theoretical bases for predicting, 229–30
questionable research practices (QRPs).
    See also research integrity;
    specific questionable practices
  causes of, 13–20
  chrysalis effect, 263
  as difficult to detect, 262
  effectiveness of, 262
  embracing methodological rigor, 280–81
  empirical research questions about
    specific, 8–12
  frequency of, 261–62
  general discussion, 281–83
  increase in, evidence on, 111–12

questionable research practices (QRPs). (*cont.*)
  increasing transparency in reporting, 278–80
  motivation to engage in, 14–15, 275–78
  number of scientists engaging in, 94–95, 299
  overview, 260–63
  pitfalls of meta-analysis, 155
  prevalence in literature, 95–102
  proposed solutions, 20–33
  recommendations to reduce, 273–81
  reducing motivation to engage in, 275–78
  in review process, 270–73
  scope, prevalence, and effect of, 263–73
  system processes encouraging and facilitating, 273–74, 282–83
  unreported changes to methods, 267
  unreported changes to results, 268–70
  unreported changes to theory and hypotheses, 264–67

racial stereotype threats, 237–38
racism, unconscious, 239
radiation experiments involving prisoners, 383
Raine, A., 385, 386
Ramirez, G., 78
Randomized Controlled Trial Registry (AEA), 50–52, 52*f*, 54
reaction norms, 105
recertification, 27
registered replication reports (RRRs), 168
registered reports, 167–69, 276, 351
registration, study, 50–52, 52*f*, 59–61
Rein, M., 407–8
rejection region, 183
replicability crisis in psychological literature. *See also* crisis narrative about science; questionable interpretive practices
  arguments about overstated nature of, 74–80
  benign neglect approach to, 84–86
  emergence of, 71–72
  honest conservative labeling proposal, 86–88
  meta-analyses to correct for, 81–84
  overview, 70–71, 224–25
  recent evidence of widespread published error, 72–74
  suggestions for dealing with, 81–88
replicability of research. *See also* non-replicability of research
  accountability related to, 416
  causes of problematic behaviors, 18–19
  empirical research questions about, 11
  improving peer review by prioritizing, 365–66
  increasing transparency through data sharing, 279–80
  pre-analysis plans and, 58
  proposed solutions to increase, 30–33
  stimulus sampling connections to, 205–6, 218–19
reporting biases, 228. *See also* selective reporting
reporting index tests, 48–49
Reproducibility Initiative in Cancer Biology, 107
Reproducibility Initiative in Psychology (RIP), 107–8
reproducibility paradox, 105
Reproducibility Project: Psychology (RP:P), 365–66, 416n.7
reputation, of psychology, 84
research boards. *See* institutional review boards
research design, role in type III errors, 317–18
researcher biases, stimulus sampling connections to, 206
researcher degrees of freedom, 280, 298. *See also* questionable research practices
research integrity. *See also* credibility crisis in psychological literature; crisis narrative about science; *specific problematic behaviors*
  conference overview, 3
  general discussion, 34–35
  investigating empirical research questions, 33–34
  issues in scientific practice, 3–6
  need for empirical research, 7–8
  overview, 1–2

possible solutions, 6–7
questions about causes of problematic behaviors, 13–20
questions about proposed solutions, 20–33
questions about questionable practices, 8–12
research quality
  improving peer review by prioritizing, 365–67
  and reduction of publication bias, 352
research syntheses. *See* meta-analyses
restrained p-hacking
  general discussion, 308–10
  overview, 300*f*, 301–2
  predicted effects of, 305, 306*f*
  significance rates for, 314*t*
  susceptibility to across empirical literatures, 305–6
results
  publishing good research with bad, 276–77
  questionable research practices related to, 268–70
  reproducibility of, 105
  section for, in journals, 25
results-blind peer review, 25, 58–59, 351, 352–53
retention of information by social psychology students, 144–46, 145*t*, 146*t*
Rethinking Informed Consent in Bioethics (Manson & O'Neil), 388–89
retractions, 6–7, 25–26, 27–28, 109–10
review process, questionable research practices in, 270–73. *See also* literature reviews; peer review
rewards
  for transparency, 22–23
  uncoupling, to reduce questionable research practices, 275–78
Richard, F. D., 302
right answer to wrong problem. *See* type III errors
right problem, wrong answer to. *See* type IV errors
rights of research subjects, protecting. *See* institutional review boards

rigor
  criticism based on, in peer review, 360
  embracing methodological, 280–81
  selective calls for, 231, 235–36
RIP (Reproducibility Initiative in Psychology), 107–8
risk of bias assessment, in systematic reviews, 159–60, 161
risks, institutional review board assessment of, 373–74, 376
Rodgers, J. L., 218–19
Rogalin, C., 347–48, 348*t*
Romano, J. P, 50
Rosenthal, R., 47, 127–29, 142–43, 143*t*, 145–46, 146*t*, 162, 324–25
Rosnow, R., 324–25
Roth, B., 349
rounding of p-values, improper, 99
Royall, R. M., 185
RP:P (Reproducibility Project: Psychology), 365–66, 416n.7
RRRs (registered replication reports), 168
Ryan, A. M., 348–49

Sackett, P. R., 237–38
salami slicing, 111–12
sample size, relation to effect size, 268–69, 342
sampling. *See* stimulus sampling; subject sampling
Sanna, L., 3–4
scaled up studies, 30
Schervish, M. J., 185
Schmader, T., 238
Schmitt, D. P., 328–29, 332
Scholl, B. J., 249
school grades, correlation between intelligence tests and, 349
Schuler, J., 78
Schwartz, S., 321–22, 323–24
Schwarz, N., 266, 267, 299
science, erosion of open nature of, 84–86
science, relationship between public and
  brief history of implicit bias research, 397–99
  challenges to managing, 405–12
  failures in flow of scientific information, 400–1

science, relationship between public and (*cont.*)
  future of, 414–17
  general discussion, 417–18
  idea entrepreneurs, 405
  implicit bias research today, 412
  overview, 396–97
  persuading audience, 406–10
  psychology of selling, 410–12
  public access to research, 401–2
  tragedy of the scientific commons, 413–14
  viral science, 401
  wicked problems, 402–4
Science for the Public (Boston Foundation), 400
science research. *See also* credibility crisis in psychological literature; crisis narrative about science; *specific areas of research integrity*; *specific problematic behaviors*
  conference overview, 3
  general discussion, 34–35
  investigating empirical research questions, 33–34
  issues in scientific practice, 3–6
  need for empirical research, 7–8
  overview, 1–2
  possible solutions, 6–7
  questions about causes of problematic behaviors, 13–20
  questions about proposed solutions, 20–33
  questions about questionable practices, 8–12
scientific culture
  causes of problematic behaviors, 15
  enhancing transparency in, 25–26
  overview of issues in scientific practice, 4
  solutions based on, 6–7
  solutions targeting, 31–33
scientific misconduct. *See also specific misconduct*
  increase in prevalence and impact, evidence on, 109–12
  number of scientists engaging in, 94–95
  prevalence in literature, 95–102
  as red herrings, 260–61

scientific myths, creation of, 226–28
"scientific" property of probability, 178–79
scope of authority of institutional review boards, 375–76
secondary sources, research reported in. *See* dissemination of social psychology research findings
selection bias, 154, 156. *See also* publication bias
selection for statistical significance
  evidence for, 342–44
  general discussion, 353
  overview, 338–42, 340f
  procedures for reducing, 349–53
  versus selection on inference, 346–47
selection models, as bias-correction tools, 163–65
selection on inference
  evidence for, 344–49, 348t
  general discussion, 353
  overview, 339–42, 340f
  procedures for reducing, 349–53
selective calls for rigor, 231, 235–36
selective reporting
  and creation of scientific myths, 228
  empirical research questions about, 8–10
  overview, 4
self, in power of research transmission, 406
selling, psychology of, 410–12
sequence, as part of stimulus definition, 215
sequential method for controlling FWER, 49
sex discrimination suit against Berkeley, 232
sexual partners, gender differences in desired number of, 328–30, 332
sexy-hypothesis testing, 75–76
Shaikh, A. M., 49
SHARKing, 264–65
Sharma, Y. S., 331
Sherif, M., 127–29, 131–33, 145–46, 146t
Sherman, R., 80
Shrout, P. E., 218–19
sign (type S) errors, 321–22, 323–24
significance testing, frequentist, 181–82, 183–84. *See also* p-values

Silberzahn, R., 344–45
Simmons, J. P., 43–44, 72, 164n.5, 280, 412
Simmons, S., 345
Simonsohn, U., 40–41, 46, 295, 299, 304–5, 309, 314
simple narrative, relation to problematic behavior, 18
Simpson's paradox, 232–33
simulation, investigating research questions with, 34
single-stimulus studies, 211–13, 216, 217–18
skepticism
  as component of intellectual diversity, 244–45
  embracing, 242–44
Smaldino, P. E., 281
small-study biases, 101–2
Smeeters, Dirk, 3–4
Smith, J. L., 235–36
Smith, M. L., 154, 156–57
social desirability biases, 235–36
social influence, complexity of, 130
social priming, 76–77
social psychology. *See* dissemination of social psychology research findings; research integrity; *specific aspects of research integrity*
Social Psychology (Aronson, Wilson, & Akert)
  accuracy of experiment presentation in, 129–30, 132–33, 134–35, 136–38, 139, 140–41, 142–44
  as frequently used textbook, 124–25, 126t
  selection of core experiments in, 125–29
Social Psychology (journal), 73
Social Psychology (Kassin, Fein, & Markus)
  accuracy of experiment presentation in, 129–30, 132–33, 134–35, 136–38, 139, 140–41, 142–44
  as frequently used textbook, 124–25, 126t
  selection of core experiments in, 125–29
Social Psychology (Kenrick, Neuberg, & Cialdini)
  accuracy of experiment presentation in, 129–30, 132–33, 134–35, 136–38, 139, 140–41, 142–44
  as frequently used textbook, 124–25, 126t
  selection of core experiments in, 125–29
Social Psychology (Myers)
  accuracy of experiment presentation in, 129–30, 132–33, 134–35, 136–38, 139, 140–41, 142–44
  as frequently used textbook, 124–25, 126t
  selection of core experiments in, 125–29
social science research. *See* research integrity; *specific aspects of research integrity*; *specific misconduct*
social support, role in obedience studies, 136–37
software, Bayesian analysis, 197–98, 198f
solutions to wicked problems, public expectations for, 402–4
specification curve, 46–47
specification searching, 42–45. *See also* publication bias; transparency
specific practices, to limit questionable interpretive practices, 242, 246–50
Spencer, S. J., 237
spin, and creation of scientific myths, 228
standardized test scores, racial stereotype threats and, 237–38
Stanley, T. D., 48, 166–67
Stapel, D., 3–4, 72–73
Starbucks, 396, 416
statistical analysis plans, 52–53
statistical assumptions
  generalizing Type IV error, 325–27
  role in type III errors, 317–18
  and type III error definitions, 323–24
statistical evaluation errors. *See* type IV errors
statistical inference. *See also* epistemic errors
  Bayesian estimation, 193–97, 195f
  Bayesian software, 197–98, 198f
  Bayesian testing, 190–91
  Bayesian testing with likelihood ratios, 192–93, 193f
  Bayesian updating, 188–89
  Bayes' theorem, 179–80
  defined, 180
  frequentist estimation criticisms, 188

444 INDEX

statistical inference (*cont.*)
  frequentist estimation overview, 186–87
  frequentist inference origins, 181–82
  frequentist testing basics, 183–84
  frequentist testing criticisms, 184–86
  general discussion, 198–99
  limiting questionable interpretive practices, 242–43
  mathematical likelihood, 191
  overview, 175–76
  "scientific" property of probability, 178–79
  types of probability, 176–78
statistical methods. *See also* Bayesian statistical approaches; epistemic errors
  analysis and replication of stimulus samples, 218–19
  improved analytical methods, 45–50
  overview, 37
  pre-analysis plans, 52–61
  publication bias, 38–42
  and replicability crisis in psychological literature, 74–75
  results-related questionable research practices, 269
  specification searching, 42–45
  subgroup analysis, 44–45
Statistical Methods for Research Workers (Fisher), 182
statistical power
  effects of raising, 313, 314*t*
  measuring in literature, 102–4
  reform to fix p-hacking, 309
statistical significance. *See also* p-hacking; p-values; selection for statistical significance
  limiting questionable interpretive practices, 242–43
  pitfalls of meta-analysis, 153
  results-related questionable research practice, 268–69
statistical validity, need for attention to in peer review, 360–61
status bias, 361–63
Steele, C. M., 237–38

stereotypes
  gender, 234–35
  inaccurate, as phantom fact, 240
stereotype threat, 237–38, 348–49
Sterling, T. D., 38
Stern, C., 246–47, 248
stimulus sampling
  analysis and replication of stimulus samples, 218–19
  choosing right number of stimuli, 216–18
  connections to research integrity, 205–8
  general discussion, 220
  how stimuli are defined, 214–16
  importance of good stimulus samples, 208–10
  improving, 213–20
  limiting questionable interpretive practices, 244
  media psychology example, 210–13
  observing multiple stimuli in natural settings, 219–20
  overview, 203–5
stochastic probability, 176–77
storytelling, research transmission through, 406
Strack, F., 78
strategic approaches to limit questionable interpretive practices, 242–46
strategic p-hacking
  general discussion, 308–10
  overview, 300*f*, 300–2
  predicted effects of, 303–5, 304*f*
  significance rates for, 313, 314*t*
  susceptibility to across empirical literatures, 305–6
stress, myth regarding ulcers as caused by, 226–27
Stroebe, W., 78
strong causality, 397, 407–8
strong inference, 248–49, 250
students, dissemination of research to. *See* dissemination of social psychology research findings
Student t-test, 325–26
study registration, 50–52, 52*f*, 59–61
study selection for meta-analysis, 154

subgroup analysis, 10, 27, 44–45, 164–65
subjective subtype of epistemic probability, 178
subjects, protection of human. *See* institutional review boards
subject sampling, 203, 214, 216–17, 218, 220
suboptimal research behaviors. *See* research integrity; *specific suboptimal behaviors*
superstitious beliefs, 408
surveys about scientist engagement in misconduct, 94–96
Swidler, A., 402–3, 406
synthesizing research, 338. *See also* meta-analyses; publication bias
syphilis experiments, 378–79
systematic maps (evidence map or gap map), 160
systematic reviews, 159–62

Takavarasha, K., 53
Tate, C., 328–30
teacher expectations experiment
  accuracy of presentation in textbooks, 142–43, 143*t*
  as core social psychology experiment, 127–29
  retention of information by students, 145–46, 146*t*
technology, in stimulus sampling, 210, 219–20
Tennant, J. P., 357
TESS (Time-sharing Experiments for the Social Sciences), 38–39, 343–44, 349–50
testing
  Bayesian, 190–93, 193*f*
  frequentist, 181, 183–86
  intelligence, correlation between school grades and, 349
  racial stereotype threats and performance, 237–38
Tetlock, P. E., 401, 410
Tett, G., 413
textbooks. *See also* dissemination of social psychology research findings
  causes of problematic behaviors, 19–20
  increasing accuracy of information in, 29–30
  knowledge of research in, 6
THARKing, 264–65
theoretical bases for predicting questionable interpretive practices, 229–30
theoretical diversity, as component of intellectual diversity, 245
theoretical importance of findings, and replicability crisis, 75–77
theories
  explicit statements regarding falsification of, 250
  procedural errors of data analysis, 319–20
  questionable research practices related to, 264–67
  role in type III errors, 317–18
  testing, criteria for, 247–48
  unreported changes to, 264–67
theory implementation errors. *See* type III errors
theory pruning, 277
thinking about research, changing, 7
Thinking Fast and Slow (Kahneman), 76
third-party evaluation, 30–31
37 cultures dataset, 330–31
Thompson, P. A., 301–2
three-parameter selection model (3PSM), 165
time series analysis, 34
Time-sharing Experiments for the Social Sciences (TESS), 38–39, 343–44, 349–50
tone, in peer review, 359–61
Top10 technique, 166n.6
t-prime (Welch t′) correction, 325–26
tragedy of the scientific commons, 413–14
training
  to ensure replicable interventions, 30–31
  implicit bias, 396, 399, 403
  reducing questionable research practices through, 277–78
translation of research for public. *See* public, relationship between science and

transparency
  causes of problematic behaviors, 14, 15–16
  evidence on problems with current body of research, 37–45
  future directions for research, 61–62
  improved analytical methods, 45–50
  overview, 4, 36–37
  pre-analysis plans, 52–61
  proposed solutions, 20–26
  publication bias, 38–42
  in reporting, increasing, 278–80
  specification searching, 42–45
  stimulus sampling connections to, 208
  study registration, 50–52, 52f
  subgroup analysis, 44–45
treatment, unintentional errors related to, 30–31
tribalism in science, 413
Trikalinos, T. A., 342–43
trim and fill, 162–63
true effect, 48
Truman, Harry, 409–10
trust in science, 413
truth, current state of, 414
t-tests, 41–42, 325–26
Tukey, J. W., 318–19
Turner, E. H., 41
Tuskegee syphilis experiments, 378–79
Tversky, A., 397–98
Twain, M., 260
21-word statements, 22
two-sample t-test, 325–26
two-step review process, 276
type I errors (false positives)
  in frequentist testing, 183
  overview, 317
  prevalence in literature, 102–4
  related to stimulus sampling, 211–12
  statistical misunderstandings related to, 74–75
  type III or IV errors leading to, 334
type II errors (false negatives)
  in frequentist testing, 183
  overview, 317
  versus procedural error of data analysis, 320
  related to stimulus sampling, 211–12
  type III or IV errors leading to, 334

type III (implementation) errors
  commonality among definitions, 323–24
  definitions of, 317–18, 321–22
  improving science by use of, 334–35
  overview, 316–17
  related to stimulus sampling, 212
  specific examples of, 327–31
type IV (evaluation) errors
  existing definition of, 324–25
  generalizing to all cases of errors of statistical assumptions, 325–27
  improving science by use of, 334–35
  need for, 324
  specific examples of, 327, 332–34
type M (magnitude) errors, 323–24
type S (sign) errors, 321–22, 323–24

ulcers, scientific myths about, 226–27
Umesh, U. N., 324–25
uncertainty. See also probability
  acknowledging and recognizing, 242–44
  embracing intellectual diversity to resolve, 244–46
  model, improved analytical methods regarding, 46–48
  role in science, 176
unconditional p-hacking
  general discussion, 308–10
  overview, 299–300, 300f, 301
  predicted effects of, 303f, 303
  significance rates for, 313, 314t
  susceptibility to across empirical literatures, 305–6
unconscious racism, 239. See also implicit bias research
under-sampling of stimuli, 211
understanding, errors related to, 319–20, 321. See also epistemic errors
unethical behavior in research. See research integrity; *specific types of unethical behavior*
unintentional errors
  empirical research questions about, 11
  proposed solutions, 26–31
United Nations
  International Covenant on Civil and Political Rights, 372n.8, 382–83
  role in international research, 387–88, 389

universalism, 361–62
universities, dissemination of findings in. *See* dissemination of social psychology research findings
University of California, Berkeley, 232
University of Southern California (USC), 385, 386
unjustified conclusions, 228–29. *See also* questionable interpretive practices
unreported changes
  to methods, 267
  to results, 268–70
  to theory and hypotheses, 264–67
Unresponsive Bystander, The (Latané & Darley), 140–41
unreviewed preregistration, 167–69
updating, Bayesian, 188–89
urban legends, 406–7
utilitarian approach, of institutional review boards, 373–74

validity, need for attention to in peer review, 360–61. *See also* construct validity; credibility crisis in psychological literature; external validity
van Aert, R. C. M., 155, 164–65
van Zelst, M., 276n.5
variables, overlooked, role in replicability crisis, 77–80
variance, stimuli, 209–10
Vietnam, breast cancer research in, 384–85
viral science
  defined, 401
  general discussion, 417
  persuading audience, 406–10
  psychology of selling, 410–12
  tragedy of the scientific commons, 413–14
volume of stimuli, 214–15
voluntary informed consent. *See* informed consent
von Mises, L., 177
Vosgerau, J., 48

vote-counting method, 158–59
vulnerable populations, research involving, 378–84

Walmart v. Dukes et al., 408–9
Walton, G. M., 238
Wänke, M., 78
Ward, Robert, 380
Wasserstein, R. L., 243
weapons effect on aggression experiment
  accuracy of presentation in textbooks, 138–39
  as core social psychology experiment, 127–29
  retention of information by students, 145–46, 146*t*
Welch t' (t-prime) correction, 325–26
Westfall, J., 218–19
Westfall, P. H., 49
wicked problems, 402–4
Williams, J. C., 235–36
Williams, W. M., 233–34, 233*t*, 235–36
willingness to engage in questionable research practices, 8–9
Willowbrook School case, 380
Wilson, B. M., 86
Wilson, T. D., 124–30, 126*t*, 132–33, 134–35, 136–38, 139, 140–41, 142–44
Winship, C., 407–8
Wixted, J. T., 86
Wolfe, C. T., 237
World Health Organization (WHO), 387–88, 389
"wow" effects/papers, 13–14, 32, 231, 236–39
Wright, P. M., 264–65
wrong answer to right problem. *See* type IV errors
wrong problem, right answer to. *See* type III errors

Young, S. S., 49

Zenter, M., 331
Zigerell, L. J., 348–49